MINDFULNESS- AND ACCEPTANCE-BASED BEHAVIORAL THERAPIES IN PRACTICE

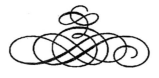

Guides to Individualized Evidence-Based Treatment

Jacqueline B. Persons, *Series Editor*

Providing road maps for managing real-world cases, volumes in this series help the clinician develop treatment plans using interventions of proven effectiveness. With an emphasis on systematic yet flexible case formulation, these hands-on guides provide powerful alternatives to one-size-fits-all approaches. Each book addresses a particular disorder or presents cutting-edge intervention strategies that can be used across a range of clinical problems.

Mindfulness- and Acceptance-Based Behavioral Therapies in Practice

Lizabeth Roemer
Susan M. Orsillo

Series Editor's Note by Jacqueline B. Persons

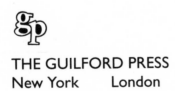

THE GUILFORD PRESS
New York   London

To Josh, Paul, Sarah, and Sam
with love and gratitude

© 2009 The Guilford Press
A Division of Guilford Publications, Inc.
72 Spring Street, New York, NY 10012
www.guilford.com

Printed in the United States of America

This book is printed on acid-free paper.

Last digit is print number: 9   8   7   6   5   4   3   2

Library of Congress Cataloging-in-Publication Data

Roemer, Lizabeth, 1967–
    Mindfulness- and acceptance-based behavioral therapies in practice / by Lizabeth Roemer, Susan M. Orsillo.
        p. ; cm.—(Guides to individualized evidence-based treatment)
    Includes bibliographical references and index.
    ISBN 978-1-59385-997-8 (hardcover: alk. paper)
    ISBN 978-1-60623-999-5 (paperback: alk. paper)
    1. Acceptance and commitment therapy.   I. Orsillo, Susan M., 1964–   II. Title.   III. Series.
    [DNLM: 1. Behavior Therapy—methods. 2. Awareness. 3. Patient Acceptance of Health Care—psychology. WM 425 R715m 2009]
    RC489.C62R64 2009
    616.89′142—dc22
                                                                        2008016226

\# 226279627

About the Authors

Lizabeth Roemer, PhD, is Professor of Psychology at the University of Massachusetts–Boston, where she is actively involved in research and clinical training of doctoral students in clinical psychology. In collaboration with her students, her research examines basic processes that may underlie clinical problems, such as the role of emotional acceptance, emotional suppression, emotion regulatory strategies, and mindfulness in a range of clinical presentations. Dr. Roemer has published over 70 journal articles and book chapters, coedited two books, and coauthored two books.

Susan M. Orsillo, PhD, is Professor of Psychology at Suffolk University in Boston, Massachusetts. Her current research focuses on the role of emotional response styles, most notably experiential avoidance, in maintaining psychological difficulties. In collaboration with her doctoral students in clinical psychology, she has developed a number of prevention and treatment programs that integrate acceptance and mindfulness with evidence-based behavioral approaches. Dr. Orsillo has published over 70 journal articles and book chapters, coedited two books, and coauthored two books.

Together, Drs. Roemer and Orsillo have developed an acceptance-based behavioral therapy for generalized anxiety disorder. They are currently examining its efficacy as well as mediators and moderators of change in a study funded by the National Institute of Mental Health. Their forthcoming self-help book, *The Mindful Way through Anxiety: Break Free from Chronic Worry and Reclaim Your Life*, draws from their decade of research in this area to provide guidance to people struggling with anxiety.

Series Editor's Note

This volume is the latest in the series Guides to Individualized Evidence-Based Treatment, which aims to facilitate the transportation of evidence-based therapies from research and academic communities to the frontlines of clinical settings.

Lizabeth Roemer and Susan M. Orsillo aid the busy clinician by providing in this volume a thoughtful synthesis of several of the important and increasingly popular mindfulness- and acceptance-based behavioral therapies, including acceptance and commitment therapy, mindfulness-based cognitive therapy, mindfulness-based relapse prevention, integrative behavioral couple therapy, and dialectical behavior therapy. The authors offer us their distillation of the essential principles and elements of this new group of behavioral therapies.

Drs. Roemer and Orsillo present a general model that proposes that many problems and disorders for which our patients seek treatment result from three related mechanisms: a maladaptive relationship to internal experience (such as fusion, judgment, and/or lack of awareness), experiential avoidance, and behavioral constriction. The authors show the clinician how to use the general model as the foundation for an individualized case formulation and treatment plan that addresses the unique details of each patient's symptoms and problems. They show the therapist how to use the individualized case formulation to understand the relationships among a patient's multiple disorders and problems and to select treatment targets and interventions. They describe and offer numerous examples of interventions that are designed to help individuals accomplish their treatment goals by altering their relationship to their internal experience, reducing experiential avoidance, and promoting valued action. The authors also describe how to integrate other evidence-based therapies into this therapy and how to account for cultural factors. The result is a therapy that clinicians can use in a flexible way to address a wide range of clinical phenomena.

The approach to acceptance-based behavioral therapy described in this book is supported by data from randomized controlled trials showing that the therapies on which the approach is based provide effective treatment for individuals and couples who have a wide range of clinical disorders and problems. The approach presented here is also evidence based in the sense that the clinician collects data to monitor the progress of every client.

This volume provides a wonderful balance of hands-on clinical detail, conceptual clarity, scholarship, and reliance on the empirical literature. I am delighted to include this book in the Guides to Individualized Evidence-Based Treatment.

JACQUELINE B. PERSONS, PhD
San Francisco Bay Area Center for Cognitive Therapy

Preface to the Paperback Edition

We are pleased that Guilford has decided to release a paperback version of *Mindfulness- and Acceptance-Based Behavioral Therapies in Practice* in order to make it even more afford-able for clinicians. This book is a culmination of our shared journey as researchers, clini-cians, supervisors, and human beings, exploring the ways that mindfulness- and other acceptance-based strategies can enhance behavioral approaches to reducing suffering and enriching life. We wrote the book in order to share what we have learned from our own research, clinical work, and personal exploration; from other researchers and practitioners; and from the therapists and clients with whom we have worked over the years about how to integrate these approaches and use them flexibly in therapy. Since that time, we have continued to see the benefits of this approach in our research, in our conversations with clinicians who have read the book, and in our own lives. We hope readers will continue to find the practical, conceptually and evidence-based suggestions in this book useful in their practice, their research, and their lives.

We have just completed a self-help book based on the principles presented here, *The Mindful Way through Anxiety: Break Free from Chronic Worry and Reclaim Your Life*, to be published by Guilford in 2011. We were inspired by how accessible Mark Williams, John Teasdale, Zindel Segal, Jon Kabat-Zinn, Christopher Germer, and Ronald Siegel have made a mindfulness approach to psychological growth and healing in their books (*The Mindful Way through Depression, The Mindful Path to Self-Compassion,* and *The Mindfulness Solution*) and hope that our book will help individuals who struggle with anxiety in its various forms to find their own strength and freedom and re-engage in living satisfying lives. Audiotapes of many of the exercises presented in both of our books are now avail-able for download at *www.mindfulwaythroughanxietybook.com*. We hope these resources will be helpful for your clients.

The explosion of interest in mindfulness- and acceptance-based approaches to ther-apy has continued to grow since the publication of this book. We attempt to place our work within the context of this constantly growing field in the Introduction to this book and address important issues of commonalities and distinctions across approaches. We also acknowledge those who have influenced and informed our work in the Introduc-tion. We remain extremely grateful to each of these individuals for their vital contributions to our understanding of how best to help people struggling with their internal experiences.

Since the book was published, we have had the opportunity to speak to many groups of clinicians across the United States and internationally about the approach we present here. We thank each of these clinicians, and all those we have not met yet, for their continual, earnest efforts to help those who are struggling, their thoughtfulness in approaching clinical work, and their consistent desire to expand their practices in order to optimally help their clients. Clinicians from a range of backgrounds regularly tell us that they find our approach similar to things they already do, but that it provides them with a structure and a way of thinking about their work that is new. This is a particularly gratifying response for us. We are pleased that our approach resonates with approaches developed from the clinical wisdom and experience of people from such disparate backgrounds, and also pleased that people find that our work can support and deepen their practices. We hope you will find it similarly useful.

We also thank the countless graduate students and new psychologists across the United States and the world who have shared their enthusiasm and excitement for this approach with us, as well as their own ideas and experiences. You help to keep this work alive for us and we look forward to the many important contributions you will all make to our understanding of how to best help people make the most of their lives.

Acknowledgments

This book is a culmination of our collaborative work over the past 14 years, and we are grateful to the large number of people who have facilitated and supported its development in a wide range of ways. We thank Kitty Moore and Jacqueline Persons for their invitation to write the book, their encouragement and support throughout the process, and their valuable editorial feedback, which led to this final product. We also thank Hillary Brown for her diligent and careful copyediting, Paul Gordon for his beautiful cover design, and everyone else at The Guilford Press for their help in getting the book to its final form. We are deeply grateful to Laura Allen and Sarah Hayes-Skelton for their skill and care in overseeing our treatment grants, without which we could not possibly have written this book. The insights that they and the other therapists we have supervised over the years have shared with us have shaped our understanding in significant ways, all of which is reflected in these pages. We have had the privilege of working directly with clients and supervising therapy with clients who have continually taught and inspired us with their willingness to open up to their pain and their courage to make changes in order to live more meaningful lives. We thank them for all they have taught us as psychologists and as human beings. As we mention in the Introduction, our work has been inspired and influenced by a number of clinical psychologists and Buddhist writers; we are grateful to each of them for their efforts and their wisdom. In particular, we thank our postdoctoral mentor, Brett Litz, for personally and intellectually challenging us, for kindling our interest in emotion, and for introducing us to one another. We are grateful to David Barlow, Bonnie Brown, and the faculty, students, and staff of the Center for Anxiety and Related Disorders for generously supporting our work, and to the National Institute of Mental Health for supporting our work and this book with Grants Nos. MH63208 and MH074589.

In addition, I (Lizabeth Roemer) want to thank Sue, first and foremost. There are no words to describe the ways that our collaboration and friendship has strengthened, expanded, and nourished me and my work throughout these past 14 years. Her wisdom, kindness, conscientiousness, insightfulness, and care create and enrich our shared work and continually inspire me. With her steadfast support, I am far more able to engage my life in ways that matter to me. I am also eternally grateful to my graduate school mentor, Thomas Borkovec, for all of his teachings, his continuing guidance and nurturance, and the model he provided of integrating science and practice, to which I continue to aspire. I have had the amazing luck of working with a team of exceptional graduate students over the years (Kim Gratz, Matthew Jakupcak, LaTanya Rucker, Kristi Salters-Pedneault, Yonit Schorr, Matt Tull, Darren Holowka, Heidi Barrett-Model, Shannon Erisman, Cara Fuchs, Lindsey West, Mike Treanor, Kathleen Sullivan-Kalill, Jess Graham, and Lucas Morgan), whose enthusiasm, intellectual curiosity, insights, and care continually teach, enrich, and motivate me. I am grateful also to my friends and colleagues Alice Carter, Sarah Hayes-Skelton, Karestan Koenen, Doug Mennin, Carolyn Pepper, Karen Suyemoto, and Amy Wagner, who influence my work and help to sustain my spirit; to my parents, whose many forms of ongoing love and support included taking my school-age writing efforts seriously; and to all the other friends and family who enrich my life. And last, but far from least, I thank my partner, Josh Bartok, whose wisdom, love, and care immeasurably enhanced both the content of this book and the process of writing it, as they enhance the content and process of my life each day.

I (Susan Orsillo) am deeply indebted to Liz, my coauthor, collaborator, and friend. Liz brings clinical sensitivity, passion, scientific rigor, and integrity to our shared work, and I am extremely grateful for all I have learned from her. Her tremendous generosity, compassion, and encouragement help me to navigate the daily challenges inherent in trying to live consistently with my personal and professional values. Several mentors have influenced my personal and professional growth and deserve recognition, most notably Robert McCaffrey for his loyalty and support, Richard Heimberg for introducing me to treatment research and teaching me how to mentor, and Brett Litz as noted above. I am thankful to Sonja Batten and Jenn Block-Lerner for the clinical sensitivity and wisdom they have brought to my understanding of acceptance and mindfulness and for their personal and professional support. I thank my talented and enthusiastic team of graduate students (Stephanie Berube, Deborah Glick, Justin Hill, Aviva Katz, Meredith Klump, Jonathan K. Lee, Susie Michelson, Christina Theodore-Oklota, and Pete Vernig), whose intellectual curiosity, hard work, and willingness continually to grow as professionals provide daily inspiration and support for my work. I am appreciative of my fabulous colleagues Lisa Coyne, Gary Fireman, Amy Marks, David Pantalone, Tracey Rogers, Elisabeth Sandberg, and Lance Swenson, who make coming to work each day stimulating and fun. I am grateful to all my friends and family for their sustaining care. Finally, I thank my husband, Paul, for more than 20 years of unwavering encouragement, support, friendship, and love, and my children, Sarah and Sam, for helping me connect with the peace, wisdom, and joy of living in the present moment.

Contents

Introduction

Our hope in writing this book is to give clinicians and clinicians-in-training a helpful framework and guidelines for conducting psychotherapy that uses mindfulness- and acceptance-based behavioral approaches with clients with diverse clinical presentations. This book is different from typical treatment protocol books in that we do not present a standardized protocol nor do we focus on a single type of acceptance-based behavioral therapy. In our work developing a manualized treatment for clients with a principal diagnosis of generalized anxiety disorder (along with a range of comorbid disorders; Roemer & Orsillo, 2007; Roemer, Orsillo, & Salters-Pedneault, 2008), we found it helpful to integrate material from a range of evidence-based interventions that emphasize acceptance and mindfulness (e.g., acceptance and commitment therapy [ACT]: Hayes, Strosahl, & Wilson, 1999; dialectical behavior therapy [DBT]: Linehan, 1993a; mindfulness-based cognitive therapy [MBCT]: Segal, Williams, & Teasdale, 2002) along with other behavioral and cognitive interventions that have received extensive empirical support. We use a similar approach here in describing how to develop an acceptance-based behavioral case conceptualization and flexibly apply the central elements of this range of interventions (drawing also from integrative behavioral couple therapy [IBCT]: Jacobson & Christensen, 1996; and mindfulness-based relapse prevention [MBRP]: Witkiewitz, Marlatt, & Walker, 2005) to therapy with clients presenting with a range of clinical issues. Our approach is similar to the stance one might take in conceptualizing and treating a case from a cognitive-behavioral perspective, drawing from a range of empirically supported treatment packages and flexibly applying methods in a way that meets the individualized needs of a particular client.

Our thinking in this area has been informed and shaped by a wide array of valuable sources, and we cannot possibly accurately or sufficiently acknowledge them all, although we do our best to note the most proximal sources for the specific suggestions we make. One of the most exciting aspects of treatment work is the way that ideas from very different contexts can overlap and intermingle. Thus, although our work is most directly influenced by behaviorally and cognitively oriented clinical psychologists (e.g., David H. Barlow, Thomas D. Borkovec, Andrew Christensen, Steven C. Hayes, Richard G. Heimberg, Neil S. Jacobson, Marsha M. Linehan, Brett T. Litz, G. Alan Marlatt, Zindel

V. Segal, John D. Teasdale, and J. Mark G. Williams), we also draw explicitly from the work of experientially oriented psychologists (e.g., Leslie S. Greenberg) and integrationists (e.g., Douglas S. Mennin), as well as psychological and Buddhist writings on mindfulness (e.g., Pema Chodron, psychologists from the Institute for Meditation and Psychotherapy, Jon Kabat-Zinn, and Sharon Salzberg), and we likely draw implicitly and in ways we do not recognize from a host of other sources (including more relationally oriented psychologists such as Paul Wachtel).

DEFINING THE APPROACH

When we use the term *mindfulness*, we refer to "an openhearted, moment-to-moment, non-judgmental awareness" (Kabat-Zinn, 2005, p. 24). This construct, drawn from Buddhist traditions but used here in a secular context, refers to being able to pay attention in the present moment to whatever arises internally or externally, without becoming entangled or "hooked" by judging or wishing things were otherwise. When using mindfulness in psychotherapy, we are often particularly focused on mindful awareness of internal experience. That is, we help our clients observe the rise and fall of their thoughts and feelings without clinging to highly valued ones or trying to banish painful ones. For us, this cultivation of mindfulness is therapeutic because it helps promote *acceptance* of internal experience and diminish avoidance. As we discuss in Chapter 1, experiential avoidance, or avoidance of internal experiences such as thoughts, emotions, images, and physiological sensations, may promote and perpetuate a wide range of clinical problems. Acceptance may serve to lessen these difficulties. Although the term *mindfulness* is sometimes used to refer specifically to treatments that incorporate extended sitting meditation practices (such as mindfulness-based stress reduction [MBSR]), we use it here to refer to the use of a broad array of formal and informal practices, as discussed in Chapter 6.

In our work, we use the terms *acceptance-based behavioral therapies (ABBTs)* and *mindfulness- and acceptance-based behavioral therapies* to define a range of approaches that explicitly emphasize altering clients' relationships to and avoidance of internal experience as a central mechanism of therapeutic change. There has been much debate in the field as to how these approaches should be classified, whether they are novel or simply another version of more traditional cognitive-behavioral approaches, and whether specific approaches are meaningfully similar or distinct. Perhaps a more central question, which is just beginning to be explored empirically, is whether acceptance and mindfulness processes are mediators of change in therapy. To date, the empirical literature does not provide clear answers to these questions. Behavioral and cognitive therapies have evolved significantly, and there is much variability across applications that may or may not be clinically meaningful. We feel that acceptance-based behavioral approaches share a great deal with the full range of behavioral and cognitive therapies and that many elements of the latter treatments implicitly or explicitly encourage acceptance of internal experiences (e.g., exposure-based interventions cultivate nonavoidance of anxiety symptoms; see Chapter 10 for a more extensive discussion of overlap among approaches and potential for integration). What may be unique and meaningful about ABBTs is the central, explicit, consistent focus on targeting the nature of clients' relationships to internal experiences and the strategies designed to do so. This explicit focus may be a more efficient and robust way of facilitating this change, although more research is needed to support this premise. In addition, an explicit focus on enhancing the client's ability to live a meaningful, valued life may be a unique aspect of these approaches that more directly targets quality of life, although this claim is not yet empirically supported because research in this area is in its infancy. Therefore, rather than claiming that ABBTs are either new or old, we present our understanding of how these approaches may be used effectively, based on research and our clinical experience.

We are concerned that debates over whether ABBTs add something new will devolve into extreme stances that minimize the strong behavioral foundation we see as central to ABBTs or narrow the range of approaches to cognition that characterize cognitive-behavioral therapies (CBTs). In our view, acceptance-based behavioral approaches to treatment, such as ACT and DBT, are part of the evolution of the CBT tradition, not something that exists outside of it. As such, they share a great deal with CBT approaches, while at the same time there are some distinctions that may prove clinically important.

Naming approaches is always problematic. Names serve to highlight similarities and downplay distinctions among approaches with similar names and maximize distinctions and downplay similarities among differently named treatments. We highlight the role of acceptance-based elements (which are often cultivated through various forms of mindfulness practice) and an emphasis on action or behavior in describing our approach to treatment, but this focus is not intended to ignore or obscure the relationship of acceptance-based approaches to aspects of cognitive therapy (such as the process of noticing thoughts, seeing thoughts as not definitively true, and promoting a more flexible relationship with one's thoughts). We feel that the term *cognitive* applied to therapy in common discourse has become narrowly associated with efforts to *change* thoughts in ways that may differ from some of the approaches described here, which is why we do not use the word "cognitive" in the name of these therapies. Nonetheless, many cognitive strategies may promote the kinds of change we describe as therapeutic in this book. We also feel that the cognitive aspect overshadows the behavior aspect in cognitive-behavioral therapy in many circles; we retain the term *behavior* because we feel experience and behavior are primary in these approaches to treatment.[1] We also see the therapeutic relationship, as well as other relationships in the client's life, as important sources of therapeutic change, even though we do not use "relational" or "interpersonal" in the name. Furthermore, although we think there are important commonalities among the approaches we group as ABBTs, we do not wish to discount the specific aspects of each approach (ACT, DBT, etc.) that their developers emphasize. These may be important elements of change.

We see *valued action* (Hayes, Strosahl, & Wilson, 1999), a central element of ACT, as a particularly important part of our work from an acceptance-based behavioral orientation. Consistent with behavior therapy in general, valued action emphasizes behavioral change as part of therapy, but clients choose behavioral goals by connecting those goals to what matters most to clients, or what clients *value*. *Value* here refers to personal importance rather than moral judgment. As we describe in Chapters 7 and 8, therapy can assist clients in exploring the ways in which they would like to act in relationships, at work or at school, and when caring for themselves or contributing to their commu-

---

[1] This emphasis on experience is also clearly evident in all descriptions and demonstrations of MBCT, providing an example of how choices in naming, in this case ours, can suggest distinctions that are inaccurate.

nity. Therapy then assists in overcoming barriers to behaving in ways consistent with those values.

We have also found cultivation of *self-compassion* (as a contrast to judgments and criticism that often arise in response to clients' own thoughts and feelings) to be an important aspect of these treatments. Clients are encouraged to cultivate kindness and care toward their own experience, seeing any thoughts, feelings, and sensations that arise as part of the human experience rather than a sign of their pathology, weaknesses, or limitations. We describe this process in more detail in Chapter 6.

CURRENT STATUS OF EMPIRICAL SUPPORT FOR MINDFULNESS- AND ACCEPTANCE-BASED BEHAVIORAL THERAPIES

The field is still in the early stages of investigating the efficacy, effectiveness, and underlying mechanisms of these approaches to treatment. As we write this book, many trials are underway that will help us determine which presenting problems may be most efficiently addressed by these approaches, which clinical problems will be more effectively addressed by using mindfulness- or acceptance-based strategies as an adjunct to other treatment approaches, and if there are any clinical presentations for which mindfulness- and acceptance-based approaches are contraindicated. Although an extensive review of this literature is beyond the scope of this book (and would quickly go out of date), we want to give an overview of the current status of empirical support to provide guidelines for using the approaches we describe here.

Randomized controlled trials are one way of determining the efficacy of a treatment. Participants are randomly assigned to receive the treatment under investigation or a comparison condition (which may be delayed treatment, treatment as usual, or some other active specific treatment), and outcomes are assessed to see whether the treatment in question is associated with reliable improvements in clinically relevant outcomes. In the absence of active control conditions, these designs can only tell us that a treatment is better than nothing, not that something specific about the intervention is efficacious. In Tables I.1–I.5, we present a summary of the studies investigating the efficacy of mindfulness- and acceptance-based behavioral therapies for clinical problems. We exclude studies of nonclinical participants, or participants with medical rather than psychological presenting problems, but those trials also inform our understanding of the potential utility of these approaches in promoting psychological well-being.[2] Again, this overview is not an extensive, critical review. For clarity of presentation, we omit many important methodological details (such as dropouts, specific measures used, and validity and reliability indices).

These treatment approaches appear to show promise in the treatment of anxiety and depressive disorders (see Table I.1); however, several caveats should be noted. While one study found that an ABBT (ACT) was comparable to cognitive therapy (CT) in treating a range of clients at a counseling center (Forman, Herbert, Moitra, Yeomans,

---

[2]For instance, Jain et al. (2007) found that students randomly assigned to a mindfulness meditation condition reported a significant decrease in reports of distraction and rumination compared to students in either a somatic relaxation or control condition, suggesting that a treatment using mindfulness alone may have an incremental effect on this clinically relevant symptom.

TABLE 1.1. Randomized Controlled Trials Examining Mindfulness- and Acceptance-Based Behavioral Therapies for Anxiety and Depressive Disorders

Reference	Presenting problem	No. of clients	Racial/ethnic makeup	Treatment	Comparison	No. of sessions/format	Findings/limitations[a]
Woods, Wetterneck, & Flessner (2006)	Trichotillomania	25[b]	96.4% White	ACT plus habit reversal training	Wait list (WL)	10 Individual	• Greater decreases in hair pulling, depression, anxiety, and experiential avoidance at post in ACT vs. WL. • Findings generally maintained at 3-month follow-up, although increase in one measure. • No diagnostic assessments of outcome. • No comparison to active treatment. • Treatment included an efficacious treatment; effects could be due to that.
Koszycki et al. (2007)	Social anxiety disorder (SAD)	53[c]	Not reported	MBSR	Cognitive-behavioral group therapy (CBGT)	MBSR = 8 plus all-day retreat CBGT = 12 Group	• Greater improvements in symptoms of SAD and clinician-rated improvement in CBGT vs. MBSR, although both conditions improved. • Comparable, clinically significant reductions in reports of depression and disability, and improvement in quality of life. • Response rates greater in CBGT vs. MBSR (66.7% vs. 38.5%). • No follow-up assessments. • No diagnostic assessments of outcome. • No report of fidelity to protocol or competence ratings. • MBSR delivered by a layperson; no social anxiety–specific content.
Roemer et al. (2008)	Generalized anxiety disorder (GAD)	31[c]	87% White	ABBT for GAD	WL	16 Individual	• Greater improvements in symptoms, diagnostic status, quality of life, and proposed mechanisms of change in ABBT vs. control. • 75% of those treated met criteria for high end-state functioning. • Improvements maintained over 9-month follow-up. • No comparison to active treatment.

(continued)

TABLE 1.1. (continued)

Reference	Presenting problem	No. of clients	Racial/ ethnic makeup	Treatment	Comparison	No. of sessions/ format	Findings/limitations[a]
Forman et al. (2007)	Counseling center clients (33.7% depressive disorder, 31.9% anxiety disorder)	101[c]	64% White, 13% Black, 11% Asian, 3% Latino	ACT	CT	Approx. 15 Individual	• Both groups experienced similar large decreases in symptoms and improvements in clinician-rated functioning. • 62% "recovered" for depressive symptoms, 55% for anxiety symptoms, 38.3% for functioning. • No diagnostic assessments of outcome. • No manuals used, but adherence and competence were assessed as good.
Zettle & Rains (1989)	Women who reported moderate to severe levels of depression on the Beck Depression Inventory, Minnesota Multiphasic Personality Inventory, and Hamilton	31[b]	Not reported	Comprehensive distancing (an early version of ACT)	CT (two different versions)	12 Group	• All groups experienced similar improvements in depressive symptoms at post and 2-month follow-up. • No diagnostic assessments. • No assessment of competence; cannot be sure that CT was administered with competence.
Teasdale et al. (2000)	Recovered recurrently depressed clients	145[c]	99% White	MBCT	Treatment as usual (TAU)	8 Group	• Participants with three or more previous major depressive episodes were less likely to relapse in the MBCT vs. TAU condition (40% vs. 66% during the 120-week study period). • No condition differences with participants who only had two prior episodes. • Not balanced in amount of therapy contact.

Study	Sample	N	Race/Ethnicity	Condition 1	Condition 2	n	Format	Outcomes
Ma & Teasdale (2004)	Recovered or remitted recurrently depressed clients	75[c]	100% White	MBCT	TAU	8	Group	• Participants with three or more major depressive episodes were significantly less likely to relapse in the year following treatment in MBCT vs. TAU condition (36% vs. 78%). • No condition differences with participants who only had two prior episodes. • Not balanced in amount of therapy contact.
Lynch et al. (2003)	Older adults with major depressive disorder	34[b]	85% White, 9% African American, 6% Hispanic American	Medication (MED) + modified DBT	MED	28	Group skills + telephone coaching, no individual	• Only the MED + DBT condition showed a decrease in reports of depressive symptoms on the Beck Depression Inventory. • More participants in remission at 6-month follow-up in DBT + MED (75%) vs. MED alone (31%). • Many other comparisons did not reveal significant differences between groups, but this may have been due to small sample size. • No diagnostic assessments of outcome. • Not balanced in amount of therapy contact.
Lynch et al. (2007)	Older adults with elevated depression scores; at least one personality disorder. Failed to respond to an 8-week MED trial	35[b]	85.7% White	MED + DBT	MED	24	Group and individual	• Both groups reported similar improvements in depression. • MED + DBT associated with greater reductions in interpersonal sensitivity and interpersonal aggression than MED alone, maintained at follow-up. • No diagnostic assessments of depression. • Not balanced in amount of therapy contact. • DBT not adapted for depressed older adults; adaptation could improve outcome.

[a] All differences reported reflect statistically different effects, unless otherwise noted.
[b] Completer sample, on which analyses were conducted.
[c] Intent-to-treat sample, on which analyses were conducted.

7

& Geller, 2007), another found that a cognitive-behavioral group therapy that specifically targeted social anxiety disorder was more efficacious in targeting symptoms of social anxiety than a general mindfulness intervention (MBSR), even though both led to improvements in functioning (Koszycki, Benger, Shlik, & Bradwejn, 2007). An ABBT for generalized anxiety that integrates disorder-specific and behavioral strategies shows promise, although it has not yet been compared to an active intervention (Roemer, Orsillo, & Salters-Pedneault, 2008). While an ABBT (MBCT) had an impressive effect on reducing relapse among individuals in remission from recurrent depression (with three or more previous episodes—Ma & Teasdale, 2004; Teasdale et al., 2000), we do not yet know its efficacy with symptomatic individuals,[3] and it does not seem beneficial for individuals with only two prior episodes. On the other hand, DBT seems to be efficacious in reducing depressive symptoms among older adults with a current mood disorder who do not also present with a personality disorder (Lynch, Morse, Mendelson, & Robins, 2003). An early version of ACT seemed comparable to CT in treating women with depression (Zettle & Rains, 1989), but the absence of independent ratings as to the competency with which CT was delivered and diagnostic assessments limits our ability to draw strong conclusions from this study. We suggest that clinicians draw from the evidence-based literature in treating anxiety and depressive disorders. Minimally, treatment should include some disorder-specific content, such as psychoeducation about depression and anxiety (as we discuss in Chapter 5). We agree with Teasdale, Segal, and Williams's (2003) suggestion that applications of these treatments be grounded in a clear formulation of their relevance to clients' specific presenting problems. Furthermore, given the strong efficacy data for behavioral therapies, we suggest integrating behavioral strategies into any mindfulness-based approach. Treatment strategies such as interoceptive exposure for panic disorder, social exposures for social anxiety, and behavioral activation or CT for active depressive symptoms should be part of any initial treatment plan. We integrate these strategies within an acceptance-based behavioral model (as discussed specifically in Chapter 10). Progress should be repeatedly monitored, and an absence of response to these strategies warrants further incorporation of mindfulness- and acceptance-based strategies. In addition, clients who refuse exposure-based interventions may be particularly well suited for an acceptance-based behavioral approach, which may help prepare them for exposure exercises.

Preliminary evidence is also beginning to accrue supporting the efficacy of mindfulness- and acceptance-based approaches in the treatment of substance dependence and eating disorders (although treatments for eating disorders have not yet been compared to an active control condition; see Table I.2). Interestingly, a comprehensive validation comparison condition that combined acceptance-based elements of DBT with a 12-step program also had encouraging findings, although DBT was associated with greater abstinence in the latter parts of therapy (Linehan et al., 2002). In addition to the randomized controlled trials (RCTs) listed in the table, a recent study examined the effects of a vipassana meditation course offered to individuals in prison on substance abuse and psychosocial outcomes (Bowen et al., 2006). Participants in the course dem-

---

[3]One nonrandomized study did find that MBCT was associated with a significant reduction in residual depressive symptoms among individuals whose depressive episode had remitted (Kingston, Dooley, Bates, Lawlor, & Malone, 2007), while another has shown that individuals with active, treatment-resistant depression show decreases in symptoms when in an MBCT group, although no control group was used in this study, so causality cannot be concluded (Kenny & Williams, 2007).

onstrated significantly less substance use and psychiatric symptoms than those who participated in treatment as usual in a medium-security prison. ABBT (specifically ACT) also shows promise in reducing rehospitalization among individuals with psychotic symptoms, suggesting that it may be a beneficial adjunctive treatment approach among individuals with clinically significant psychotic symptoms (see Table I.3). DBT appears to be efficacious in reducing suicide attempts, medical risk, substance use, and rehospitalization among individuals with borderline personality disorder (BPD), and preliminary evidence suggests that an acceptance-based behavioral group therapy alone can reduce deliberate self-harm among these individuals (see Table I.4).

Finally, integrative behavioral couple therapy (IBCT), a treatment that incorporates acceptance and change strategies, has shown promise with distressed heterosexual married couples, yielding effects comparable to or better than traditional behavioral couple therapy (an empirically supported intervention for couples' distress); these gains are maintained over a 2-year follow-up period (see Table I.5). In addition, a mindfulness-based relationship enhancement intervention improved relationship satisfaction among happy, nondistressed couples (compared to a wait list control), and reports of mindfulness practice were associated with increased relationship happiness and reduced relationship stress among couples in the treatment (Carson, Carson, Gil, & Baucom, 2004).

Thus, research suggests that mindfulness- and acceptance-based behavioral therapies hold promise for individuals and couples with a range of presenting problems, from significant, chronic conditions to milder presentations. For more severe problems, incorporating other interventions such as pharmacotherapy (e.g., for serious mental illness) is warranted, as are more intensive versions of these treatments (such as DBT, which consists of 12 months of both group and individual therapy). These strategies have also been shown to reduce stress, enhance well-being, and promote health, even among those who are already functioning well (e.g., Shapiro, Astin, Bishop, & Cordova, 2005; Williams, Kolar, Reger, & Pearson, 2001). Clients can use what they learn in treatment to maintain and enhance their well-being following termination of treatment and when they are no longer symptomatic.

Although considerably more research is needed on the efficacy of these treatment approaches and adaptations for underserved populations, some of these trials suggest they may be beneficial for individuals from economically disadvantaged (e.g., Koons et al., 2001; Linehan et al., 1999) or racial minority (e.g., Gaudiano & Herbert, 2006) backgrounds. (See Chapter 11 for a discussion of cultural considerations in using ABBTs.) A number of studies have also investigated the efficacy and effectiveness of ABBTs and more traditional mindfulness-based treatments for individuals with a wide range of physical disorders (for examples of ACT treatment studies, see Gregg, Callaghan, Hayes, & Glenn-Lawson, 2007, and Lundgren, Dahl, Melin, & Kies, 2006; for a meta-analysis of studies of mindfulness-based treatments, see Grossman, Niemann, Schmidt, & Walach, 2004), suggesting that these approaches may also be beneficial for people with physical health problems with comorbid psychological presentations.

We present our suggestions for how to incorporate mindfulness- and acceptance-based behavioral approaches into clinical practice in the context of this evolving empirical basis. Throughout the book, we provide examples of handouts and homework assignments and include clinical examples (either composites or with significantly altered descriptive information) to illustrate different presentations and responses to therapy.

TABLE I.2. Randomized Controlled Trials Examining Mindfulness- and Acceptance-Based Behavioral Therapies for Substance-Related and Eating Disorders

Reference	Presenting problem	No. of clients	Racial/ethnic makeup	Treatment	Comparison	No. of sessions/format	Findings/limitations[a]
Linehan et al. (1999)	Women with borderline personality disorder (BPD) and substance use disorder (SUD)	28[c]	78% European descent, 7% African American, 4% Latina, 11% other	DBT adapted for substance abuse	TAU	1 year DBT = weekly group, individual, and coaching calls	• Greater proportion of drug and alcohol abstinent days in DBT vs. TAU condition at post and 4-month follow-up. • Greater number of clean urinalysis (UA) results in DBT vs. TAU condition at post and follow-up. • Greater gains in global and social adjustment in the DBT vs. TAU condition at follow-up. • Not balanced in amount of therapy contact.
Linehan et al. (2002)	Women with BPD and opiate dependence	28[c]	66% White, 26% African American	DBT for substance abuse + opiate agonist	Comprehensive validation therapy + 12-step + opiate agonist	1 year Weekly group and individual and coaching/sponsor	• Decreases in opiate-positive UA results in both conditions; these decreases were maintained better from 8–12 months in the DBT condition. • Fewer opiate-positive UAs in DBT vs. TAU at 12 months. • Similar opiate-positive UAs at 4-month follow-up (27% DBT; 33% CVT + 12-step). • Reductions in psychopathology in both conditions at post and follow-up. • Greater dropout in DBT vs. CVT + 12-step.
Hayes, Wilson, et al. (2004)	Polysubstance abuse or dependence, with a recent relapse while on methadone	73[d] (69 at follow-up)	87% White	ACT + methadone maintenance (MM)	MM alone Intensive 12-step	16 weeks ITSF and ACT	• More UAs negative for opiates in ACT (61%) vs. MM (28%) at 6-month follow-up. • More UAs negative for any drugs in ACT (50%) vs. MM (12%) at follow-up.

Study	Sample	N	Demographics	Treatment	Comparison	Dosage	Outcomes
					facilitation (ITSF) + MM	both 32 individual and 16 group sessions	• No difference in UAs negative for opiates in ITSF (50%) vs. ACT or MM. • More UAs negative for any drugs in ITSF (38%) vs. MM at follow-up, no difference from ACT. • Reduced sample (due in part to high attrition) limited ability to detect any difference in active treatments. • ACT and MM not balanced in amount of therapy contact.
Gifford et al. (2004)	Nicotine-dependent smokers with at least 12-month history	62[d] (55 at follow-up)	77% White, 7% Native American, 7% Hispanic	ACT (in individual and group form)	Nicotine replacement therapy (NRT)	7 weeks ACT 7 individual and 7 group sessions	• Higher quit rates in ACT (35%) vs. NRT (15%) at 12-month follow-up. • Quit rates still low in ACT. • Not balanced in amount of therapy contact.
Telch, Agras, & Linehan (2001)	Binge-eating disorder (BED)	34[b]	94% White	DBT for BED	WL control	20 Group	• Reduction in binge episodes in DBT vs. WL. • More women abstinent (for 4 weeks) in DBT (89%) vs. WL (12.5%) at post. 56% abstinent at 6-month follow-up. • No comparison to active treatment.
Safer, Telch, & Agras (2001)	Women with one or more binge–purge cycles per week (80.6% bulimia nervosa)	31[c]	87.1% White	Adapted DBT	WL control	20 Individual	• Reduction in bingeing and purging in DBT vs. WL. • More women abstinent in DBT (28.6%) vs. WL (0%). • No follow-up assessment. • No comparison to active treatment.

[a]All differences reported reflect statistically different effects, unless otherwise noted.
[b]Completer sample, on which analyses were conducted.
[c]Intent-to-treat sample, on which analyses were conducted.
[d]Participants with complete assessment data, on which analyses were conducted.

TABLE I.3. Randomized Controlled Trials Examining Mindfulness- and Acceptance-Based Behavioral Therapies for Psychotic Disorders

Reference	Presenting problem	No. of clients	Racial/ethnic makeup	Treatment	Comparison	No. of sessions/ format	Findings/limitations[a]
Bach & Hayes (2002)	Hospitalized with psychotic symptoms	70[b]	80% White, 12% Hispanic, 4% African American	ACT + TAU	TAU (included therapy on the unit and medication)	4 Individual (+ TAU)	• Slower rates to rehospitalization in ACT vs. TAU over 4-month follow-up. • 20% in ACT rehospitalized by follow-up, 40% in TAU (significance not analyzed). • Greater decrease in believability ratings in ACT vs. TAU. • No assessment of adherence. • Not balanced in amount of therapy contact.
Guidiano & Herbert (2006)	Hospitalized with psychotic symptoms	40[c]	88% African American	ACT (4 sessions) + enhanced TAU (included medication and therapy)	ETAU with ind. contact added and balanced therapy contact hours	1–5, average of 3 Individual	• Greater decrease in distress over hallucinations in ACT vs. ETAU. • Greater improvement in social functioning in ACT vs. ETAU. • More participants with clinically significant improvement in ACT (50%) vs. ETAU (7%). • 28% in ACT rehospitalized by 4-month follow-up, 45% in ETAU; difference not significant. • No assessment of adherence possible. • Small sample size may mask significant difference in rehopitalization rates.

[a]All differences reported reflect statistically different effects, unless otherwise noted.
[b]Sample with complete assessment data, on which analyses were conducted.
[c]Intent-to-treat sample, on which analyses were conducted.

Given the centrality of a coherent case conceptualization in responsive, individualized, evidence-based practice, we begin by presenting a conceptualization of clinical difficulties that highlights why these approaches may be beneficial (Chapter 1), methods for assessing clinically relevant factors (Chapter 2), and how to develop a case conceptualization to guide treatment (Chapter 3). In Chapters 4–8, we describe the central elements of ABBTs, including setting the stage for treatment, psychoeducation, mindfulness- and acceptance-based strategies, and valued action. We then discuss how to monitor progress, prevent relapse, and effectively terminate therapy (Chapter 9) as well as how to integrate other approaches into an ABBT approach to treatment (Chapter 10). Finally, we discuss relevant cultural considerations and suggest other readings in this area (Chapter 11). For those interested in further mindfulness resources, we provide suggestions of books that we, our therapists, and our clients have found particularly useful (see the Appendix).

Over the last 10 years, we have found our research and clinical work in this area to be challenging, exciting, inspiring, and personally meaningful. We sincerely hope that you will find our efforts to share our clinical experiences, along with those of many other clinicians and researchers operating from a mindfulness- and acceptance-based behavioral perspective, to be personally and professionally relevant.

TABLE I.4. Randomized Controlled Trials Examining Mindfulness- and Acceptance-Based Behavioral Therapies for Borderline Personality Disorder

Reference	Presenting problem	No. of clients	Racial/ethnic makeup	Treatment	Comparison	No. of sessions/format	Findings/limitations[a]
Linehan, Armstrong, Suarez, Allmon, & Heard (1991) Linehan, Heard, & Armstrong (1993)	Women with BPD and parasuicidal acts	44[b]	Not reported	DBT	TAU	1 year Group, individual, and coaching	• Fewer parasuicide acts in DBT vs. TAU throughout treatment year. • Better retention in therapy in DBT vs. TAU. • Fewer days in hospital in DBT vs. TAU during treatment year. • No differences in depression, hopelessness, suicidal ideation at post. • At 12-month follow-up, better employment performance, better social and global adjustment, and fewer psychiatric hospitalizations in DBT vs. TAU. • Conditions not balanced on amount of therapy contact.
Turner (2000)	BPD with recent suicide attempt	24[c]	79% White, 17% African American, 4% Asian American	DBT with psychodynamic techniques	Client-centered therapy (CCT)	1 year (49–84 sessions) Individual with 6 group sessions	• Greater improvements in suicide/self-harm in DBT vs. CCT. • Greater reductions in hospitalizations in DBT vs. CCT. • No follow-up assessment. • No assessments of adherence or competence.
Koons et al. (2001)	Women veterans with BPD (at VA)	20[b]	75% White, 25% African American	DBT	TAU	6 months DBT + individual, group, and coaching	• Greater decreases in suicidal ideation, hopelessness, and depression in DBT vs. TAU. • Decrease in parasuicidal acts greater in DBT vs. TAU at $p < .10$. • No follow-up assessment. • Small sample size may have masked some differences. • Comparable individual contact across conditions; more group in DBT.

Study	Population	N	Treatment	Comparison	Ethnicity	Format/Duration	Findings
Verheul et al. (2003) Van den Bosch, Koeter, Stijnen, Verheul, & Van den Brink (2005)	Women with BPD	58[c]	DBT	TAU	97% Dutch nationality	12 months DBT = individual, group, and coaching	• Greater decrease in self-mutilating and self-damaging acts in DBT vs. TAU; sustained at 6-month follow-up. • Greater decrease in alcohol consumption in DBT vs. TAU; sustained at follow-up. • Better therapy retention in DBT vs. TAU. • Conditions not balanced on amount of therapy contact. • Authors note nonsignificant increase in symptoms during follow-up; booster sessions might be beneficial.
Gratz & Gunderson (2006)	Women with BPD and history of deliberate self-harm	22[b]	Acceptance-based emotion regulation group (draws from ACT and DBT) + TAU	TAU	100% White	14 weeks Group	• Greater reductions in deliberate self-harm, anxiety, depressive symptoms, and symptoms of BPD in ER + TAU vs. TAU. • No follow-up assessment. • Conditions not balanced on amount of therapy contact.
Linehan et al. (2007)	Women with BPD and past suicidal behavior	101[c]	DBT	Community treatment by experts (CTBE)	87% White, 5% other, 4% African American, 2% Asian American	1 year Standard DBT format Supervision group added for CTBE	• Greater reductions in suicide attempts, medical risks associated with suicide attempts and self-injury, psychiatric hospitalizations, and emergency room visits in DBT vs. CTBE across treatment and 12-month follow-up. • Improvements in depression and suicidal ideation in both conditions. • Fewer dropouts or change in therapists in DBT vs. CTBE. • More group contact in DBT vs. TAU.

Note. ER, emotion regulation.

[a]All differences reported reflect statistically different effects, unless otherwise noted.

[b]Completer sample, on which analyses were conducted.

[c]Intent-to-treat sample, on which analyses were conducted.

TABLE I.5. Randomized Controlled Trials Examining Mindfulness- and Acceptance-Based Behavioral Therapies for Couples' Distress

Reference	Presenting problem	No. of clients	Racial/ethnic makeup	Treatment	Comparison	No. of sessions/ format	Findings/limitations[a]
Jacobson, Christensen, Prince, Cordova, & Eldridge (2000)	Heterosexual married couples with clinically significant distress	21 couples[b]	Not reported	Integrative behavioral couple therapy (IBCT)	Traditional behavioral couple therapy (TBCT)	Maximum of 26 sessions Couples	• Due to reduced power, no statistical analyses conducted. • Both husbands and wives in IBCT reported greater improvements in satisfaction and decreases in distress than those in TBCT (medium to large effect sizes for group differences). • 70% of couples in IBCT and 55% of couples in TBCT were recovered. • Both treatments performed with equal competence and adherence. • No follow-up assessment.
Christensen et al. (2004) Christensen, Atkins, Yi, Baucom, & George (2006)	Heterosexual married couples with serious and chronic distress	134 couples[b]	Husbands: 79.1% White, 6.7% African American, 6% Asian or Pacific Islander, 5.2% Latino Wives: 76.1% White, 8.2% African American, 5.2% Latina, 4.5% Asian or Pacific Islander	IBCT	TBCT	Maximum of 26 sessions Couples	• Couples in both treatments showed improvements in marital satisfaction across treatment. • Recovery or reliable improvement at post: 71% in IBCT, 59% in TBCT (not statistically different). • Couples in both treatments initially showed a deterioration in adjustment over 2-year follow-up; this reversed and gradually increased. • Couples in IBCT deteriorated less and began to recover more quickly than those in TBCT. • 69% of couples in IBCT and 60% of couples in TBCT still recovered or reliably improved at 2-year follow-up.

[a]All differences reported reflect statistically different effects, unless otherwise noted.
[b]Intent-to-treat sample, on which analyses were conducted.

ONE

An Acceptance-Based Behavioral Conceptualization of Clinical Problems

Maya, a college student, came to therapy because she was experiencing intense anxiety that was making it difficult for her to get her school assignments done and take exams. She reported worrying that she would fail out of school and never be able to support herself or help support her aging parents. She described herself as an anxious person and saw her anxiety as evidence that she was "weak." Maya recounted numerous methods and strategies she had tried to make herself feel less anxious and more self-confident. Although she described some periods of her life during which she felt better, overall she felt as if her attempts to control her anxiety had failed. When asked about avoidance, Maya was able to give many examples of situations she avoided, such as calling her parents because she knew they would ask about school. When asked about her social life, she described not having time to make friends because she needed to spend time on her schoolwork, and it took her so long to get it done. Upon further questioning, she also noted that she "felt uncomfortable" when she was with groups of people, which also contributed to her avoidance of socializing. Maya said she was so busy with schoolwork that she did not have much time to feel lonely or sad, although, upon questioning, she was able to recall times she had briefly felt this way when she wasn't "keeping herself busy." She also described periods of binge eating followed by restricted eating. Maya wanted to reduce her binge eating but saw her restricted eating as one of her few strengths.

Our treatment of Maya would begin by developing an understanding of how her experiences and behaviors are linked and understandable, even though they may seem compartmentalized and confusing to her. We would collaborate with Maya in developing a conceptualization and use it as a foundation for designing an individualized treatment plan; it would be based in the overarching conceptual model that underlies acceptance-based behavioral approaches to treatment and is presented in this chapter. Defining this underlying model is critical because the model serves as the foundation for an individualized formulation of a particular client's difficulties. The model also

provides a starting point from which we choose specific assessment strategies and clinical methods and a touchstone to which we return repeatedly to evaluate the course and
progress of therapy.

The model contains three main elements, each of which relates to the others. First,
clinical problems are seen as stemming from the way that clients (and humans in general) often *relate to their internal experiences*. This relationship can be characterized as
"fused" (Hayes, Strosahl, & Wilson, 1999), entangled (Germer, 2005), or "hooked"
(Chodron, 2007) and is distinguished by an overidentification with one's thoughts, feelings, images, and sensations. In other words, everyone feels sad from time to time, but
a client who is fused with her internal experience may define herself by that sadness;
for example, Maya defines herself as "weak" due to her anxiety. This overidentification or fusion with internal experiences can set off a cascade of problematic responses.
Anxiety is no longer viewed as a natural emotion that ebbs and flows; instead, it is
seen as a defining or all-encompassing state, which can lead to it being judged and
viewed as intolerable and unacceptable. The second element of the model is *experiential
avoidance*, or emotional, cognitive, and behavioral efforts to avoid or escape distressing thoughts, feelings, memories, and sensations (Hayes, Wilson, Gifford, Follette, &
Strosahl, 1996). Clients engage in experiential avoidance hoping to improve their lives,
but it often paradoxically leads to further distress or diminished quality of life (e.g.,
Hayes et al., 1996). Experiential avoidance is closely tied to the ways clients relate to
their internal experiences. If a client is fused with an emotion and sees that emotion as
potentially overwhelming and dangerous, he or she may be highly motivated to engage
in strategies aimed at avoiding or changing that internal experience. In Maya's case,
whenever she experiences anxiety, she views it as a reflection of her inherent weakness,
is threatened by it and tries to get rid of it, but her efforts often fail, further fueling her
sense of herself as weak. Self-monitoring reveals that Maya eats to soothe her anxiety
but then experiences more anxiety due to fears of weight gain, which she tries to control
by restricting her eating. Thus, both of these behaviors seem to serve an experientially
avoidant function. The final element of the model is *behavioral restriction or constriction*,
which occurs when individuals who are struggling with internal experiences fail to
engage in actions consistent with what matters most to them (i.e., valued action; Wilson
& Murrell, 2004), further perpetuating their distress and dissatisfaction. When internal
experiences are negatively judged and seen as dangerous, action is motivated more by
an attempt to avoid unpleasant states than by a desire to engage in fulfilling behaviors.
Maya has come to avoid many aspects of social support, including being with friends
and talking to her parents, because she commonly experiences anxiety in these contexts.
Her occasional feelings of sadness may signal that she is not living her life in a way that
is meaningful and satisfying (i.e., values-consistent), yet she avoids these feelings by
working hard, further perpetuating the cycle.

Acceptance-based models have been presented in detail by several clinical theo-
rists/researchers, such as Hayes, Strosahl, and Wilson (1999); Linehan (1993a); Segal and
colleagues (2002); and Jacobson and Christensen (1996; see Hayes, Follette, & Linehan,
2004, for a book-length review). In this chapter, we (1) draw together elements of these
approaches, as well as traditional cognitive-behavioral approaches, to highlight what
we consider the central elements of an acceptance-based behavioral conceptualization,
(2) briefly review some of the research that supports this model, and (3) illustrate how

this model can be applied to specific clinical problems. We conclude with an overview of how this model translates into intervention and continue in the next two chapters with discussion of how this model guides individual treatment planning, assessment, and delivery.

Our approach to understanding problematic clinical behaviors is based in a behavioral conceptualization. That is, we understand responses to be learned through both associations and consequences, and we work to identify the function of problematic responses to determine strategies for intervention. We see human difficulties as arising from a combination of biological predispositions, environmental factors, and learned habits that lead to a host of reactions and behaviors that occur automatically, without awareness or apparent choice. Learning happens in several ways. We can learn through *direct experience*. For instance, a woman who was raped might learn an association between the smell of specific cologne and danger, which motivates her to avoid others with that same scent. We also learn through consequences that consistently follow particular behaviors, either reinforcing or punishing them and, thus, altering their frequency, as when an individual continues to drink excessively because of the stress-relieving properties of alcohol. Learning also occurs through *modeling and observation*, such as seeing the reactions and behaviors of our parents or siblings, and through *instruction*, such as being told to act in certain ways or not to show certain emotions. These learned patterns of behaviors often serve a useful function, particularly in the short term; however, as contexts change or new behaviors become available to us, certain patterns may no longer serve us well. This is particularly the case when we have come to respond inflexibly (i.e., having the same response in a wide range of contexts). For instance, we might learn from our family to "put on a happy face" when we feel distressed, and this behavior might be adaptive if our parents punish us any time we display sadness or anger, such as through criticism or inattention. However, overlearning this response (i.e.., doing it rigidly and inflexibly) is typically maladaptive. Masking our distress in a romantic relationship could interfere with the development of true intimacy or leave us unable to clearly express our needs and desires. We might even learn to mask our distress so quickly and consistently that we lose awareness of our own emotional state, which limits our ability to benefit from the function of emotions.

A central problem, then, is the habitual, insensitive (to context), and automatic nature of these responses. From an acceptance-based behavioral model, three types of habitual responses are seen as clinically important targets for intervention. First, learned qualities of awareness (particularly awareness of internal experiences) are seen as both a cause and a consequence of clinical problems and an important focus of treatment. Awareness can be severely diminished (a common feature of automatic responding), narrowly focused on unpleasant cues and events, or judgmental and critical. Second, the experientially avoidant function of many overlearned behaviors can be problematic. That is, clinically relevant behaviors such as avoiding certain situations, alcohol use, overeating, and general inaction may be maintained specifically because they serve the function of temporarily reducing, eliminating, or avoiding distressing thoughts, feelings, or sensations. Finally, the shift away from engaging in actions that are of value to the individual (and sometimes toward impulsively and automatically engaging in actions that are not valued, due to their experientially avoidant function), is thought to contribute to distress and diminish quality of life.

RESTRICTED, ENTANGLED, FUSED INTERNAL AWARENESS

Limits in Internal Awareness

Many clinical theories highlight the potential role of deficits in internal, or experiential, awareness in psychological difficulties and the role of increased awareness in promoting psychological well-being.[1] Consistent with these models, from an acceptance-based behavioral perspective, deficits in awareness may manifest in several ways that indicate clinical problems (these different ways may co-occur in the same individual). First, clients are often *unaware* of their internal experiences, not recognizing emotional, cognitive, or physiological responses that precede problematic behaviors (e.g., alexithymia). Clients may also *misunderstand* their internal responses, labeling physiological sensations as hunger when they in fact reflect distress or mistaking one threatening emotion (such as anxiety) for another, more personally acceptable one (such as anger). Diminished or inaccurate awareness reduces clients' ability to use their emotional responses functionally and may lead them to react in ways that are puzzling to them. For instance, a chronically lonely client may tell you that he does not attend social events because he does not enjoy them, when, in fact, he is avoiding them due to his unrecognized anxiety and would very much like to be more socially engaged. Another client may surprise herself by responding aggressively to a coworker because she did not realize she had felt resentment and anger due to her coworker's repeated apparent slights and disrespectful tone. Although Maya was very aware of her anxious internal experiences, she had more trouble noticing and identifying her experience of sadness, so that she was not conscious of the ways her life was unsatisfying to her. In sum, individuals may either avoid or engage in undesired behaviors due to their lack of emotional awareness, and this impaired awareness may interfere with individuals' ability to choose to act rather than react to situations.

Lack of emotional awareness, like many clinically relevant characteristics, is probably learned. Individuals may be taught by their parents to distrust their emotional reactions, such as when a parent tells a child not to be afraid in a threatening situation or dismisses feelings of sadness over a loss or disappointment (Linehan, 1993a). If a parent habitually responds to a child in this way, the child may come to rely on external sources to "know" how he or she is feeling in a particular situation. Children may be punished for being "emotional" and rewarded for being "rational," or "calm, cool, and collected," which teaches them to ignore their internal experiences in the hope that negative emotions will pass.

Difficulties with the Quality of Internal Awareness

Clients with limited awareness of the nuances of their emotions can also simultaneously report a heightened awareness of their general distress, which can be confusing to them and their therapists. For instance, individuals with panic disorder are hyperaware of their physiological sensations, individuals with generalized anxiety disorder (GAD) are painfully aware of their worry, and individuals with depression are very aware of their

---

[1]Darren Holowka, in his dissertation, suggests that experiential awareness may be a common factor across diverse forms of psychotherapy (Holowka, 2008; Holowka & Roemer, 2007).

negative mood state; however, this awareness differs significantly from the awareness that psychotherapy aims to cultivate. First, this awareness may not be *clear*, in that individuals may perceive they are generally distressed but not be able to pinpoint specific and subtle shifts in their emotional, physiological, or cognitive state. For instance, a client might describe a panic attack that lasted 2 weeks (which is not physiologically possible) or feeling "bad," without a clear sense of whether he feels sadness, anger, fear, or a blended emotion. Individuals' awareness may be *critical, judgmental,* or *reactive*. For instance, a client with recurrent depressive episodes might notice her sadness and be very distressed that she is sad again, think her sadness is a sign that a debilitating depression is returning, and feel alarmed by its occurrence. These reactions likely perpetuate and worsen the sadness, possibly leading to depression, rather than promoting adaptive functioning. Maya provides an example of this kind of quality of awareness. She was very aware of any signs of anxiety and responded to them with self-judgment and criticism, further perpetuating her anxiety. Awareness can also become *narrowed*, or *selective*. For instance, individuals with anxiety disorders may be so aware of a potential threat that they do not notice other cues in their environment that signal safety, or they may be so focused on their anxious responding that they do not detect the occurrence of positive emotional responses. This selective attention to anxiety further exacerbates their sense that their anxiety is unchanging and pervasive.

All of these examples of ways in which the quality of experiential awareness can be problematic can be thought of as aspects of a larger category of *overidentification*, or *"fusion"* (Hayes, Strosahl, & Wilson, 1999) or *"entanglement"* (Germer, 2005), with one's internal experience in a way that inhibits adaptive functioning. Different acceptance-based approaches use different terms to identify this quality and emphasize somewhat different aspects of it, but they share a conceptualization of this "hooked" relationship as a source of suffering or clinical problems and an important target of intervention. These models are consistent with traditional behavioral models of "fear of fear" (Goldstein & Chambless, 1978), distress about emotions[2] (Williams, Chambless, & Ahrens, 1997), interoceptive conditioning (e.g., Barlow, 2002), cognitive theories of anxiety sensitivity (e.g., Reiss, Peterson, Gursky, & McNally, 1986), and metacognitive beliefs (e.g., Wells, 1995), each of which suggests that negative reactions to or appraisals of internal experiences explain how these experiences progress from natural human responses that ebb and flow to more rigid patterns of problematic responding. Although a detailed discussion of these models is beyond the scope of this book, some are highlighted due to their potential utility in clinical formulations.

Reactivity to and Judgment of Internal Experiences

Many models of clinical problems note that internal responses become problematic due to individuals' reactions to these responses rather than the responses themselves (e.g.,

---

[2]Although the terms *fear of fear* and *fear of emotion* have been used in the literature, these concepts are more accurately labeled "anxiety of" or "distress about" fear and other emotions, in that they describe an anticipatory or reactive process with a longer duration than fear (Barlow, personal communication; see Barlow, 1991, for a discussion of the role of anxiety/dysthymia in response to the experience of basic emotions in emotional disorders).

Barlow, 1991; Borkovec & Sharples, 2004).[3] While a whole range of internal responses may naturally come and go for all of us, humans have also developed an ability to respond to these experiences in certain ways that may lead them to become more rigid, "sticky," or inflexible, resulting in clinical problems. For instance, models of panic note that panic attacks are common across the population, but only some people develop panic disorder, and these seem to be the individuals who experience anxious apprehension about future panic attacks (Barlow, 1991). Relatedly, behavioral models suggest that individuals with panic disorder have learned to experience anxiety in response to their bodily sensations (interoceptive conditioning; Barlow, 2002). This distress or apprehension seems to be the crucial element of panic disorder, and successful treatments target it directly; successfully treated individuals continue to experience panic sensations but no longer experience heightened anxiety in response to these sensations. The reactive awareness of bodily sensations that characterizes individuals with panic disorder is also narrowed, so that they focus solely on arousal sensations and may have limited emotional awareness. For instance, a recent study found that individuals who reported a high level of panic symptoms reported more negative emotional responses and more emotional avoidance efforts in response to a positively valanced film clip than did individuals not prone to panic (Tull & Roemer, 2007); thus, these individuals may respond to all kinds of arousal symptoms with anxiety rather than discriminating between sources of that arousal.

Acceptance-based models that emphasize *mindfulness* (a construct drawn from Buddhist traditions but used in secular contexts for health promotion and intervention purposes—e.g., Kabat-Zinn, 1990; Segal et al., 2002), which has been defined as "open-hearted, moment-to-moment, non-judgmental awareness" (Kabat-Zinn, 2005, p. 24), similarly emphasize the significance of reactions to one's experiences, highlighting the role that judgmental, critical awareness may play in human suffering or clinical problems. Often, clients present with habitual judgments of themselves or their responses as being "weak," "crazy," "irrational," or "stupid." As they notice their internal experiences, they react with critical judgments, prompting efforts to avoid these experiences. These judgments may stem from the way caregivers responded to them growing up. In fact, clients are often able to recognize that the critical words they use to describe their responses are the same words a parent habitually used in criticizing them. These judgments may also stem from, or be perpetuated by, the perception that others do not seem to have the same internal reactions (because they cannot observe others' internal experiences). Maya may not recognize that her friends and family also experience anxiety in certain contexts. She may have heard her parents or others refer to people who expressed anxiety as "weak," leading her to view her own anxiety that way. This kind of judgment is likely to keep her from sharing her experiences of anxiety with others, which will also keep her from learning that others have similar experiences.

Although clients often report beliefs that this kind of self-critical stance helps motivate them to change, it seems more likely that this perspective contributes to distress and impairment. Linehan's (1993a) classic model of borderline personality disorder highlights the etiological role of an invalidating environment on subsequent dysregulated

---

[3]Christensen and Jacobson (2000) note a similar process in couples. They distinguish between *initial* problems (such as a difference in desired frequency of sexual activity) and *reactive* problems (the difficulties that emerge from each member of the couple's attempts to cope with this problem, such as hostility, withdrawal, and accusation).

emotion, cognition, and behavior. Individuals then learn to invalidate their own experience, further contributing to their dysregulation. The presence of a judgmental, self-critical stance (and the absence of self-compassion) can be seen as a causal or maintaining factor in a wide range of presenting problems (see Neff, Rude, & Kirkpatrick, 2007, for evidence of association between self-compassion and psychological well-being). For instance, when individuals feel sad and become critical of their responses, this negative view of themselves may decrease their motivation to make behavioral changes or engage fully in their lives. Individuals with social anxiety commonly engage in self-judgment that may exacerbate their fears of others' judgments, reduce their willingness to engage in various actions when they may be judged, and increase their sense of being unsafe in the world due to some kind of personal failing. Maya's criticisms of herself for experiencing anxiety exacerbate her fears that she will be unsuccessful, heightening rather than lessening her anxiety.

Entangled or Fused Awareness

Broadly, acceptance-based models that emphasize mindfulness highlight a quality of awareness that leads to suffering and contrast it with a quality of awareness that can be more freeing. According to these models, we commonly become "hooked" into our internal experience, partly by seeing it as more indicative of reality than it is and partly by judging it and disliking it and wanting it to be other than it is. Thus, rather than just experiencing anger, we have anger, a dislike of anger, and a wish for anger to go away.[4] Rather than experiencing a fearful response, we define ourselves as a fearful person. Paradoxically, these responses hook us more to the very emotions we are trying to avoid.

Wishing internal experiences were other than what they are is natural, given how unpleasant certain emotional, cognitive, or physiological reactions can feel and our common socialization experiences (e.g., being told, "don't worry, be happy").[5] Yet this desire for our internal experiences to be other than they are, particularly when we attach to it and act from it, is thought to increase their unpleasantness without diminishing the experiences themselves. Hayes, Strosahl, and Wilson (1999) describe a similar process in their description of *clean* versus *dirty* emotions. Clean emotions are those we have in response to an event, while dirty emotions arise from our strong desires and efforts to make clean emotions go away, which only add to our distress.

The human tendency to mistake transient internal experiences for indications of permanent truth or reality is a likely cause of or contributing factor to these desires to feel or think other than we do. For instance, if we feel anxiety about an upcoming presentation and have the thought that we are not capable of doing it, we may take that thought as an indication that we cannot do the presentation. When we feel hurt by a comment from our partner and have the thought that she does not really care about us,

---

[4]Shame in response to anger or other emotional reactions to environmentally elicited emotions are examples of what Greenberg and Safran (1987) refer to as secondary emotions, or emotions that occur in response to adaptive primary emotions. They suggest these types of emotional responses are particularly important targets of therapeutic intervention.

[5]Mindfulness-based models similarly note the ways that approaching external events by judging or wishing they were otherwise leads to suffering. We discuss this aspect of mindfulness in the section on behavioral constriction.

we may take this as an indication of her true, lasting feelings. Conversely, we may take our own transient experience of anger toward and absence of affection for our partner as an indication of our true feelings and fear that the relationship is over. When we experience sadness and consider ourselves defined by this experience, we can develop a stigmatized sense of ourselves as damaged. This fusion between our experience and our perception of reality makes internal experiences particularly powerful and likely underlies our desire for them to be other than they are. If the thought that our partner does not really care about us were just a thought, that would arise and fall naturally and did not necessarily reflect reality, it would not be so aversive and distressing.[6]

Hayes and colleagues (e.g., Hayes, Strosahl, & Wilson, 1999) have written extensively about the role that cognitive fusion may play in psychological problems and the process through which this fusion develops. Relational frame theory (RFT; Hayes, Barnes-Holmes, & Rosche, 2001) suggests that humans continually derive relations among events, words, feelings, experiences, and images as we engage with our environment, interact with others, think, observe, and reason. These relations result in internal stimuli (e.g., images, feelings, thoughts, memories) taking on the functions of the events to which they are linked. That is, a memory of a painful event can elicit the same reactions as the event itself, and thoughts and feelings can provoke reactions comparable to the external contexts with which they have been paired. Relational learning has an adaptive component. For instance, it allows us to imagine situations in order to anticipate our potential reactions to them and make choices without having to actually experience each option before us. We can describe our experiences to another person, and that person can vicariously imagine our subjective experience. In these ways, we can learn far beyond our direct experience, increasing our potential and flexibility exponentially. Relational learning also sets the stage for fusion between internal experiences and the events they reflect, such that internal experiences come to elicit anxiety, sadness, anger, or distress, as if the events themselves were actually happening. This fusion can prompt experiential avoidance, similar to the modern learning theory of panic described above, in which interoceptive conditioning (i.e., conditioning to internal sensations) leads bodily sensations to be associated with anxiety and distress, resulting in panic disorder. The responses themselves are not problematic, but a fused experience of them is. The anxiety Maya experiences around her schoolwork or in social situations is not problematic on its own, but her reactions to any anxiety symptoms that arise make the anxiety more distressing and pervasive, creating difficulties for her.

Fusion or entanglement has been identified as an important component in depressive relapse. Segal and colleagues (2002) suggest that depression results from learned patterns of negative thinking and ruminative response styles activated by a negative mood state. These habits of processing information feed on themselves, dropping mood lower and lower and making it more difficult to recover. The inability to see thoughts as just thoughts (in other words, to step back, or *decenter*, from these thought processes and observe them) is a key element of this depressive spiral. Objective awareness at

---

[6]It is important to note that thoughts do not have to be clearly false for *defusion* or *decentering* to be beneficial. While models underlying cognitive therapy often suggest that the irrationality of thoughts is central to clinical problems, acceptance-based models emphasize the problematic nature of relating to thoughts in a specific way, taking them as unchanging realities rather than reactions to a given moment. In this context, a fused relationship to a thought that accurately reflects a momentary reality would still be problematic in that it would preclude a flexible, choice-based adaptive mode of responding.

any point would help alter the trajectory and allow for more flexibility in behavioral responding. Thus, in this model, *critical* negative awareness characterizes depression and the *absence of a more decentered, disentangled* awareness of this negative thought process perpetuates it. Studies have found that successful cognitive therapy increases this decentering (Teasdale et al., 2002), suggesting it may be an active ingredient in both cognitive and acceptance-based behavioral interventions.

EXPERIENTIAL AVOIDANCE

One of the most clinically relevant consequences of a fused, entangled relationship with internal experiences is that it is likely to lead to rigid efforts to alter or avoid internal experiences, or *experiential avoidance*. Hayes, Strosahl, and Wilson's (1999) seminal work on the role of experiential avoidance in clinical problems provides an important cornerstone for acceptance-based behavioral models. In highlighting the importance of considering the function, rather than the form, of clinical presentations, Hayes and colleagues suggest that many diverse clinical problems can be understood as serving the function of experiential avoidance. Behaviors such as substance abuse and deliberate self-harm and symptoms such as worry or rumination may all be strategies aimed at altering the form or frequency of internal experiences (thoughts, feelings, sensations, images). That is, these are all (ultimately unsuccessful) attempts to reduce or eliminate unwanted, distressing internal experiences. These avoidance efforts often seem to have paradoxical effects, resulting in increases in both the targets of avoidance (e.g., the unwanted thoughts, feelings, or sensations) and more general psychological distress (for reviews, see Purdon, 1999; Salters-Pedneault, Tull, & Roemer, 2004) and interfering with quality of life. Sometimes these effects occur in different channels of responding. For instance, in one experiment, instructing participants to conceal their emotional expression while watching an emotional film clip resulted in a paradoxical increase in physiological activation (Gross & Levenson, 1993, 1997). People can easily become stuck in a cycle, with their efforts to avoid distress actually increasing it and fueling further avoidance efforts. A host of studies have demonstrated significant relationships between reports of experiential avoidance and reports of a wide range of clinical problems (see Hayes, Luoma, Bond, Masuda, & Lillis, 2006, for a review), and experimental studies have shown that individuals instructed in experiential acceptance demonstrate reduced subjective distress following laboratory stressors compared to those who are instructed in experiential suppression (e.g., Eifert & Heffner, 2003; Levitt, Brown, Orsillo, & Barlow, 2004). Maya reported intense efforts to keep others from recognizing her anxiety, which may have heightened her arousal and distress. She also described trying to push anxious thoughts out of her head but finding that they frequently returned even more intensely.

   Experiential avoidance efforts are likely robust and difficult to change for many reasons. First, experientially avoidant responses are often initially negatively reinforced by an immediate reduction in distress. That is, actions aimed at reducing distress likely lead to an initial reduction in distress, and this removal of an unwanted stimulus increases the frequency of the behavior that preceded it. A commonly held understanding of excessive substance use provides a particularly salient example of this process (e.g., Marlatt & Witkiewitz, 2005). Although substance use can have numerous apparent negative consequences in the long term, it typically results in an initial mood shift that is experienced as pleasant and stress reducing. This consequence is highly reinforcing, particularly for individuals who experience a great deal of distress and/or have particularly negative reactions to their distress. Thus, the behavior is likely to continue, although its long-term consequences (e.g., disruptions in relationships and other areas of functioning, heightened tolerance, withdrawal symptoms in the absence of use, and the failure to effectively process or resolve the distress that is habitually avoided) all perpetuate and increase distress. Similar models have been presented for restricted eating (e.g., Heffner, Sperry, Eifert, & Detweiler, 2002) and deliberate self-harm (Chapman, Gratz, & Brown, 2006). Maya's pattern of both bingeing and restricting her eating fits this model. She describes an initial reduction in anxiety when she eats excessively, but her anxiety increases as she begins to worry about her weight. She then restricts her food intake, again lowering her anxiety but making her emotionally vulnerable due to reduced nutrition, increasing her risk of becoming distressed and overeating again.

In addition to the natural consequences that serve to maintain and perpetuate experientially avoidant strategies, social forces likely maintain these strategies as well. Although several psychological (e.g., Hayes, Strosahl, & Wilson, 1999; May, 1996) and Buddhist (e.g., Chodron, 2001) theorists have noted the ubiquity of emotional pain, we often get the message from other people that we should be able to control our emotional distress through sheer willpower. Also, it can seem to us that others are successfully avoiding their emotional pain because we do not have access to their experience. Maya commented that her peers and siblings do not experience the same anxieties that she does, but she was able to recognize that these individuals may also be unaware of her anxiety, given her tendency to conceal it. In addition, avoidance or escape behavior can be functional, making it harder for us to notice its ineffectiveness in reducing internal distress. Avoiding and escaping threatening environmental contexts is evolutionarily adaptive and functional, but our inability to escape internal experiences permanently (fueled by our ability to imagine and remember) renders these same strategies futile, and, in fact, harmful when directed at internal responses.

Experiential avoidance is also ubiquitous because our fused, entangled relationships with our internal experience naturally motivate these efforts. If anxious sensations are experienced as equivalent to impending disaster and negative thoughts about ourselves are experienced as indicators of reality, motivation will be very high to avoid these sensations and thoughts. If, on the other hand, these experiences are seen as rising and falling, each no more true or permanent than the last, then the strong urge and effort to avoid and escape them will be diminished. Conversely, every attempt to avoid them may strengthen the danger associated with them, contributing to the cycle and prompting further avoidance efforts.

Research, theory, and clinical observation suggest that experiential avoidance may be a useful way to conceptualize a host of clinical presentations. In addition to the behavioral symptoms described above that serve an experientially avoidant function, some common internal processes may also reflect efforts at experiential avoidance. The avoidance model of worry (Borkovec, Alcaine, & Behar, 2004) posits that chronic excessive worry (repeatedly considering potential negative outcomes in the future) may in part function to reduce physiological arousal. Although worry itself is a troubling internal experience that individuals often want to get rid of, studies have shown that worry actually serves a positive function by reducing physiological arousal in response to fearful images or situations (e.g., Borkovec & Hu, 1990). This negatively reinforcing property of worry increases its frequency. People are likely to keep worrying because it has this relieving physiological effect, even if they are unaware of that effect. However, worry also perpetuates threatening associations by interfering with the complete processing of feared events. Someone who is anxious about socializing with coworkers at lunch may decrease her arousal in this situation if she is preoccupied throughout lunch by her worries about an upcoming dental appointment, but this prevents her from learning that, although socializing with colleagues can elicit some feelings of fear, it can also be pleasant and fearful feelings diminish over time. Ruminative processes in depressed individuals may serve a similar function, reducing deeper levels of sadness and pain but maintaining generalized negative mood states.

Clients with a range of clinical problems also engage more purposefully in efforts to avoid internal experiences. For instance, individuals with obsessive–compulsive disorder describe their cognitive rituals as a strategy that reduces distress in the moment, but the impairing anxiety and fear is maintained over time. Clients with posttraumatic stress disorder attempt to avoid thoughts, feelings, and memories associated with the traumas they have experienced. Although they may gain some short-term relief from these efforts, they find that the recollections return repeatedly, perhaps more often because of these efforts to push them away. Individuals with substance dependence or abuse problems try to ignore thoughts and urges to use, only to find them returning more strongly. Couples in distressed relationships may engage in repeated efforts to push away anger, hurt, or worry in response to their partner, only to find these reactions return more intensely.

Experiential avoidance can also help explain clinical presentations where avoidance is less obvious. For instance, Toni and Janelle described a pattern of interaction in which, during stress, Toni expressed anger and irritation, while Janelle withdrew, became "numb," and expressed little emotion. Toni experienced Janelle's withdrawal as rejection, prompting further anger, while Janelle experienced Toni's anger as threatening, prompting further withdrawal. Delving more deeply into each partner's experience revealed that Toni first experienced anxiety and fear of rejection. She found this vulnerability threatening and avoided it through anger, lashing out at Janelle. Her anxiety was heightened when Janelle withdrew, prompting further angry outbursts. Janelle similarly feared rejection and tried to reduce her distress by withdrawing and "shutting down" emotionally; her distress was increased by Toni's angry behavior. This shared understanding can help Toni and Janelle cultivate empathy for one another (given the shared experience they are having, despite very different behavioral manifestations; Jacobson & Christensen, 1996). They can then build from this shared understanding to develop alternative ways to approach and respond to one another, at times tolerating increased distress but eventually working toward a more effective resolution for both of them.

Complexities of Experiential Avoidance

Experiential avoidance is a key part of an acceptance-based behavioral model because rigid efforts at experiential control appear to have a host of clinically relevant consequences, suggesting it is a useful target for intervention. Before describing these consequences in more detail, it is important to note that, in certain contexts, efforts to modify internal experience may not be problematic or harmful. Unfortunately, the apparent success of these strategies can fuel and maintain maladaptive efforts at internal control.

Skillful application of acceptance-based behavioral therapy relies on a clear understanding of the complexities of experiential control and the contexts in which trying to influence our internal experiences might be beneficial versus harmful.

In many cases, efforts to *modulate* our internal experiences can be beneficial. For instance, we might focus on our breathing prior to a public speaking engagement and find it reduces our heart rate slightly, allowing us to present material more effectively to our audience. On the other hand, this focused breathing may have no effect on our heart rate or even increase it. We might find that we keep thinking about a mistake we made at work or something we wish we had not said to a friend and choose to turn our attention to a movie or a book in an effort to reduce our rumination. This distraction might lead to some relief, or we might find that our minds return to the event repeatedly, regardless of what we try to bring our attention to. If we are able to allow for the possibility of *any* of these consequences of our behavior, there is no harm in engaging in actions that might modulate or alter our internal experiences. When they work, they might allow us to expand our awareness, gain additional perspectives, have new experiences, and increase flexibility. If we can accept it when they do not work, we can continue living our lives with the internal experiences we were unable to alter.

Problems can arise when we begin to try rigidly to *eliminate* or *avoid* distressing internal experiences and when this goal becomes a prominent motivator of our behavior, either consciously or not (experiential avoidance often becomes an automatic process). These habitual, rigid efforts are problematic in that they (1) often do not work, (2) interfere with the function of emotional responses, (3) perpetuate a problematic relationship with internal experiences, and (4) impair functioning. As reviewed above, efforts to avoid or suppress our thoughts or feelings are often unsuccessful and instead increase the targets of suppression or avoidance. They are most likely to be ineffective when we most want them to work; in fact, our efforts may worsen our distress rather than ameliorate it. Maya's experience studying for exams highlights this process. As she experiences anxious thoughts and sensations, she tries to put them out of her mind, telling herself to focus on the material. She finds that the more she tries to calm herself and the more strongly she wants the anxiety to go away, the more anxious and out of control she feels. This makes it harder for her to study effectively, further increasing her anxiety.

Consequences of Avoidance

Avoidance or suppression of naturally occurring emotional responses (i.e., *primary emotions*, according to Greenberg & Safran, 1987, or emotions that stem naturally and functionally from a particular context) can exacerbate emotional distress and interfere with successful emotional processing. Extensive research on exposure-based treatments for anxiety disorders reveals the importance of clients experiencing their fear during exposure to feared stimuli, so that they can fully access their fearful associations and incorporate new, nonthreatening associations (Foa & Kozak, 1986). For instance, clients who display more intense facial fear expressions (Foa, Riggs, Massie, & Yarczower, 1995) and those who report higher subjective anxiety ratings (reflecting higher emotional engagement; Jaycox, Foa, & Morral, 1998) in the first session of exposure therapy achieve better results from such treatment. Avoidance or distraction inhibits this new learning of nonfearful associations. Thus, experiential avoidance is likely to maintain distress rather than allow emotional responses to run their course and new learning to evolve. Maya's pervasive anxiety may result in part from her repeated efforts to suppress or limit her anxious experience, which likely interfere with the natural ebb and flow of her anxious and fearful responding so that she does not experience the natural decline that would accompany continued exposure to threat cues.

Experiential avoidance can also interfere with other aspects of the functional value of emotional responses. Emotions provide important information regarding our interaction with our environment, telling us when our needs are being thwarted, when a threat is present, or when we have lost something of value (e.g., Frijda, 1986; Greenberg & Safran, 1987; Linehan, 1993a, 1993b). Our emotional responses help us communicate our needs to others in the form of expressions that occur rapidly and automatically. Habitual, rigid avoidance of our emotional responses is likely to interfere with our understanding of our interactions with others as well as of our own needs and desires. For instance, a client who is avoiding his chronic feelings of sadness and disappointment by distracting himself with alcohol might be missing the information this sadness can provide him, such as his dissatisfaction with his current job and a need to explore ways to improve this situation or pursue another job. Similarly, Maya's constant focus on her work is keeping her from noticing the sadness and loneliness that might motivate her to cultivate her social and familial relationships.

Experiential avoidance can also affect our judgments of or reactions to our internal awareness. One study revealed that instructions to suppress specific thoughts led to reports of increased anxiety in response to these thoughts (Roemer & Borkovec, 1994). Another found that individuals who were told to control physiological sensations rated their sensations as more distressing than those who were encouraged to accept them, even though the intensity of the sensations was similar across groups (Levitt et al., 2004). Repeated efforts to eliminate specific thoughts, emotions, sensations, and memories is likely to lead to increased negative judgments of these internal events when they recur, prompting heightened efforts to avoid them. It is easy to engage in a cycle in which reactivity to internal experiences leads to control efforts that increase reactivity to these experiences. Maya's critical response to her anxious symptoms is likely worsened by her repeated, unsuccessful efforts to reduce these symptoms, making them seem more threatening and pervasive.

Experiential avoidance may also promote more critical reactions to our internal experiences because it inhibits our ability to receive validation from others. A common strategy for avoiding distress is to conceal our emotional responses. In addition to the effect this may have on our physiological arousal (possibly heightening it; Gross & Levenson, 1993), masking our distress makes it impossible for others to respond empathically to our experience or share their own similar struggles. External validation is one way to cultivate self-compassion (recognizing the humanness of our responses), while concealing distress can heighten our sense that our struggles are unique, making it easier to judge and criticize these experiences.

Experiential avoidance also occludes and narrows awareness. Attempts to reduce and avoid distress are likely associated with a tendency to direct attention away from internal experiences. This lack of attention can reduce the clarity of one's internal awareness, making it harder to respond effectively. For instance, if Maya becomes angry at her parents after they make critical comments about her school performance but is uncomfortable with her anger, she may only briefly note her reaction and then shift her attention toward internal and external efforts to avoid this experience of anger. As a result, she will likely continue to feel activated and reactive in some way, but she may no longer be aware of what prompted this reaction. She may misinterpret her response as more anxiety, which could hinder her ability to change the situation that elicited her anger. Thus, reduced, limited, or "muddy" internal awareness may be a result of habitual experiential avoidance.

Finally, experiential avoidance often leads to behavioral avoidance or behavioral engagement that interferes with individuals' broader functioning. In addition to the more obvious costs (behaviors such as substance use, overeating, or self-harm), experiential avoidance can subtly impact behavior by preventing individuals from engaging fully in their relationships, pursuing careers with meaning to them, or effectively dealing with stressful life contexts. Again, rigidity is the central problem—efforts to reduce distress may promote functioning in many contexts, but rigid avoidance efforts at the expense of life-enhancing goals may lead to restricted, unsatisfying lives.

BEHAVIORAL CONSTRICTION:
FAILURE TO ENGAGE IN VALUED ACTION

Acceptance-based behavioral models focus particularly on the behavioral costs of experiential avoidance, which are sometimes prominent and sometimes subtle. Behavioral costs take the form of behaviors that temporarily reduce distress (like cleaning, hair pulling, dieting, or smoking) and avoidance of behaviors for fear of emotional distress. Avoidance can be obvious, as when Jack, a Vietnam veteran with posttraumatic stress disorder (PTSD), isolates himself in his home to avoid the anxiety he experiences in crowds or with other people, or it can be much more subtle, as when Leia appears engaged in her work, volunteers for numerous organizations, and has a broad social network but avoids slowing down to notice what is really important to her, leaving her with a general sense of dissatisfaction that she is unable to address effectively. Similarly, Maya is focused on her schoolwork and does not avoid it, despite the anxiety it elicits, but she avoids contact with people in her life and is unaware of the effect this is having on her. She may also have lost contact with why schoolwork is important to her and may continue her academic pursuits because it is what she "should" be doing. The behavioral cost of experiential avoidance is a particularly important focus of treatment because it emphasizes the way that difficulties interfere with individuals' lives.

Ironically, behavioral efforts to control, eliminate, or avoid negative internal experiences often perpetuate distress. A man who wants an intimate relationship but fears rejection may not engage in actions that would put him in situations where he might be rejected by a potential partner. While this serves the immediate function of reducing his risk of being rejected, it also increases the chance that he will not find a partner. He has effectively protected himself from the immediate risk of rejection, but he has increased his long-term risk of loneliness and general dissatisfaction. Often, these restrictions in behavior happen automatically so that, although clients feel the pain associated with their restricted lives, they are not aware of the role they play in perpetuating it.

Sometimes avoidance is evident in the quality of actions rather than their occurrence. For instance, in our work with clients with generalized anxiety disorder, we have often found that they seem to be engaging in the areas of life that matter to them (e.g., jobs they value, spending time with their children). When clients begin to monitor their activities carefully, however, it becomes clear that they are not fully present when they are engaging in these actions. Instead, they are worrying about what may happen next, in another domain. Similarly, clients may distract themselves or hold back emotionally in certain contexts as a way of avoiding distress from potential rejection or hurt. For instance, Dex, a client who feared abandonment, went through the motions of developing a new relationship but kept himself distant emotionally when he was with his partner as a way of avoiding this feared outcome. This distancing could have provoked separation, which he would have experienced as abandonment, confirming his fear and reinforcing the behavior. All of these forms of disengagement can limit clients' satisfaction and success in various areas, further driving experiential avoidance and perpetuating distress.

Another way in which clients might unintentionally diminish their satisfaction is by applying the same judgmental, rigid way of responding to external situations as they do to their internal experience. Acceptance- and mindfulness-based approaches highlight the role that judgment of external events can play in suffering. Repeatedly wishing that things were other than they are (e.g., one's partner was different, one's colleagues were different) can prolong distress and interfere with effective action. Linehan (1993b) gives the example of choosing to become stuck in an angry and frustrated state when driving behind someone who is going too slowly in the fast lane of the highway. She suggests that an alternative would be to notice that the person is driving more slowly than you would prefer and switch to another lane, without getting caught up in how that person should be driving differently. This kind of rigid attachment to the way things or people *should* be is often a factor in the difficulties people have. Bringing awareness to this way of relating to our world can help us make more effective choices.

Hayes, Strosahl, and Wilson (1999) highlight the ways that habitual patterns of experiential avoidance may lead individuals not to attend to the way they want to be living their lives. Instead, they make choices based on avoiding distress. In essence, individuals choose avoidance-based rather than approach-based paths, interfering with their ability to approach the lives they want to be living. Often, these "choices" happen outside of awareness. Individuals overlearn patterns of engaging in or avoiding behaviors and are not aware that other, less behaviorally restrictive options are available. An important first step of treatment is bringing awareness to behaviors so that intentional choices rather than reactive behaviors can begin to influence individuals' actions.

GOALS AND METHODS OF INTERVENTION

Drawing from the model presented above, ABBTs aim to (1) alter individuals' relationships with their internal experiences, (2) reduce rigid experiential avoidance and increase flexibility and choice, and (3) increase action in valued directions. The methods used to achieve each of these goals are described in detail throughout the book. Below, we provide a brief overview.

Altering relationships with internal experiences includes expanding and clarifying internal awareness to counter the restricted or occluded awareness that individuals often experience. In addition, an emphasis is placed on cultivating a nonjudgmental, compassionate relationship with experiences as they arise to reduce reactivity, fear, and judgment, which have been found to increase distress, motivate experiential avoidance, and interfere with functioning. Finally, this goal includes cultivating an experience of thoughts, feelings, and sensations as naturally occurring and transient and reducing an experience of them as indicators of a permanent truth. For instance, Maya, who habitually experiences physiological sensations of anxiety and interprets these as evidence of her fragility, vulnerability, and inability to cope, would engage in a range of practices designed to help her notice the sensations as they arise, feel compassion for herself for experiencing them, see them as overlearned physical sensations that elicit a range of reactions but that do not define her, and expand her awareness to notice other experiences and sensations that co-occur with anxiety as well as the way that anxiety-related sensations subside over time.

Several types of interventions can be used to assist in meeting this goal. *Psychoeducation* (described in depth in Chapter 5) helps clients understand the nature of internal experiences (specifically the function of emotions) and the role that these types of relationships to internal events can play in sustained distress and restrictions in their lives. *Self-monitoring* can help enhance clients' awareness of their internal experiences, especially the way these experiences rise and fall and their connection to contexts and behaviors. Understanding is not sufficient for changing these overlearned, deeply ingrained relationships. Therefore, significant time is devoted to a range of *experiential practices* that assist in cultivating new ways of relating to internal experiences. These mindfulness- and acceptance-based strategies are described in depth in Chapter 6. Clients engage in both formal (specific, planned practice of a particular technique) and informal (applying skills to daily living) mindfulness practice, both within and between sessions. While standard practices may be most beneficial to begin with (in order to help clients develop the basic skills of attending, noticing, and allowing intentionally), they can be developed over time to target specific aspects clients find challenging. Other acceptance-based, or defusion, strategies are drawn from ACT, such as labeling thoughts and feelings to bring awareness to them as separate, rather than fused, experiences.

The second goal of treatment is *reducing efforts at experiential avoidance while increasing choice and flexibility*. This includes bringing awareness to the way that a range of behaviors and symptoms may function as efforts to avoid or escape internal distress. Clients are also encouraged to practice and learn how to choose, rather than react, in a potentially evocative situation, reducing the role that experiential avoidance plays in determining their actions. Developing a new, unentangled relationship with internal experiences will naturally decrease the habitual pull to rigidly avoid or escape distressing experiences. Cultivating a curious, inviting stance toward internal experience will help reduce experientially avoidant tendencies.

Many of the methods described above also target this goal of treatment. Psychoeducation presents examples of how trying to control internal experiences can increase difficulties. We encourage clients to look to their own experience to see whether this is true for them. We help clients increase flexibility by noticing how, although thoughts, feelings, and sensations seem to pull for particular actions, we can separate them and choose responses rather than reacting. Monitoring helps clients see how experiential avoidance affects their lives and identify early cues to contexts in which to practice an accepting, rather than avoidant, response. Mindfulness- and acceptance-based practices help develop the skill of acceptance, increasing clients' flexibility in the ways they respond to contexts that elicit intense reactions.

Finally, ABBTs emphasize the goal of *increasing valued action*. This includes refraining from actions that may be very tempting in the moment (often because they serve an experientially avoidant function) but are not in line with the way the client wants to live his or her life and engaging in actions that matter to the individual but have been avoided. Important components of this goal include identifying and clarifying what matters to the individual, bringing awareness to moments when choices could be made based on these values, and engaging in action in desired directions.

All the methods that promote the first two goals also serve this goal, in that engaging in chosen action is facilitated by an unentangled, defused relationship to one's experience and an ability to choose a nonexperientially avoidant response. In addition, psychoeducation and monitoring help bring a client's attention to what is important to him or her, to set the stage for chosen action. Writing exercises serve to clarify values, as does mindfulness practice. Nonreactive, decentered awareness can allow one to *reflectively* see what matters, rather than *reflexively* endorsing values based on societal pressure or fears (Shapiro, Carlson, Astin, & Freedman, 2006). Finally, between-session behavioral exercises, in which actions are chosen and planned for, engaged in, and reviewed, allow clients to expand their behavioral repertoire and engage more fully in their lives. These behavioral changes often elicit new types of problematic relationships with internal experiences and impulses that promote experiential avoidance, feeding back into the previous two goals.

CONCLUSION

ABBTs draw from this conceptualization of clinical problems by developing an individualized case formulation that highlights the way a client's presenting problems can be explained by the model. Goals for treatment target each of these three elements (and their interrelationships), and intervention strategies are chosen to meet these goals. In the next chapter, we present assessment methods that can be used to develop an individualized case conceptualization and treatment plan based on this model. We also describe in detail the intervention strategies that specifically target problematic relationships with internal experiences, experiential avoidance, and behavioral constriction (i.e., failure to engage in valued actions).

TWO

Clinical Assessment of Relevant Domains

The first step to working with a client from an acceptance-based behavioral perspective is to conduct a comprehensive assessment of the nature and extent of the client's presenting problems, psychological status, attitudes toward internal experiences (e.g., emotions, physical sensations), common coping strategies (including experiential avoidance), quality of life, and previous experience in treatment. Not only is a careful and systematic assessment critical to developing an accurate case conceptualization and an informed treatment plan, but it also helps validate the client's experience and develop a strong therapeutic alliance.

In this chapter, we focus primarily on the assessment strategies to be used in the initial sessions, but ongoing assessment throughout therapy (discussed in Chapter 9) is essential as it provides important information about the potential efficacy of the intervention, encourages a rapid response to unproductive strategies, facilitates change by providing feedback, motivates both the client and therapist, enhances accountability, and demonstrates the effectiveness of treatment to relevant third parties (Woody, Detweiler-Bedell, Teachman, & O'Hearn, 2004).

Below is a description of each of the domains that are important to assess when working with a client from an acceptance-based behavioral perspective. In order to make this chapter useful for therapists working with a wide variety of clients, we have been overinclusive in describing potential targets of assessment. In our own practice, we select a subset of these measures based on the needs of the individual, usually including at least one measure from each domain.

Although many of the domains can be assessed through the use of a careful clinical interview, we also underscore the importance of using self-monitoring between sessions to gather information about the unique pattern of symptoms and problem behaviors experienced by clients. Additionally, we make some recommendations about the use of specific interviews and questionnaires that may provide valuable information throughout the assessment process. In our selection of instruments, we have tried to heed the advice of Woody and her colleagues (2004) in that we focus on measures we find to be highly *applicable* (in that they assess constructs that are important and meaningful to the client and that guide treatment), *acceptable* (brief and user-friendly), *practical* (minimal cost, easy to score and interpret), and *psychometrically sound* (reliable, valid, and sensitive to change).

SYMPTOM-BASED ASSESSMENT

Broad Overview of Presenting Concerns

We start the assessment process by trying to get a sense of the client's presenting concerns, desired life directions, and current factors that motivated him or her to seek treatment. Typically, this initial report will include a description of psychological symptoms (e.g., difficulty concentrating, hyperarousal), current emotional state (e.g., sad, anxious, angry), and difficulties in functioning that are impacting quality of life (e.g., interpersonal conflicts, problems at work, diminished physical health and well-being). Persons (1989) and Woody and colleagues (2003) suggest that, early in the assessment period, clinicians develop a comprehensive problem list, which can be used to identify, prioritize, and manage all of the client's current difficulties. For example, Derek initially presented with complaints about depression, including depressed mood, fatigue, difficulty sleeping, decreased appetite, and difficulty concentrating. He also noted that he was quite irritable both at work and with his partner. His partner was also distressed about Derek's lack of sexual interest and was threatening to leave the relationship. Derek described spending most of his free time watching television and playing video games. He also admitted to smoking marijuana almost every night and on the weekend in order to "get through" his leisure time. Derek had missed 10 days of work over the previous 3 months due to unspecified illnesses (colds, headaches, etc.) and had been given a written warning that he could not have any additional unexcused absences over the next 6 months. We worked with Derek to create a problem list (Figure 2.1). When a client presents with multiple complaints and concerns, it can be difficult to know where to begin in treatment. As discussed in Chapter 3, the acceptance-based case conceptualization aims

---

- Sad mood
- Fatigue
- Difficulty sleeping
- Decreased appetite
- Difficulty concentrating
- Irritability
- Decreased sexual interest
- Diffuse somatic complaints
- Marijuana use
- Limited recreational activities
- Limited social contact
- Relationship difficulties
- Attendance issues at work
- Interpersonal conflict at work

FIGURE 2.1. Derek's problem list.

to propose an underlying mechanism that accounts for the problems enumerated on the problem list and tie them together in a way that will guide treatment.

We also make an effort to learn about the client's cultural identity. A culturally sensitive approach to assessment is aimed at ensuring that the client's problems are accurately understood and defined, taking into account cultural norms and expectations, informing the development of an appropriate treatment plan that adequately meets the needs of the client, and demonstrating respect for the client's culture in an attempt to promote a strong therapeutic alliance (Tanaka-Matsumi, Seiden, & Lam, 1996). The therapeutic relationship is a critical component of ABBT that is assumed to foster an environment in which the client can begin to develop a self-accepting and self-compassionate stance. ABBTs require a significant commitment on the part of the client as extensive between-session practice with mindfulness and valued actions is encouraged. In our experience, a strong therapeutic relationship increases engagement in and compliance with therapeutic activities.

As discussed in more depth in Chapter 11, understanding a client's cultural identity can inform many facets of ABBT. Cultural factors can play a significant role in how one views one's emotions, how emotions are viewed by one's family members, and the types of values (e.g., individualistic or interdependent) that are personally held. Attention to how external forces such as economic disadvantage and oppression affect a client informs the conceptualization of the client's presenting issues and the choice of therapeutic strategies. Inquiring about culturally specific sources of support can help communicate respect and identify naturally occurring supports that can be drawn on in later behavioral interventions (Hays, 2008). Hays describes a multidimensional approach to assessing culture that includes attention to the client's (1) age and generational influences, (2) developmental and acquired disabilities, (3) religion and spiritual orientation, (4) ethnicity, (5) socioeconomic status, (6) sexual orientation, (7) indigenous heritage, (8) national origin, and (9) gender.

Once we have a sense for our clients' cultural identity and presenting problems, we ask them specifically to describe the ways they would be living life differently if the presenting problems were not serving as obstacles. Often, clients present to therapy in such distress and despair that they can only focus on the frequency and intensity of their painful experiences. However, behavioral change aimed at increasing valued life activities is an essential component of ABBTs. Therefore, both informal and formal methods of assessing valued directions are indicated.

Finally, as a way of assessing readiness for change, we encourage clients to talk about the internal and external factors that motivated help seeking. Obviously, clients who come to therapy independently are typically more motivated than those encouraged (or required) to seek treatment by others. However, we often share with our clients our view of motivation. While some assume motivation to be a trait or personality feature, we conceptualize motivation from a behavioral perspective. Simply put, we believe clients are motivated to change when the positive rewards of change seem more reinforcing than the negative consequences of engaging in change efforts. For instance, Maria was a client diagnosed with borderline personality disorder who described herself as a lazy procrastinator with no motivation to pursue a career. Further discussion uncovered that the shame and self-disgust she felt about her limited employment history prevented her from even considering the type of career she could potentially want.

From this perspective, we welcome and expect clients who feel both disconnected from the rewards associated with making a life change and painfully aware of the obstacles to making this change to present with ambivalence. The goal of ABBT is to increase the salience of positive rewards of change by helping clients access what is personally meaningful about their goals for treatment and decrease the size and magnitude of obstacles by changing the relationship clients have with their internal experiences.

Once we have a broad overview of these presenting issues, we delve deeper into the assessment process by more systematically assessing a variety of domains.

Psychopathology

Hayes and his colleagues (1996) criticized the widely held medical syndromal model of psychopathology, citing the high rates of comorbidity, low treatment utility, and frequent irrelevance of the diagnostic model to the types of presenting problems typically seen in clinical practice. As an alternative, he and his colleagues proposed a dimensional, functional approach to psychopathology that assumes that many forms of psychopathology are best conceptualized as experiential avoidance. While we support this perspective, for a number of practical and clinically relevant reasons (e.g., insurance requirements, ease of communication between providers, validation of clients' experiences, appropriateness of treatment recommendations given current standards of practice), we continue to assess our clients to determine whether or not they meet criteria for specific Axis I disorders, according to the *Diagnostic and Statistical Manual of Mental Disorders*, Fourth Edition (DSM-IV).

Often, we find that a structured or semistructured interview helps us learn more about the specific symptoms and struggles that our clients experience. In several cases, a systematic assessment has revealed the presence of important life events and/or symptoms that a client may not otherwise readily share. For instance, given the high comorbidity between major depressive disorder (MDD) and posttraumatic stress disorder (PTSD), it is common for clients to present with symptoms of MDD who may also have significant trauma histories and related symptoms that can go undetected. Similarly, clients may be embarrassed to disclose their dependence on illegal substances or their thoughts about suicide unless they are directly asked about such problems in a compassionate and professional manner.

For many of the clients we see, the Anxiety Disorders Interview Schedule for DSM-IV (ADIS-IV; DiNardo, Brown, & Barlow, 1994), can be a useful guide for comprehensively evaluating DSM-IV anxiety and mood disorders. The Structured Clinical Interview for DSM-IV Axis I Disorders, Clinician Version (SCID-CV; First, Spitzer, Gibbon, & Williams, 1996) is also an efficient, clinical tool that assesses those DSM-IV diagnoses most commonly seen by clinicians (mood, psychotic, substance use, anxiety, eating, and somatoform disorders) and includes the diagnostic criteria for these disorders with corresponding interview questions.

There are also a number of global and symptom-specific questionnaires that can be used to provide more information about the nature and severity of psychological symptoms experienced by the client. The Depression Anxiety Stress Scales—21-Item Version (DASS-21; Lovibond & Lovibond, 1995) is a 21-item measure that yields separate scores of depression, anxiety (i.e., anxious arousal), and stress (e.g., tension). The Brief Symptom Inventory (BSI; Derogatis & Spencer, 1982) can also be a useful questionnaire measure for assessing overall psychological distress. The BSI provides information about a client's symptom report on nine primary symptom dimensions and yields three more global indices of psychological functioning.

Potentially Harmful Behaviors

Engagement in self-injurious and impulsive behaviors, such as deliberate self-harm (e.g., cutting, burning), substance misuse, unsafe sexual practices, and compulsive spending, gambling, and eating, can be a form of experiential avoidance that is important to assess. For many clients, these behaviors are also associated with significant shame, which means they are frequently underreported. It can be clinically useful to routinely ask clients whether or not they use alcohol, drugs, food, or potentially dangerous activities as a way to cope with their emotional pain. Directly asking about embarrassing and risky behaviors in a matter-of-fact way demonstrates acceptance and validation and increases the probability that clients will be willing to disclose such information.

It can also be useful to overestimate the frequency of potentially harmful behaviors during questioning to get a more accurate self-report. For example, during a phone screening, a client named Rochelle was asked how many drinks she consumed each day and answered, "about one or two"; however, during the clinical interview, she was presented with an overestimate—"So, do you typically have about six to seven drinks a day?"—and she disclosed that she was averaging about four to five drinks per day.

In addition to asking about frequency of certain behaviors, it can also be useful to inquire about their consequences. The CAGE (Mayfield, McLeod, & Hall, 1974) is a short and simple way to screen for problematic alcohol use. The client is asked if he or she should cut (C) down on drinking, if others are (A) annoyed by his or her drinking, if he or she has ever felt (G) guilty about drinking, and whether he or she ever has an (E) eye-opening drink in the morning. While two affirmative responses are typically suggestive of the presence of an alcohol use disorder, even one positive response merits further exploration.

Clients who have a low threshold for tolerating emotional pain may also be at heightened risk for suicidal behavior. Chiles and Strosahl (2005) provide a compelling discussion of how the assessment of suicidal behavior must include both ethically and legally responsible risk assessment and a therapeutically efficacious means of offering the client hope. They underscore the importance, when exploring suicidal ideation and intent with a client, of validating the client's emotional pain, allowing for an open discussion of suicidal thoughts, and most notably reconceptualizing suicidal behavior as an attempt to solve problems that are seen as intolerable, inescapable, and interminable. For instance, Angel was a client who was seen for clinically significant symptoms of PTSD. Given his long history of being involuntarily hospitalized for suicidal ideation, he was hesitant to share his suicidal thoughts with a therapist, which paradoxically increased the intensity of thoughts, his feelings of isolation, and ultimately the probability that he would be rehospitalized. During an assessment meeting, Angel's new therapist shared his view that people engage in all sorts of behaviors that they know are harmful because they find their emotional pain so intense. The therapist normalized suicidal thoughts by suggesting that suicide often seems like the only option to someone who is in significant distress. He encouraged Angel to talk openly about his thoughts and feelings and offered Angel the possibility that he could learn new problem-solving skills (e.g., acceptance and tolerance of emotional pain, behavioral activation) through ABBT as an alternative to suicide.

A number of individual and situational factors should be assessed to inform the clinician of the potential targets for treatment to decrease suicidality, including cognitive style (e.g., inflexibility), problem-solving style (e.g., deficit in skills), emotional pain and suffering, emotionally avoidant coping style, interpersonal deficits, self-control deficits, and environmental stress and support (Chiles & Strosahl, 2005). The Reasons for Living Inventory (Linehan, Goodstein, Nielsen, & Chiles, 1983) can be used to measure a range of beliefs (social and coping beliefs, responsibility to family, child-related concerns, fear of suicide, fear of social disapproval, and moral objections) that may be important in preventing a client from attempting suicide.

RELATIONSHIP TO INTERNAL EXPERIENCES

Awareness of Emotional Experience

A critical part of our assessment involves exploring the client's relationship to his or her internal experiences (e.g., emotions, thoughts, internal sensations). First, we pay attention to the level of awareness and specificity with which clients describe their emotional state. Often, clients present to therapy with a nonspecific complaint of general negative affect and struggle significantly to convey a more nuanced description of their current emotional state. In these cases, it can be useful to ask the client to complete a mood adjective checklist such as the 36-item Mood Adjective Check List (MACL; Nowlis, 1965) or the 20-item Positive and Negative Affect Schedule (PANAS; Watson, Clark, & Tellegen, 1988) at different points in the day. Not only does this assessment provide valuable information about range of affect, but it also begins to give clients a more complex vocabulary to describe their internal experience.

Many clients begin therapy unaware of the moment-to-moment fluctuations in mood they are experiencing. For instance, we once worked with a client, Sharon, who described a panic attack that lasted approximately 2 weeks. Despite the fact that the human body is physically incapable of sustaining such a high level of arousal for that long, Sharon's experience was that her fear and arousal was constant. In this case, a very simple monitoring sheet can be used as a way of teaching a patient like Sharon to notice the variations in her mood. A rating scale ranging from 0 to 100 can be given to the client so that he or she can indicate the intensity of an experienced emotion several times a day—in the morning, afternoon, evening, and before bed (see Form 2.1, p. 51). In order to improve the validity of such an assessment, it is important to spend some time creating personalized behavioral anchors for the rating scale. The client can be asked to think of a situation in which he or she experienced no anxiety at all (0), moderate anxiety (50), and severe anxiety (100). When completing the daily assessment measure, the client can consider his or her current emotional state relative to the emotions evoked in those anchor situations when making a numerical rating.

Similarly, clients are often unaware of specific situational triggers that elicit particular emotions. Once again, individualized self-monitoring sheets can be developed to better assess these domains (see Form 2.2, p. 52). For example, a client can be asked to notice the emergence of two or three strong emotions each day. When the client experiences one of those emotions, he or she can be asked to note the day and time, the situation, the emotion elicited, and any accompanying thoughts or physical sensations.

While an interview and self-monitoring may reveal difficulties in identifying and describing emotions, there are also questionnaires that assess this response style. For instance, the Twenty-Item Toronto Alexithymia Scale (TAS-20; Bagby, Parker, & Taylor, 1994) is a questionnaire that measures the construct of alexithymia. Alexithymia is characterized by difficulties identifying and describing emotions, a tendency to minimize emotional experience, and a pattern of focusing attention externally. Items such as "I am often confused about what emotion I am feeling" and "I often don't know why I am angry" are rated on a 5-point scale ranging from 1 ("strongly disagree") to 5 ("strongly agree"). The TAS-20 yields an overall score and scores for three subscales: Difficulty Describing Feelings, Difficulty Identifying Feelings, and Externally Oriented Thinking.

The Difficulties in Emotion Regulation Scale (DERS; Gratz & Roemer, 2004) is a 36-item measure that can provide comprehensive information about various aspects of a client's emotion regulation (discussed in more depth below). Two specific subscales of this measure directly measure awareness of emotions (e.g., "I pay attention to how I feel") and clarity of emotions (e.g., "I am confused about how I feel").

Mindfulness

ABBTs aim to increase mindfulness, thus assessment of this construct is essential. Awareness of emotions is a key feature of mindfulness; therefore, some of the measures discussed in these sections can be used to measure both constructs, but there are other components to mindfulness beyond awareness. Baer, Smith, Hopkins, Krietemeyer, and Toney (2006) reveal mindfulness to be a multifaceted construct consisting of five distinct elements: observation of and attention to one's internal experience, description and labeling of one's experience, the ability to engage in activities with awareness and without distraction, the allowing and nonjudging of experience, and nonreactivity to inner experience. While many of these facets of mindfulness can be assessed through clinical interview and some of the self-monitoring exercises noted above, there are also a growing number of questionnaires that can be quite useful in assessing the different elements of mindfulness.

The Mindful Attention Awareness Scale (MAAS; Brown & Ryan, 2003) is a 15-item scale that measures a single factor of mindfulness: the general tendency to be attentive to and aware of present-moment experiences in daily life. Items such as "It seems I am 'running on automatic' without much awareness of what I'm doing" are rated on a 6-point scale ranging from "almost always" to "almost never." While this measure is helpful in assessing awareness, it does not tap into many of the other important elements of mindfulness.

Several other measures of mindfulness are designed to capture more of its facets. For instance, the Freiburg Mindfulness Inventory (FMI; Bucheld, Grossman, & Walach, 2001) is a 30-item questionnaire that assesses nonjudgmental present-moment observation and openness to negative experiences. The Kentucky Inventory of Mindfulness Skills (KIMS; Baer, Smith, & Allen, 2004) is a recently developed 39-item scale designed to measure four of the five aspects of mindfulness described above: observation, description, acting with awareness, and accepting without judgment. There is also preliminary support for the development of a 39-item measure, the Five Facet Mindfulness Questionnaire (FFMQ; Baer et al., 2006), which includes items from all of the measures described above.

Fusion with Internal Experiences

The model driving ABBT proposes that being fused with or hooked by your internal experiences drives attempts at experiential avoidance. Thus, one of the goals of therapy is to help clients decenter or defuse from their thoughts, emotions, images, and physical sensations. One potentially useful way to assess an individual's fusion with his or her own thoughts and feelings is to ask him or her to rate the believability of different thoughts and internal experiences that arise. While there are no general measures to assess this construct, researchers have developed content-specific measures that ask individuals to rate the believability of the content of depressive thoughts (Zettle & Hayes, 1987), hallucinations and delusions (Bach & Hayes, 2002), and stigmatizing attitudes (Hayes, Bissett, et al., 2004).

The Thought–Action Fusion Scale (TAFS; Shafran, Thordarson, & Rachman, 1996) is a 19-item scale that has been used primarily with obsessive–compulsive disorder (OCD) but it may be useful more generally as a measure of cognitive fusion. The TAFS taps into two components: (1) the belief that thinking about an unacceptable or disturbing event will increase the probability that it may occur, and (2) the belief that having an unacceptable thought is almost the moral equivalent of carrying out an unacceptable action. Items such as "Thinking of cheating in a personal relationship is almost as immoral to me as cheating" and "If I think of a relative/friend being in a car accident, this increases the risk he/she will have a car accident" are rated on a 5-point scale ranging from 0 (disagree strongly) to 4 (agree strongly).

Distress Related to Internal Experiences

There are also a number of questionnaires that have been specifically developed to assess how distressed a client is by his or her internal, particularly emotional, experience. Anxiety sensitivity, or "fear of fear," is a construct common in panic and other anxiety disorders. The Anxiety Sensitivity Index (ASI; Reiss et al., 1986) is a 16-item questionnaire that measures reactivity to anxiety-related symptoms. Items such as "It scares me when my heart beats rapidly" are rated on a 5-point scale ranging from 0 ("very little") to 4 ("very much"). The Affective Control Scale (ACS; Williams, Chambless, & Ahrens, 1997) is a 42-item questionnaire that extends the "fear of fear" construct to include distress about anxiety, depression, anger, and positive affective states. Sample items include "It scares me when I am nervous" (anxiety subscale), "Depression is scary to me—I am afraid that I could get depressed and never recover" (depression subscale), "I am afraid that letting myself feel really angry about something could lead me into an unending rage" (anger subscale), and "I worry about losing self-control when I am on cloud nine" (positive affect subscale). Responses are scored on a 7-point scale ranging from 1 ("very strongly disagree") to 7 ("very strongly agree").

CURRENT AND PAST COPING STRATEGIES

General Coping Strategies

A core assumption of ABBT is that internal and external attempts to control or escape uncomfortable thoughts, feelings, images, and sensations create significant psychological distress and interfere with life satisfaction. Therefore, a careful assessment of the coping strategies that a client uses when experiencing psychological distress is critical to the development of an effective program of treatment. We start this assessment process by asking the client to describe the ways that he or she has tried to cope with the presenting problems (typically painful thoughts and feelings). We specifically ask about the use of internal control strategies such as imagery, distraction, self-talk, wishful thinking, and experiential avoidance. However, rather than simply assessing the general use and utility of these strategies, we ask the client to offer specific examples of times when he or she used an internal control strategy and the short- and long-term outcomes. Self-monitoring is also a useful method for assessing the frequency and effectiveness of particular strategies (see Form 2.3, p. 53).

For example, one client we worked with, Bob, reported that distraction was a very effective coping strategy that he was able to use when feeling extremely anxious. A more comprehensive evaluation revealed that this strategy was often ineffective and associated with long-term negative consequences. Bob described using distraction as a way of managing his anxiety during an interaction with his supervisor at work. Although he initially judged the strategy to be helpful, a more detailed analysis of the situation revealed that, while his anxiety was decreased in the moment, his sleep was disturbed for the next three nights as he ruminated on the interaction. Furthermore, it became clear that Bob did not encode or retain the information his supervisor had tried to provide him during the interaction. Therefore, Bob had to ask his supervisor to repeat the information in a subsequent encounter, which left him feeling embarrassed and stressed.

Similarly, Mary reported that positive self-talk was an effective strategy for dealing with her dysphoric mood. She described several situations in which she had successfully "talked herself out of" her depression. Mary was asked to monitor her mood over the course of the week and to use the self-talk strategy whenever she felt sad. In the subsequent session, she described several instances in which she tried to use the strategy, but her mood did not improve. With further assessment, Mary came to notice that there did not seem to be a consistent relationship between the use of positive self-talk and improved mood.

Specific Measures of Experiential Avoidance

Because experiential avoidance is so important to conceptualization and treatment from an acceptance-based behavioral perspective, we also typically administer at least one questionnaire specifically aimed at assessing this form of coping. The Acceptance and Action Questionnaire (AAQ; Hayes, Strosahl, et al., 2004) is the most widely used self-report measure of experiential avoidance, tapping into both the unwillingness to remain in contact with particular feelings and thoughts and the unwillingness to act intentionally while experiencing distressing private events. Items such as "I'm not afraid of my feelings" are rated on a 7-point scale from 1 ("never true") to 7 ("always true"). Several versions of this measure are available. The most common is the nine-item scale, which has demonstrated adequate psychometric properties (Hayes, Strosahl, et al., 2004). There are also two 16-item versions of the scale that have shown some promise in measuring underlying processes that may change as a function of treatment. Because each of these three versions has psychometric strengths and weaknesses, many clinicians opt to use a 22-item version that combines all of the items from the three versions into one measure. Finally, a 10-item version of the AAQ (the AAQ-II) that aims to address some of the problems of earlier versions (e.g., complexly worded items, low internal consistency) is currently under development (F.G. Bond, personal communication).

The Thought Control Questionnaire (TCQ; Wells & Davies, 1994) is a 30-item instrument aimed at assessing the effectiveness of strategies used to control unpleasant and unwanted thoughts. Items such as "I punish myself for thinking the thought" and "I tell myself not to be so stupid" are rated on a 4-point scale ranging from 1 ("never") to 4 ("almost always"). Although the TCQ measures five factors that correspond to different strategies for controlling unwanted thoughts (distraction, social control, worry, punishment, and reappraisal), punishment and worry most clearly relate to the construct of experiential avoidance. The White Bear Suppression Inventory (WBSI; Wegner & Zanakos, 1994) is another measure aimed at assessing strategies to control thoughts. Specifically, this 15-item self-report measure assesses the tendency to avoid and suppress one's unwanted thoughts. Items such as "I always try to put problems out of mind" are rated on a 5-point scale ranging from 1 ("strongly disagree") to 5 ("strongly agree").

Emotion Regulation

Emotion regulation is a broad concept that has been used to describe one's ability to modulate (e.g., Gross, 1998), monitor, and evaluate one's emotional state (e.g., Thompson, 1994). Although this construct is likely highly related to both general coping strategies and mindfulness, it can also be useful to specifically assess it.

Gross and John (2003) developed the 10-item Emotion Regulation Questionnaire (ERQ) designed to assess individual differences in the habitual use of two emotion regulation strategies: cognitive appraisal (e.g., "I control my emotions by changing the way I think about the situation I'm in") and suppression of emotional expression ("I control my emotions by not expressing them"). Each item is rated on a 7-point scale ranging from 1 ("strongly disagree") to 7 ("strongly agree"). Kashdan and Steger (2006) modified this measure to develop the eight-item State Emotion Regulation Questionnaire to assess strategic attempts to modify mood during the day. This adapted measure may be useful in providing clients and therapists with some individualized information about the relationship between the emotion regulation strategies used by a client in different situations and his or her subsequent emotional response.

As described earlier, the Difficulties in Emotion Regulation Scale (DERS; Gratz & Roemer, 2004) is a comprehensive measure of emotion regulation. The scale provides a total score as well as six subscale scores measuring difficulties in aspects of emotion regulation, including acceptance of emotions (e.g., "When I'm upset, I become embarrassed for feeling that way"), ability to engage in goal-directed behavior when distressed (e.g., "When I'm upset, I have difficulty getting things done"), impulse control (e.g., "When I'm upset, I lose control over my behaviors"), and access to strategies for regulation (e.g., "When I'm upset, I believe that there is nothing I can do to make myself feel better") in addition to the awareness of emotions and clarity of emotions subscales described earlier. Participants indicate how often each item applies to themselves on a 5-point Likert-type scale, with 1 as "almost never" (0–10%) and 5 as "almost always" (91–100%). Scores are coded such that higher scores indicate greater difficulties in emotion regulation.

Assessing Strengths

While these assessments of problematic ways of responding to internal experiences are an important part of a comprehensive assessment, we also make an effort to assess ways that clients are able to cope effectively and the strengths that they draw on. As described in the previous chapter, clients often come to treatment with narrowed, critical views of themselves resulting from fusion with their distressing internal experiences. Asking specifically about strengths can help broaden their perspective so that they also attend to parts of their lives that are rewarding. This information helps the therapist plan early behavioral assignments that are most likely to be successful and reinforcing, supporting future change efforts.

QUALITY OF LIFE

Domains of Functioning

As discussed in Chapter 1, the explicit goal of ABBT is to improve clients' quality of life fundamentally and significantly. While this goal is implicit in any form of therapy, ABBT uses a number of clinical methods to help clients engage in behaviors that are consistent with personally relevant values. Therefore, a careful assessment of clients' behavior and satisfaction in multiple life domains is highly recommended. We commonly ask our clients to describe their current school/occupational functioning, noting any issues with attendance, performance, or dissatisfaction. We assess the size and quality of clients' social support networks, particularly attending to signs of isolation, lack of intimacy in relationships, or conflictual relationships. Additionally, we ask how our clients spend their free time and specifically assess for the presence of hobbies, leisure activities, and spiritual and community interests.

Physical health and well-being are also important targets of assessment. While we routinely assess for the presence of significant medical conditions, there are a number of other important health indicators that are related to life satisfaction. For example, according to the Institute of Medicine, 50 to 70 million Americans chronically suffer from a sleep disorder. A recent poll by the National Sleep Foundation (2007) revealed that two-thirds of women experience sleep problems at least a few nights a week. Among those reporting poor sleep, 80% report feeling stressed out and anxious, and 55% report feeling unhappiness, sadness, or depression within the past month. Additionally, poor sleep is associated with less time spent with friends and family and decreased sexual activity.

The relationship between sleep and mental health is complex and reciprocal. Psychological disorders such as MDD and PTSD are characterized by sleep disturbances; lack of sleep contributes to poor mood, attention, and concentration; and prescribed (psychotropic medications) and nonprescribed (drugs and alcohol) substances impact sleep frequency and quality. Furthermore, deficits in sleep can intensify the presence of negative emotions and reduce the positive effects of goal-enhancing activities (Zohar, Tzischinsky, Epstein, & Lavie, 2005).

There are several methods one can use to assess sleep quality. The Pittsburgh Sleep Quality Index (PSQI; Buysse, Reynolds, Monk, Berman, & Kupfer, 1989) is a 19-item self-report measure of sleep quality and disturbances. Another brief self-report measure is the 19-item Sleep Scale from the Medical Outcomes Study (Hays & Stewart, 1992). In addition to these questionnaire measures, a sleep diary, in which participants self-monitor their daily sleep/wake patterns, has been shown to be a reliable assessment instrument (Rogers, Caruso, & Aldrich, 1993).

Diet and exercise are also important components of quality of life worth assessing. Even when eating concerns are not a presenting problem, poor nutrition and erratic eating patterns can threaten a client's health and well-being. Sexual functioning is often overlooked as a component of quality of life. A large epidemiological survey conducted in the United States (Laumann, Paik, & Rosen, 1999) found that 43% of female and 31% of male respondents experienced some form of sexual dysfunction. Problems in sexual functioning can negatively impact mood and strain intimate relationships. Although many clients are uncomfortable discussing their sexuality, we have found that it can be quite normalizing to ask about satisfaction in this important life domain as part of a comprehensive assessment of quality of life. Furthermore, a questionnaire, such as the Derogatis Sexual Functioning Inventory (DSFI; Derogatis & Melisaratos, 1979), can be administered to get an overall sense of a client's functioning in this area.

The Quality of Life Inventory (QOLI; Frisch, Cornwell, Villanueva, & Retzlaff, 1992) is an excellent tool to help the therapist get an overall sense of a client's satisfaction across several important domains. Respondents rate the importance of (on a 3-point scale) and current satisfaction with (on a 6-point scale) 16 areas of life (health, self-esteem, goals and values, money, work, play, learning, creativity, helping, love, friends, children, relatives, home, neighborhood, and community). An overall quality of life score is obtained in addition to a weighted satisfaction profile for the 16 areas assessed.

Values

Wilson and Groom (2002; as cited in Wilson & Murrell, 2004) developed the Valued Living Questionnaire (VLQ), which requires clients to assess the *importance* of 10 commonly valued domains of living on a scale of 1–10: family, marriage/couples/intimate relations, parenting, friendship, work, education, recreation, spirituality, citizenship, and physical self-care. Next, clients are asked to estimate, using a scale of 1–10, how *consistently* they have behaved in accord with each of the values during the past week. The VLQ is primarily used as a clinical tool to identify areas of living that might end up being targets for treatment.

Wilson and Murrell (2004) describe three clinically notable profiles that can be extremely informative to the therapist. The first common profile reflects a high discrepancy between ratings of importance and ratings of consistency in one or more valued domains. For example, a client who is currently out of work on disability due to symptoms of MDD and who highly values being challenged and contributing in the workplace might rate this domain as highly valued and inconsistently pursued. Clients with this profile are likely to report significant psychological distress and to appear immobilized with regard to moving forward and making changes in valued domains.

Another pattern worth noting is one of extremely low importance scores across most or all valued domains. For instance, a client who is extremely isolated, with a history of social rejection, might uniformly rate family, intimate relations, parenting, and friendship as all unimportant. Sometimes this pattern of "not caring" may actually reflect a desire to avoid the pain associated with acknowledging a wish to be connected with others (Wilson & Murrell, 2004). In these cases, the clinician can gently explore if "not caring" is preventing the client from pursuing these important life domains.

A final notable pattern is that of extremely high total importance and consistency scores. Particularly when a client reports little psychological distress, such endorsement may reflect the client's desire to present him- or herself in a socially acceptable way (Wilson & Murrell, 2004). In our own practice, we have seen a number of clients who endorse many values as highly important and report that they are consistently acting in accordance with these values but describe significant psychological distress. In these cases, clients are often "going through the motions" of living a valued life without bringing mindfulness to their experiences. For example, Wendy was a professional with an exciting and challenging career, a solid marriage, and three wonderful children. On the surface, she seemed to be striking a balance between succeeding in her career and spending quality time with her family; however, upon more careful interviewing, it became apparent that Wendy was not bringing mindfulness and intention to her behavior in valued domains. When she was at work, although her performance was strong, she was often distracted with thoughts and feelings of guilt and worry about her family. At home, she would spend time playing with her children, but her attention was focused on thoughts about work and deadlines. Her pattern of scores on the VLQ, along with her stated distress, indicated to her clinician the importance of working with Wendy to bring mindfulness to her valued activities.

Emmons (1986) developed an assessment system aimed at assessing personal strivings, a concept similar to that of values. He defined *personal strivings* as unifying, organizing abstract constructs, such as wanting affection from others, that guide and direct everyday behavior. Using this system, each striving is rated on a number of dimensions, including value (happiness or unhappiness associated with success in the striving), clarity regarding the striving, ambivalence toward the striving, commitment, level of importance, expectancy for success, and motives for pursuing these goals.

Drawing from this measure, which is primarily used in research on personality and well-being, Blackledge, Ciarocchi, and Bailey (2007) developed the Personal Values Questionnaire for use in a clinical context. The questionnaire is designed to help clients articulate their values, to identify whether their values are intrinsically or extrinsically motivated, to rate the personal importance of each value, and to gauge commitment to the value. Values are assessed in the nine domains of living described in ACT (Hayes, Strosahl, & Wilson, 1999): family relationships, friendships/social relationships, couples/romantic relationships, work/career, education/schooling/personal growth and development, recreation/leisure/sport, spirituality/religion, community/citizenship, and health/physical well-being. Clients are asked to read a brief description of each values domain (e.g., in the friendships/social relationships domain they are asked to think about what it means be a good friend and given possible descriptions to consider, such as being supportive, considerate, caring, accepting, loyal, or honest) and then asked to articulate any personal values they may have in this domain. Next, clients are presented with nine questions about the value, each rated on a 5-point scale, that assess motivation for holding the value, the extent to which behavior is currently consistent with the value, commitment to the value, importance of the value, and whether or not it is a potential area for improvement.

Lundgren, Dahl, and Hayes (2008) have developed the Values Bull's Eye, a measure of values attainment and persistence when encountering barriers, using a series of four pictorial representations of dartboards. The first three dartboards are used to assess the extent to which clients are living consistent with their values. The client is asked to describe three deeply held, personally relevant valued directions that he or she would like to work on in therapy. The center of the dartboard (the bull's eye) represents living fully in accord with that value, and the client is asked to mark how close to the bull's eye he or she is currently living. A fourth dartboard is used to assess persistence of acting in accordance with values in the face of psychological barriers such as anxiety or sadness. The client is asked to write down individual barriers that make it difficult to live consistent with his or her values, then to indicate persistence of valued action in the face of the described barriers (with the bull's eye meaning the client always persists). The distance between the center (bull's eye) and the edge of all four dartboards is 4.5 centimeters, and scores, representing the distance between the mark and the bull's eye, can vary from 0 to 4.5, with lower scores equaling greater attainment or persistence. Values attainment is a mean of the first three dartboards; persistence through barriers is generated by the single measure.

While these measures can be helpful in obtaining a baseline assessment of values, we have also found a more in-depth assessment of values throughout treatment to be useful. We use a series of writing assignments in treatment to help our clients obtain a clearer and richer sense of their own values. These treatment strategies are discussed in Chapter 7.

PREVIOUS TREATMENT

Just as it is important to fully assess the coping strategies that the client uses to cope with difficult psychological events, it is also critical to obtain a comprehensive understanding of the client's previous experiences in therapy. We routinely ask our clients to describe their previous therapy, to note which methods and strategies they found most effective, and to describe any components they found less useful.

Cognitive-Behavioral Treatment

In our own practice, we have worked with a number of clients who have previously completed a trial of cognitive-behavioral therapy. Although acceptance-based behavioral approaches spring from this tradition, and many of the methods of traditional CBT are highly consistent with acceptance-based approaches (see Chapter 10), one should fully explore the client's experiences with CBT (for more information on the similarities and differences between CBT and acceptance-based approaches, see Orsillo & Roemer, 2005; Orsillo, Roemer, Lerner, & Tull, 2004). Acceptance-based behavioral approaches draw from, and are compatible with, CBT techniques such as self-monitoring, exposure therapy, behavioral activation, and skills training. Some ways of approaching irrational thoughts with cognitive restructuring are consistent with the ABBT goal of changing the relationship that the client has with his or her internal experiences. For example, encouraging a client to consider his thoughts as merely thoughts and not facts, to attend a party even when he is feeling anxious, and to observe what really happens in that feared situation might be part of both approaches to treatment. In contrast, other cognitive approaches may focus more on changing the content of a specific thought in order to decrease anxiety, which is less consistent with an ABBT perspective. For example, a client who is anxious at parties may be asked to try and replace the thought "I feel like a fool because I am not as educated as the other people here" with something like "I am an interesting and educated person." The rationale of CT in this case would be to reduce the frequency and intensity of uncomfortable thoughts, which would be expected to decrease anxiety and facilitate exposure to feared situations. Although symptom reduction is an obvious goal of ABBT, the emphasis in this approach is on developing an accepting and compassionate stance toward oneself and engaging in actions that are consistent with personally relevant values.

As cognitive-behavioral approaches have grown in popularity, the term has come to describe a much broader class of disparate techniques. Therefore, we find it useful to ask our clients more specifically about which elements of CBT they received (e.g., psychoeducation, cognitive restructuring, behavioral activation, skills training, relaxation training, exposure therapy). Furthermore, if they report that certain techniques were not at all useful, we probe for more detail. For example, Sheila reported that she was unwilling to consider applied relaxation training in therapy because of a previous unsuccessful trial. Upon more detailed questioning, it became clear that her previous therapy had involved listening to a tape of ocean sounds as a form of relaxation. When we were able to differentiate applied relaxation from what Sheila had previously tried, she became more willing to consider it.

It can also be useful to hear a client's thoughts about why a trial of CBT may not have been effective. For instance, we often see clients who have not benefited from previous exposure therapy. John, a Vietnam veteran with PTSD, was unwilling to try exposure therapy because his experience with this method had failed. Specifically, John had completed one session of exposure therapy, during which he became extremely aroused and agitated. Exposure therapy is an extremely powerful treatment for PTSD that can be enhanced with acceptance techniques (see Chapter 10). Therefore, while we suggested that John consider engaging in exposure therapy with us, we provided him with a rationale to address his concerns. Specifically, we explained that we would first provide him with mindfulness and defusion skills to help diminish the distress associated with the painful thoughts, images, and emotions that exposure is likely to elicit.

Often, if a client has had a positive experience with CBT, he or she may struggle a bit with some acceptance strategies, which could seem inconsistent with the cognitive model that thoughts cause emotions and that cognitive restructuring is needed to alter thoughts so that they are more "rational." A careful assessment of the specific methods that were found to be useful allows the therapist to address these apparent inconsistencies. For instance, Mark had found the cognitive restructuring he received in previous therapy useful in treating his social anxiety disorder (SAD) and he expressed concern that an acceptance-based approach to treating his GAD symptoms with the current therapist would be inconsistent with the work he had completed. We were able to draw parallels for him between the self-monitoring he completed and the development of the mindfulness skill of attention. Furthermore, we discussed the consistencies between no longer accepting certain thoughts as facts and the decentering and defusion skills of mindfulness. Rather than directly confronting Mark about whether changing the content of his thoughts was necessary for treatment, we asked him if he was willing to expand his repertoire and try some new approaches to cope with his emotions when cognitive restructuring was ineffective.

Nondirective Treatment

While the acceptance and validation aspects of ABBT are quite consistent with many nondirective, humanistic approaches to therapy, the behavioral elements of ABBT that require significant out-of-session activity are not as common to these approaches. It can be very useful for the clinician to know about a client's previous experience and satisfaction with nondirective therapies as such a history can definitely affect a client's goals and expectations for treatment. For example, Richard sought treatment with one of us (Orsillo) after terminating with a humanistic therapist he had been seeing for approximately 20 years. At first Richard was put off by the suggestion that therapy would require out-of-session work, stating that he had done homework while he was in school and he did not see the need for homework in therapy. I spent considerable time with Richard in an effort to provide an adequate and compelling rationale for out-of-session practice. A common clinical pitfall among busy therapists is to rush through the introduction of homework assignments without providing a sufficient rationale or acknowledging the challenges of fitting these tasks into already busy lives. Although it is always beneficial for the therapist to take sufficient time to talk with a client about the challenges of out-of-session practice, it is particularly important to be sensitive to these issues with clients who have engaged in a less structured and directive therapy.

Previous Experience with Mindfulness

As mindfulness, meditation, yoga, and other Eastern spiritual practices become more popular in Western culture, more and more clients will present to treatment with some history of mindfulness practice. Such experience can be quite beneficial in preparing clients to start ABBT, but sometimes clients have had negative experiences with these approaches that could interfere with psychotherapy. Once again, asking clients to fully describe their previous experience with mindfulness, what they liked and disliked about the practice, and successes and failures can be extremely informative in the development of a rationale and plan for treatment.

For example, Shoshanna, a client with features of dependent personality disorder, was enthusiastic about ABBT because she thought it was consistent with her extensive sitting meditation practice. Because the therapist assumed that Shoshanna was extremely knowledgeable about mindfulness and they were limited in the number of available sessions, she spent more time in therapy encouraging Shoshanna to engage in valued actions than she did discussing and practicing mindfulness. When it became clear that Shoshanna was not making the gains she had hoped for in therapy, she and her therapist spent some time reviewing their progress and noted that Shoshanna was struggling significantly with the mindfulness concepts of self-compassion and acceptance. Because the therapist did not fully assess Shoshanna's past experience with meditation, she was unaware that Shoshanna had little practice with these skills.

TABLE 2.1. Additional Assessment Resources

Author(s) (year)	Form	Domain	Reprints measures
Antony, Orsillo, & Roemer (2001)	Book	Anxiety	Yes
Nezu, Ronan, Meadows, & McClure (2000)	Book	Depression	Yes
Cocoran & Fischer (2000)	Book	Broad spectrum of psychological constructs	Yes
Association for Contextual Behavioral Science	Website (*www. contextualpsychology. org*)	Variety of ACT-related assessment instruments, including many that currently under development	Yes
Buros Institute of Mental Measurements	Website (*www.unl. edu/buros*)	General and comprehensive listing of psychological instruments	No

ADDITIONAL ASSESSMENT RESOURCES FOR THE CLINICIAN

While we have tried to describe the methods and measures we think are most useful when conducting a comprehensive assessment working with a client from an acceptance-based behavioral perspective, there are many other assessment resources available to clinicians. A few books and websites that we have found particularly useful in helping us identify and obtain assessment instruments are summarized in Table 2.1. It is also important to note that we have been purposively overly inclusive in our description of the potential measures and methods we might use to conduct an assessment. While all of these domains are important to assess, we believe that the therapist should choose instruments carefully and flexibly to meet the individual needs of different clients and situations.

ANXIETY AWARENESS SHEET

Please rate your anxiety (on a scale of 0 to 100, with 0 being no anxiety at all and 100 being severe anxiety) at four different times during the day. If you notice anything while rating your anxiety, feel free to jot down these observations below the form.

Rating Scale:

0	50	100
No anxiety at all, completely relaxed	Moderate anxiety	Severe anxiety

Date	Morning Time/Rating	Noon Time/Rating	Evening Time/Rating	Night Time/Rating

FORM 2.2

EMOTION MONITORING SHEET

When you notice that you are experiencing a strong emotion, please take a moment to notice and write down the situation you are in and the emotion you are experiencing. Please also record any thoughts you are having at that time and any physical sensations (e.g., heart racing, muscle tension, fatigue).

Date/Time	Situation	Emotion	Thoughts	Physical sensations

ASSESSMENT OF COPING STRATEGIES

As you have been doing, please continue to notice strong emotions that emerge in different situations and the thoughts and sensations that accompany each emotion. Also, note how you respond to the emotion (e.g., pay attention to it, try and push it away, distract yourself, try and change it, etc.) and the outcome (successful, unsuccessful, feel better, feel worse, etc.).

Date/Time	Situation	Emotions/Thoughts/Sensations	Response	Outcome

THREE

Individualized Case Formulation and Treatment Planning

As we discussed in Chapter 1, a cornerstone of treatment is a shared understanding between client and therapist of the nature of the challenges the client is facing. The individualized case formulation draws from the general acceptance-based behavioral model presented earlier but is connected to the specifics of the client's presenting concerns and experiences. This formulation is then linked to the intervention approach, both generally to the overarching goals and methods of treatment and specifically to each exercise, practice, or topic that is introduced. In this way, treatment from an acceptance-based behavioral perspective (similar to CBT interventions) is *transparent*, with the therapist sharing his or her understanding and intention with the client throughout, and *collaborative*, with the therapist incorporating the client's perspective in the formulation and selection of interventions. This formulation and treatment plan are individualized by incorporating information from the assessment methods described in the previous chapter into a general acceptance-based behavioral model, sharing this formulation with the client and adjusting it based on his or her feedback, and adapting general intervention methods to meet his or her specific presentation. In this chapter, we provide an overview of how to develop an individualized case formulation and connect it to a treatment plan. The following chapters describe in detail how therapy unfolds from an acceptance-based behavioral perspective, providing examples and exercises that can help clinicians in developing, implementing, and refining treatment plans with specific clients.

DEVELOPING A CASE FORMULATION

As Persons (1989) notes, case formulations involve identifying two levels of the presenting concern: *overt difficulties* and *underlying psychological mechanisms*. While acceptance-based behavioral approaches highlight the importance of specific underlying psychological mechanisms that are thought to play a role in a wide range of overt difficulties (problematic relationships with internal experience, experiential avoidance, behavioral constriction), they also focus on identifying and targeting overt difficulties. These are the concerns that have brought clients into treatment, and motivation for and commitment to therapy will depend on clients' perception that the proposed treatment will address these pressing concerns. Also, overt difficulties are the signs that the underlying psychological mechanisms are being activated, so identifying and monitoring them provide important information to guide the client and the therapist in opportunities to practice newly learned responses. For instance, a client who describes "shutting down" when he feels criticized by his partner may be distancing from his emotional experience (and his partner) as a way to reduce the fear and vulnerability he experiences at this threat of abandonment, although he is unaware of these underlying responses. By attending to his identified tendency to shut down (and recognizing that it is inconsistent with his stated value of intimacy in his relationship), he and his therapist can begin to explore ways he might remain open or connected in these contexts and how he can tolerate the distress that might arise. Recognizing shutting down as something that arises when he feels vulnerable may help him cultivate a wider array of responses to this situation.

The previous chapter described the essential first step in developing a case formulation: comprehensive assessment of the client's presenting concerns (overt difficulties), including symptoms, problematic behaviors, and impairments in quality of life and functioning. It should include an assessment (through either interview or self-report methods) of how the client relates to his or her internal experiences, evidence of experiential avoidance, and behavioral constriction to begin to explore potential underlying psychological mechanisms that may help explain and unify presenting concerns. When the client describes specific examples of overt difficulties, the therapist can listen for evidence of connections to specific ways of relating to, or trying to avoid, internal experiences or constrictions in living that may reveal the function of these difficulties for the individual. For instance, Ana, a client struggling with excessive alcohol use, described a period of drinking prompted by a difficult interaction with her partner in which she felt as though her partner had insulted her.

THERAPIST: What did you feel right after the insult?

CLIENT: I was just so angry!

THERAPIST: And what was your reaction to feeling that way? Did any other feelings come up or any feelings about feeling angry?

CLIENT: Well, it frightened me. I was afraid I was going to do something or say something that I wouldn't be able to take back.

THERAPIST: I see. So then you were angry and frightened. Is that something you often experience when you feel angry?

CLIENT: Yes, anger scares me. I remember when my father used to get angry and the things he would do. I don't want to be like that. I know how dangerous anger can be.

THERAPIST: It makes a lot of sense that you have that kind of reaction to your anger. What did you do when you felt frightened by your anger? How did you manage that?

CLIENT: Well, I just tried not be angry, tried to push away the feelings I was having.

THERAPIST: How did that work?

CLIENT: I just felt bad then—bad all over.

THERAPIST: Can you tell me more about that? What did you feel in your body?

CLIENT: I felt like I was jumping out of my skin. My heart was pounding. My mind was racing.

THERAPIST: So, it sounds like trying not to feel angry just left you feeling generally on edge and physically activated. What did you do then?

CLIENT: I went and got a drink to calm down a bit and try to stop feeling that way. I was still worried about what I might do.

THERAPIST: Tell me a bit about what unfolded once you started drinking.

CLIENT: Then I felt terrible about drinking!

THERAPIST: So, it was a really difficult cycle for you. Did you feel anything else besides terrible about drinking, maybe even before you felt terrible? Maybe something like relief? Or a change in your physical distress?

CLIENT: Oh, yeah—first I just felt great. As soon as I took a sip, I could feel my heart slow down; my chest loosen up a little. And my mind quieted down a little, and my head stopped pounding. It was great. Then I felt guilty that it was so great. Because I know I'm trying to stop and it isn't a good thing for me to do.

THERAPIST: Well, I can definitely see why you would take a drink in this situation.

CLIENT: Really?

THERAPIST: Sure. You're having these intense feelings that are terrifying, in part because they remind you of scary memories from your past. You try to manage them internally, and it doesn't work—you actually feel more distressed. And you know that a drink will take away some of those difficult experiences. It's pretty hard not to drink given all that.

CLIENT: Yeah, it really is. Does that mean I'll always drink?

THERAPIST: No, not at all. It's just important to be able to see why it's such a hard habit to change and to start to see the things that lead up to it, so we can find ways you can make different choices along the way. So, now we can see that your fear of your anger and your efforts to get rid of it might be important for us to attend to as a way of stopping this cycle from unfolding.

This kind of analysis can help explain a client's continual engagement in a behavior that he or she intends to refrain from (e.g., excessive drinking) and identify targets for intervention (e.g., fear of anger, the strong connection between anger and unwanted behavior, automatic efforts to suppress emotional experience). Further assessment of what matters to Ana (i.e., valued directions, described more fully below), will help identify ways she might prefer to react in this type of situation, providing further targets for intervention.

Case formulation should also include attention to the client's cultural background. Contextual factors such as ethnicity, religious background and current affiliation, sexual orientation, national origin, age and generational influences, developmental and acquired disabilities, socioeconomic status, and indigenous heritage (Hays, 2008), as well as experiences of racism and other forms of marginalization or oppression, current living context, and personal identification with various aspects of identity and background should all be considered in a case formulation. Clients' conceptualization of their difficulties may be informed by many aspects of their cultural background and other contextual factors, which should be incorporated in the resulting case formulation. Tanaka-Matsumi and colleagues (1996) provide useful guidelines for using a culturally informed functional assessment (CIFA) interview to develop a CBT case formulation; this is also helpful for developing an acceptance-based behavioral conceptualization. These issues are discussed in greater detail in Chapter 11.

Monitoring forms, as described in the previous chapter, can also be very useful in developing or enhancing a case formulation. Clients can be asked to record instances of whatever problem they present with (social anxiety, bingeing, arguments with a partner, feelings of inadequacy), to rate a specific problem at several times a day (morning, noon, dinnertime, before bed; see Form 2.1, Anxiety Awareness Sheet, p. 51, for a model), or to note particularly problematic situations or experiences they have in a given day (see Form 2.2, Emotion Monitoring Sheet, p. 52, for an example). With this very simplified type of monitoring early in treatment, clients can get accustomed to bringing therapy into their lives and start to make room for it (e.g., coming up with systems for remembering to self-monitor and problem solving any issues that arise). It also helps give both therapist and client a sense of the frequency, antecedents, and consequences of presenting problems. While reviewing these forms, therapists can ask clients specifics about what came right before a given experience and what came right after, which may begin to illustrate the way various problems interrelate and the way that acceptance-based behavioral principles may explain presenting problems. This process helps clients see the link between their overt difficulties and the proposed underlying mechanism, which helps make a connection between the treatment and their reason for coming into therapy.

A case formulation is always hypothetical. We do our best to examine the evidence and apply psychological theory and research to a client's specific, idiographic presentation in order to explain how various challenges are being maintained in a client's life to identify points for intervention that can help a client to live the life he or she chooses. It is important that this formulation be grounded in the client's experience and values while also drawing from existing nomothetic principles and evidence. We work from a therapeutic stance in which the client is seen as the expert in his or her experience, while the therapist brings some expertise in general principles of human behavior and adaptation, as well as her or his own experiences, which can be shared. The therapist and client need to collaborate in order to fit the general knowledge into the specifics of the client's experience and then, based on this formulation, to plot and constantly review and adapt a course for therapy.

Persons (1989) provides detailed guidance in developing a case formulation. Although she is describing a cognitive-behavioral case formulation, the main difference in the process of developing an acceptance-based behavioral formulation is the identification of underlying mechanisms drawn from an acceptance-based behavioral model. Thus, a useful first step is forming a problem list that includes all of the difficulties that the client presents with (drawn from the assessment described in the previous chapter). It is important to note that clients may feel one or two problems are the most central, but it is still helpful to see the full landscape of challenges the client describes. Identifying areas of strength and satisfaction is also useful in painting a full picture of the client's experience and discovering areas upon which it will be important to build.

The next step is beginning to see how the client's presenting problems interrelate. Monitoring forms, responses to interview questions, and self-report measures can provide guidance in making these connections. Therapists may want to ask clients specific questions in order to better understand these relationships (e.g., "Which usually comes first, the feelings of anxiety or depression?", "What did you notice before you began to feel sad?", "Which of these problems do you remember experiencing first in your life?"). Clearly identifying antecedents and consequences to specific instances of each difficulty (using monitoring forms or recollections of recent incidents) also helps clarify the various ways that one problem may feed another. For instance, a client reports insomnia, feelings of depression and anxiety, ruminative thoughts, and trouble expressing his needs. Closer examination of the way these difficulties unfold reveals that, when he is in a situation in which he wants something, he becomes anxious and uncomfortable due to potential conflict and then becomes further distressed by his reactions to his anxiety. He then fails to express his needs (which reduces his anxiety and discomfort) but finds himself ruminating later about what transpired and feeling sad and hopeless. He describes critical thoughts toward these ruminative tendencies and a desire to stop them and not be so "weak." These ruminative feelings and the cycle of self-criticism often occur at night, making it difficult for him to fall asleep. Identifying this sequence helps reveal the way that these different symptoms cascade into one another and begins to reveal the underlying mechanisms of critical reactions to his internal experience, experiential avoidance, and behavioral constriction (not expressing his needs), which will be targets for intervention.

As therapists formulate connections between presenting problems, they can speculate about underlying mechanisms that may explain the spectrum of concerns the client describes. Questions include: "How is this behavior maintained by the consequences that follow it?", "How does the client relate to his or her thoughts, feelings, and sensations, and how might this influence the difficulties experienced?", "How has the client's life become restricted or narrowed, and what factors promote and maintain these restrictions?", and "What actions does the client engage in that might serve to avoid distress or suffering?" Through this type of inquiry, the therapist can begin to develop hypotheses regarding the functions underlying the overt difficulties that have been identified, which will then lead to identification of targets for intervention and selection of treatment strategies. Linehan's (1993a) description of chain analysis in DBT provides an excellent guideline for this kind of inquiry and analysis.

From an acceptance-based behavioral perspective (similar to a CBT perspective), the origins of presenting problems are not targets of intervention; treatment addresses maintaining rather than etiological factors. Hypotheses regarding the origins of a problematic behavior (e.g., a learned threatening association with separation from a loved one due to early childhood separation and loss or a strong negative reaction to one's own distress due to repeatedly being told that emotions are signs of weakness), however, can help validate clients' struggles, making what have been seen as indications of being "crazy" or "unreasonable" seem instead natural and understandable. This understanding can help counteract critical, judgmental responses the client has to his or her own symptoms that are thought to worsen them. An idiographic explanation of how difficulties may have developed also provides a more salient, personal example of the humanness of the client's struggle. This type of validation may be necessary in order to promote change (Linehan, 1993a), as we describe in more detail in the next chapter.

Hypotheses regarding the origins of presenting problems can be drawn from the information clients provide in the initial assessment sessions. In addition to asking when a current problem started, it can be helpful to ask if clients remember having specific experiences in childhood, seeing caregivers having similar difficulties, or being told about these kinds of problems. Often, clients come in with some sense of how their challenges may relate to earlier experiences, or they may spontaneously report on experiences that seem functionally related to their current problems (for instance, a client who currently cleans compulsively may report feelings of depression as a child, indicating that the compulsive cleaning may be a way of avoiding these distressing feelings). Having clients recall a specific and recent emotional response and then asking whether it felt familiar can identify connections to earlier experiences that may contribute to current problems. It is important to remember that these connections are only hypotheses and that what is most important is that they provide the client with an understanding that facilitates self-validation. Also, seeing one's emotional responses, thoughts, or sensations as connected to the past can help clients understand that these experiences are phenomena that can be observed, which begins the process of disentangling from them.

Others (e.g., Hayes, Strosahl, & Wilson, 1999) note that it is important to acknowledge that we can never accurately determine the factors that have contributed to this learning, given the vast amount of influences on any one individual over a lifetime, the complexities of interactions, and the limits of retrospective report. It is important for the therapist to be cautious in that some explanations for behavior can be incomplete and uninformative. For instance, one client may develop an addiction because his father was an alcoholic whereas another client might completely abstain from alcohol for the same reason. Even if a possible explanation is hypothetical, it can be validating to a client and help him or her to understand his or her current behavior. For instance, a first step that allowed Bert to bring some self-compassion to his difficulty in identifying his emotions was acknowledging that he grew up in a family who never discussed their emotional responses.

However, in some cases, a client's historical explanation for current behavior can interfere with his or her response to treatment (Hayes, Strosahl, & Wilson, 1999; Linehan, 1993a). For instance, a client who feels damaged because she was sexually abused as a child and who believes that this abuse is what causes her impulsive behavior may feel invalidated by attempts to change her behavior. If she had the ability all along to change her impulsive behavior, perhaps the abuse was not as damaging as she assumed and perhaps she is responsible for the distress she experienced throughout her adult life. A skillful therapist will both validate the client's experience that sexual abuse is a horrific violation that has significant negative consequences and encourage the client to see that, in her current context, there may be actions she can take to improve her current level of functioning.

Thus, it is critical for the therapist to be aware of the complexities associated with deriving historical explanations for current behavior. Typically, we help clients develop a hypothetical explanation for their current concerns but encourage them to hold it lightly and focus their attention on the present rather than the past.

In the next chapter, we describe in detail how we set the stage for therapy, conclud-ing with an example of how we might share our case formulation with a client. This for-mulation should be presented tentatively so that it is clear that it consists of hypotheses and with encouragement for the client to share how well it matches or does not match his or her experience. It is also important to try to use the client's words for presenting problems and incorporate meanings and interpretations drawn from the client as well as from nomothetic models. This process is often very engaging for the client, in that he or she is able to see connections between what have felt like disparate experiences and feels heard and validated by the therapist. However, sometimes, clients disagree with part of a conceptualization or do not see the role that experiential avoidance may play in their lives. For instance, Leila described herself as very emotionally expressive and open to experience and reported experiencing feelings of despair and emptiness when her partner withdrew after Leila expressed her feelings, leading to heightened, compulsive efforts to connect to her partner (which were met with more withdrawal). She initially felt that she did not avoid internal experiences but embraced them and that what she really needed was to feel less, so that she could refrain from these problematic efforts at connection that were driven by her intense emotions.

CLIENT: I completely accept my emotional responses. I accept them too much! What I need is to accept them less and to feel less so that I stop doing these things that drive Sam away.

THERAPIST: It really feels like your emotions encourage you to behave in ways you'd rather not, so of course you want to feel less.

CLIENT: I just think I've indulged my feelings too much, and now they're so intense and out of control.

THERAPIST: What makes the feelings seem out of control?

CLIENT: The way I always go after Sam when he leaves the room. I just panic and I can't help going after him. I feel this deep sense of emptiness, and I can't stand the feeling.

THERAPIST: So, the way you act when you're upset makes the feelings seem out of control? That makes a lot of sense. Can you tell me more about your reactions when you get that feeling—you said you can't stand it.

CLIENT: Oh yeah, it's just awful. I feel so weak and vulnerable and empty and like I just can't tolerate feeling that way for one more minute. So I just run after him or say something or do anything to make that feeling go away. And then it makes everything worse!

THERAPIST: That sounds like such a hard pattern to be in. When you feel so scared, it feels like such an unacceptable feeling to you that you feel compelled to do anything, and what you tend to do actually makes it *more* likely you'll feel bad, rather than making things better. Does that sound right?

CLIENT: Exactly. That's why I have to stop feeling so much!

THERAPIST: I can really see why it would feel like that. I can't help wondering though, if another solution might be to try to address how you respond to feeling that way, how it makes you feel about yourself, and how much you want the feeling to go away. Even though it might sound backwards, I think it's possible that if you wanted to get rid of the feeling *less*, you might actually find that it gets less rather than more intense. And if you were able to have a different relationship to the very natural feelings of emptiness that come up when this person you love leaves the room, you might find that it's easier to keep yourself from doing things that you later regret because they seem to make things worse. Does it seem like it might be worth trying that out at least and seeing if it fits your experience?

CLIENT: So, you're saying that if I didn't want the feeling to go away, maybe it would on its own?

THERAPIST: Yeah, kind of. On the one hand, you will always feel some sadness or fear when someone you love pulls away from you. But I think that it may be that the way in which you have learned to react to these normal and natural feelings has made them more intense and distressing. I think for feelings as intense as these, which you've had so many times now and have become such a strong habit, learning to respond differently to them is going to take a while. But it sounds like trying to get rid of them is actually making them worse. I think that finding ways not to do that would at least keep them from getting worse.

CLIENT: Well, I guess that would be a good start at least. It's so hard to imagine not trying to get rid of these feelings though. They're so awful!

THERAPIST: I really understand how awful they feel and why you want them to go away. I think that if you're willing to spend some time gradually practicing a different way of relating to your thoughts and feelings, you may find that they are more tolerable than you imagine. In fact, you do tolerate them all the time, even though you think you can't. Because they don't go away when you try. So, really all we'll be doing is working on not trying something that wasn't working so well anyway.

CLIENT: OK, I guess we can try that. But I really can't imagine it.

THERAPIST: I know, that makes a lot of sense. At this point I am only asking you to be open to the possibility that there may be another way to respond to your emotions. Often, when we develop strong habits it almost seems like they define us in some way. It can seem impossible to imagine changes in things that seem like a big part of who we are. But, if you are willing, let's see what happens as we try this out together.

Sometimes case formulations do not fit the client's experience. A therapist may misunderstand a client's experience or imagine that a client is responding the way the therapist might respond, leading to erroneous conclusions about the way the client's difficulties fit together. Listening carefully to a client's reactions to a proposed formulation will allow the therapist to incorporate this perspective and revise the formulation accordingly. This collaboration is always important but is particularly so when a client comes from a cultural background that differs from the therapist's. The therapist should be careful not to place assumptions that are contextually based in his or her cultural background onto the client and should learn about the client's background.

EXAMPLE OF A CASE FORMULATION

To illustrate an acceptance-based behavioral case formulation, we describe in detail a hypothetical case drawn from multiple real clients. Nicole, age 16, presented for therapy at the encouragement of her mother, who was concerned about her daughter's eating habits. Nicole reported concerns about her weight (which was normal for her height) and repeated, unsuccessful efforts to diet. When asked to describe her food intake in more detail, Nicole revealed that she often "lost control" of her eating and found herself eating much more than she intended to. When prompted to describe her emotional, physiological, and behavioral responses to these "losses of control," Nicole reported initial feelings of comfort and enjoyment while eating but then intense shame and disgust with herself, and negative thoughts about herself, as well as sensations of fullness and bloating that she found uncomfortable. She described "taking care" of these problems by purging, which led to feelings of relief, followed by further feelings of shame due to concerns regarding what others might think of her actions.

Nicole also reported high levels of depressive symptoms when these were directly assessed, although she had not mentioned them initially. In response to further questioning, Nicole reported that the feelings that preceded her binge eating were often sadness or loneliness, along with thoughts that she was a "freak" and a "loser" who would never have friends or a boyfriend. She described feeling sad and lonely as a child as well. When she was asked about the ways in which she coped with her negative feelings as a child, she noted that she relied heavily on her mother for support. Upon further assessment, it became clear that her mother would often cook Nicole a favorite food or take her out for an ice cream in an attempt to cheer her up.

When the therapist asked Nicole about her social life and significant relationships, she looked down and shrugged her shoulders. She described feeling like she didn't fit in easily at school and that she spent most of her time alone. At first she said she preferred to be alone, so that no one could make fun of her or judge her behaviors (like purging) and because she felt it was important to be able to be self-sufficient. When asked more about this, she described how her mother had often highlighted the importance of relying on oneself and complimented and admired those she thought of as strong and independent. Nicole disclosed that whenever she privately experienced a desire to be with others, she took this as a sign of weakness and tried to overcome her feelings. When prompted, she admitted that, in fact, she often had feelings of wanting to share with other people, make friends, and be understood, although she was confused by and judgmental of her feelings and tried very hard not to have them.

When the therapist asked Nicole what changes she was hoping to make, she said that she wanted to stop bingeing. When asked how she thought her life would be different if she no longer binged, Nicole replied that she would lose weight and feel better about herself, stronger, and more confident. The therapist asked what would be different if she felt more confident, and Nicole paused, began to cry, and admitted that she would be able to make friends with people and develop meaningful relationships.

Nicole presented with several overt difficulties. She engaged in frequent bingeing and purging, she experienced depressive symptoms and negative views of herself, and she was socially isolated. While Nicole identified the bingeing as the main presenting problem, suggesting that treatment aimed at immediately reducing this behavior would be indicated, the therapist's case formulation led to a slightly different treatment plan.

The assessment suggested that Nicole's binge eating was preceded by feelings of sadness and loneliness. Nicole reported two historical experiences that had likely led her to have a problematic relationship with her experiences of these feelings. First, she recalled her mother saying that it was weak to rely on other people, leading Nicole to respond critically to her feelings of loneliness and frequent desires to be with other people and to want to get rid of these feelings. Also, her mother had given her food to soothe her when she felt this way as a child, leading to a learned association between eating and emotional control. The comfort she initially felt after eating reinforced the binge-eating behavior, but she subsequently experienced shame and negative thoughts, which she tried to avoid through her purging behavior. The immediate relief she felt after purging reinforced that behavior, but the long-term effects were continued thoughts and feelings that distressed her and stronger feelings of isolation, thus strengthening the cycle.

Although Nicole initially downplayed a need for social interaction, it became clear that, while she desperately wanted to enjoy being alone and to be perceived as a strong, independent woman, she longed to have friends and be intimately connected with other people. Her initial goal of feeling confident was really just a means to being able to be with other people in a way that felt more comfortable to her. This behavioral constriction in her life (not having significant interpersonal relationships) was inconsistent with her values and a source of continued suffering for her, further motivating her experiential avoidance efforts.

Sharing this formulation with Nicole could help her to see the way her behaviors made sense, even though they were also painful. This formulation identified several specific targets for intervention that differed from Nicole's initial targets. Rather than initially targeting Nicole's binge eating, the first phase of therapy would be aimed at altering the relationship Nicole had with her feelings of sadness and loneliness, helping her cultivate an open, kindly attention toward these experiences rather than judging and criticizing them. This awareness would help her to allow these experiences rather than trying to get rid of them with extreme behaviors like bingeing and purging. At the same time, Nicole and her therapist would work together to address the constriction in her social life. While Nicole thought she needed to feel differently in order to act differently (e.g., less lonely, more confident, etc.), the therapist would encourage Nicole to practice engaging in behaviors that mattered to her (like talking to people at school), regardless of how she felt at the moment. Reducing her critical reactions to her sadness and loneliness would help her refrain from experientially avoidant behavior, which would reduce the intensity of her internal responses and help her be more able to act in desired ways. Thus, Nicole's bingeing and purging behaviors would be expected to diminish as a result of targeting her relationship to her internal experience and her constricted behavior. If these behaviors did not diminish as a result of other changes, they would be more directly targeted in a later phase of therapy.

LINKING CASE FORMULATION TO TREATMENT PLANNING

The case formulation is intricately linked to treatment planning—the former identifies the underlying mechanisms thought to explain overt difficulties and the latter targets these mechanisms to help the client develop the life he or she wants to be living. Although targeting the underlying mechanisms is expected to alter the overt difficulties that brought the client to therapy, often therapy from an acceptance-based behavioral perspective involves expanding or making subtle shifts in the initial goals of therapy. If one of the mechanisms that underlies the presenting problems is the strong desire and repeated effort to reduce these problems, which paradoxically increases the problems, treatments that focus exclusively on trying to reduce these symptoms may be similarly ineffective. ABBTs aim to reduce phenomena that seem to be worsening overt difficulties, such as judgmental, critical responses to these difficulties, rigid efforts to avoid them, and constrictions in a person's life as a result of these efforts.

The case formulation provides a rationale for why altering these underlying mechanisms should help the client live a more satisfying, engaging life. If a problematic relationship with internal experiences is leading to restrictions in desired behaviors, then altering this relationship while concurrently addressing the behavioral limitations should have beneficial results. If a problematic behavior is functioning to reduce internal distress, then practicing acceptance of distress should limit the motivation for the problematic behavior, making it easier to refrain from engaging in it. As all of these proposed connections are hypotheses, clients are encouraged to work with therapists to test them by practicing the proposed intervention strategies and noticing the effects. If a proposed intervention does not have the effect hypothesized in the case formulation, the formulation is revised and retested. This process actively engages clients in treatment and provides them practice in noticing the relationship between antecedents and consequences and the way that their own reaction to their responses plays a role in how problematic these responses can become.

FOUR

Setting the Stage for Therapy

This chapter presents an overview of the information useful to both therapist and client as they prepare to commit to a course of treatment from an acceptance-based behavioral perspective. We provide a brief review of this therapeutic approach, including a discussion of the overarching goals, potential modes of therapy, number and length of sessions, types of methods and strategies used in treatment, and structure of a typical therapy session. We describe the stance we (and others) adopt when working from this approach and give guidelines for cultivating this stance and examples of how it can be explicitly modeled in session. Finally, we demonstrate how we set the stage when introducing our clients to treatment by giving our conceptualization of the client's presenting problem, providing an overview of treatment, describing alternative approaches, defining roles, and setting expectations.

BRIEF OVERVIEW OF THE TREATMENT APPROACH

Overarching Goals

As discussed in Chapter 1, we focus on three main goals typical of an acceptance-based behavioral approach to treatment when we are working with a client. The first is to *alter the relationship that the client has with his or her own internal experience*. As we often work with clients who have narrowed or limited awareness and who are judgmental and critical of their inner experience, we hope to cultivate an open, curious, compassionate, and unentangled awareness. We aim to validate and normalize the full range of emotions, thoughts, and physiological sensations and to encourage clients to observe internal events as transient experiences that do not represent pathology, threaten their sense of self, or prevent them from living a vital and meaningful life.

Our second goal is to *decrease experiential avoidance and increase choice and flexibility*. Once the client is less judgmental of and threatened by his or her internal experience, we encourage practice in turning toward and accepting thoughts, feelings, and sensations to replace the habitual response of avoiding and escaping these events. This work allows the client to develop a more expansive way of attending to both internal and external experiences that is motivated by curious engagement rather than anxious avoidance. It also allows the client greater choice and flexibility in action, rather than reactively choosing (or avoiding) actions solely on the basis of their ability to minimize distress.

Finally, our goal is to *increase behavior in valued domains*. Our assumption is that a fearful, judgmental, and avoidant stance toward internal experiences significantly restricts and limits an individual's behavior. Once an alternative stance of acceptance is cultivated, the client can more flexibly engage in relationships, work/career activities, and recreational events, significantly improving overall quality of life.

Mode of Therapy

We have typically conducted ABBT in individual psychotherapy (Roemer & Orsillo, 2005, 2007), which allows for the development of a strong therapeutic bond, with the client feeling genuinely known, accepted, and validated by the therapist. Individual psychotherapy provides a context in which the client can begin to feel simultaneously emotionally vulnerable and safe. The introduction and coverage of different topics and the shaping of new skills can be paced appropriately, taking into account the client's unique style of learning. Significant effort can be devoted to the exploration of personally meaningful goals and values.

We have also delivered different versions of this type of therapy in group settings, with clients diagnosed with GAD (e.g., Orsillo, Roemer, & Barlow, 2003) and PTSD. Many acceptance-based therapeutic approaches use a group or a combined individual and group format. Mindfulness-based stress reduction (MBSR) and mindfulness-based cognitive therapy (MBCT) are conceptualized more as classroom instruction directed by a structured curriculum and involving significant in-class practice than as therapy experiences. MBSR groups often comprise about 30 participants, while MBCT conducts classes of up to 12 participants (Segal et al., 2002). In DBT, groups are typically used for training mindfulness, emotion regulation, interpersonal effectiveness, and distress tolerance skills with clients who concurrently receive individual psychotherapy. ACT has also been delivered in a combination of group and individual sessions (Gifford et al., 2004; Hayes, Wilson, et al., 2004).

Group therapy can be very effective in validating the client's experiences and highlighting the ubiquity of painful thoughts and feelings as well as urges to control and avoid internal events. It can be easier to follow an agenda, cover specific topics, and teach general skills in a group setting, whereas in individual therapy a discussion of daily stressors and pressing concerns can sometimes take a session off track. In ACT training workshops for therapists, participants are often asked to stand honestly and genuinely in front of the rest of the participants, to disclose a personally held value, and to make a public commitment to taking actions that are consistent with that value. In our experience, using this method in group psychotherapy can be similarly powerful, moving, and motivating.

We have also encountered some obstacles in group ABBT. It can be challenging to give each client the individualized attention that may be needed for him or her to be able to personally observe and apply the broad concepts covered in group therapy. Individual obstacles and barriers can be difficult to resolve in a group setting, and less time is available for each client to explore his or her own values with the therapist.

In sum, although we have used our version of ABBT primarily in individual psychotherapy, there may also be significant benefits when these interventions are delivered in a group format, particularly when the emphasis is psychoeducation and/or skill development and practice. The ideal mode of delivery may be a combination of individual and group that combines the advantages of a strong therapeutic bond, individualized attention to promote learning, and a personalized exploration of values with the benefits of structured psychoeducation and skills building in a context that allows clients the opportunity to experience firsthand the ubiquity of human suffering and the innate capacity for healing and growth. We encourage therapists to flexibly adapt the methods described in this book to meet their practice needs.

Number and Length of Sessions

In our research on ABBT for GAD (Roemer & Orsillo, 2005, 2007), we use a standardized protocol in which we deliver therapy (after initial assessment sessions) in 14 weekly sessions, followed by two biweekly sessions. In order to encourage the early development of a strong working alliance and more rapidly engage the client in therapy, we allow 90 minutes for the first four sessions. Starting with the fifth session, a typical session runs approximately 50 to 60 minutes.

In other contexts, we have varied the number of sessions and the time allotted for therapy based on the needs of the clients and the demands of the systems. For instance, if 90-minute sessions are not feasible in a particularly clinical setting, it may be beneficial to meet with the client twice a week for the first few sessions. We have also worked with clients for whom 90-minute sessions or twice weekly contact would be considered too intense. In those cases, we slowed the pace of therapy and extended the number of sessions. As discussed in Chapter 9, an ongoing assessment of progress over the course of therapy most accurately guides decisions about the length of treatment.

Methods and Strategies

The next several chapters are devoted to providing an in-depth discussion of each of the clinical strategies used in ABBTs; here we provide a brief and general overview. Drawing from their traditional behavioral and cognitive-behavioral roots, ABBTs involve an ongoing assessment of clients' responses (thoughts, feelings, sensations, and behaviors) in particularly challenging situations using self-monitoring and self-observation. Psychoeducation provides information about the function of emotions and the relationships between internal experiences and behaviors and introduces other new concepts relevant to the clients' presenting issues. Direct experience observing and experiencing concepts is considered a required element of learning new ways of relating to internal experiences and new patterns of responding. Skills training (e.g., interpersonal effectiveness) and problem solving are often used to address particular presenting concerns. Finally, behavioral strategies such as activity scheduling and exposure assignments are used within and between sessions.

These behavioral approaches are integrated with and enhanced by strategies aimed at increasing acceptance and defusion/decentering. Formal and informal mindfulness practice and other experiential exercises are considered fundamental to the practice of ABBTs. Both the therapist and the client are encouraged to develop metaphors and stories to capture the essence of key concepts and to promote experiential learning.

Although we describe many of the methods and strategies we use to promote mindfulness, acceptance, and behavioral change separately in the following three chapters, in practice we integrate these each of these elements into every session rather than presenting them linearly. To this end, we have developed a typical structure that guides each session.

The Typical Session

As discussed, we devote several initial sessions to assessment, case formulation, and treatment planning. At the end of this chapter, we describe a typical treatment planning session during which we share our formulation and treatment plan, obtain consent from the client, and set the stage for therapy. Here we describe the structure of a typical weekly therapy session.

We ask our clients to come in at least 15 minutes prior to their scheduled session to hand in their between-session monitoring forms and/or assignments and to complete some brief self-report measures assessing their current psychological functioning and their engagement in mindfulness, acceptance, and valued activities during the previous week. Before the session starts, we take some time alone to review these measures, to read through the monitoring forms, and to prepare.

Each session begins with both the therapist and the client engaging in some form of a mindful, focusing exercise together. We follow a progression when choosing these exercises, initially focusing on mindfulness of breath and physical sensations and moving toward more challenging exercises involving the observation of emotions and cognitions in later sessions (see Chapter 6 for more on this process). We also personalize these exercises by focusing on specific skills that may be particularly challenging for a client and later by encouraging clients to choose and often lead these exercises in later sessions.

Next, we briefly review with the client out-of-session work, questions or concerns from the previous session, and any significant events that occurred in the course of the week, with a particular emphasis on any changes the client may have noticed in the relationship between his or her internal experiences and behavior and any problems or obstacles that he or she encountered. For instance, we regularly ask our clients to share what they observed about their own internal experiences over the course of the week, including the thoughts, emotions, and behavioral patterns that were elicited by particular contexts. We may ask a client to describe his or her experiences with a particular mindfulness practice, specifically noting obstacles to practice, observations that emerged from practice, and areas that may require further attention. We also regularly ask clients about opportunities taken and missed during the week to engage in personalized, valued activities and follow up on specific obstacles that may have interfered with particular actions.

During the early stages of treatment, the next portion of the session is devoted to the introduction of a new concept (e.g., the function of emotion, the problems associated with attempts at controlling one's internal experience, the basic skills of mindfulness, the differentiation of values from goals). Each of these concepts is introduced in multiple ways that are described in more depth throughout this volume. For example, we may provide some psychoeducation about the function of emotion by discussing the topic in session and providing a handout for the client to read over. We also use a metaphor and/or experiential exercise, such as drawing an analogy between the vital, communicative function of physical pain and emotional pain, to allow the client to experience the concept more personally. Finally, we ask the client to systematically observe aspects of the concept over time in his or her daily life. A client might be asked to self-monitor the emergence of strong emotions at several points during the week and to speculate about the function of the emotion in each instance. In our experience, it is the combination of these methods that seems to help clients develop a deeply personal and sustained understanding of the concepts presented in therapy.

Each session ends with the client making a commitment to practice elements of the therapy over the course of the week. Although we are flexible, depending on the particular needs of the client, we typically ask the client to commit a significant amount of time between sessions to exploring and practicing the approaches and strategies raised in therapy. We believe that mindfulness is a universal human capacity that can be cultivated to reduce suffering and increase awareness and compassion. However, there are a number of cultural and historical forces that interfere with our basic ability to use this skill; therefore, significant practice is needed to develop and maintain this nonjudgmental awareness. Given the absence of empirically derived guidance on this issue, we do not regularly prescribe a specific amount or type of practice. Instead, we encourage clients to flexibly explore different options and to observe their consequences. We also regularly ask our clients to spend time between sessions working to enhance the quality of their lives. As is discussed in more detail in Chapter 7, clients are asked to explore their values deeply, to observe obstacles to living in accordance with their values, and to take regular and consistent action in valued domains.

Although between-session practice is seen as an extremely important part of therapy, it is important to acknowledge that some clients may lead challenging lives in which it is really not feasible to set aside significant time for practice. Sometimes this inability to set aside time is due to a mistaken perception, and clients can be helped to find ways to devote time to practice, which may inevitably help them feel less time pressure in other domains of their lives; however, sometimes external demands like working multiple jobs, raising children, and commitments to other family members do make it impossible to devote focused time to between-session practice. In these cases, it is important to work with clients to find ways to incorporate therapy into daily living. Informal rather than formal mindfulness practice (described in Chapter 6) may allow clients to practice while engaging in necessary activities. For instance, one of our clients who was struggling to find a chunk of time to devote to mindfulness practice at home instead practiced during her subway commute.

THE THERAPEUTIC STANCE

When clients come to us for treatment, they are experiencing significant distress and problems in functioning. In most cases, they meet criteria for one or more psychological disorders, which suggests that they are different in some substantive way from the norm, but it has been theorized that the basic processes that underlie many forms of psychopathology (a critical and judgmental perspective toward certain internal experiences such as sadness or anger, a propensity to think about the future or ruminate about the past, a desire to avoid unpleasant feelings, and a tendency to occasionally let that desire stop us from pursuing personally relevant and meaningful activities) are universal, fundamental aspects of being human (e.g., Hayes, Strosahl, & Wilson, 1999).

This theory has two major implications for therapists. First, it impacts the way we view our clients. Although a client might present with psychopathology, he or she is not pathologically flawed in some way. Every client is assumed to have the capacity to live a vital and meaningful life. The therapist must have faith in each client's ability to tolerate painful internal experiences and to ultimately choose his or her own way. In ACT, this concept is described as developing and holding radical respect toward the client and the choices the client makes about how to live his or her life (Hayes, Strosahl, & Wilson, 1999). Hayes and colleagues describe the barriers to radical respect that can develop, particularly when a client is engaging in socially unacceptable behaviors such as substance dependence. Therapists can exert subtle and obvious pressures in therapy when they bring a priori assumptions about the "right" way for a client to live his or her life. To avoid this trap, therapists should maintain a mindful awareness of the urge to convince and control a client and be willing to act in accordance with the value of supporting the client in his or her own choices.

One exercise we sometimes use with therapists to help them to develop radical respect for their clients is to ask them to think about one or two things they would like to change about themselves. Therapists might want to act more assertive with a coworker, initiate more social activities with a neighbor, set more reasonable deadlines for finishing tasks, or exercise more frequently. Despite being experts on the importance of defusing from and accepting difficult internal states and the impact of engaging in valued actions on life satisfaction, all of us can easily identify changes that would improve our well-being but that, for one reason or another, we are not ready to pursue. It is important to keep that self-awareness in mind, particularly when we are working with a client who at a particular moment may not be willing to make a change.

Second, it suggests that we need to be vigilant about our own tendency to struggle with many of the same basic issues as our clients. Acceptance-based behavioral therapists are encouraged to move consistently toward applying the concepts and methods from this approach to their own experience and behavior in and outside of therapy. For example, if a therapist feels uncomfortable and has thoughts of her own incompetence when her client expresses anger, she might choose clinical strategies on the basis of their ability to please the client rather than on the basis of their efficacy. We recommend that therapists develop their own mindfulness practice and actively use other defusion strategies to promote awareness, acceptance, and value-driven behavior.

Drawing from the seminal work of Carl Rogers (1961), acceptance-based behavioral therapists are encouraged to develop an accurate empathic and nonjudgmental view of the client and to display this empathy, warmth, and acceptance genuinely and consistently in session. The development of this stance is influenced in part by the therapist's understanding of the ubiquitous nature of the basic processes underlying the client's presenting problems and self-knowledge of the ways in which the therapist is struggling with the same issues.

ABBT blends acceptance strategies adapted from Eastern (Zen) sources and other mindfulness, meditative, or spiritual practices with change strategies from traditional cognitive and behavioral traditions. Thus, as Linehan (1993a) has eloquently discussed, therapists are required to maintain a dialectical stance in relation to clients—simultaneously validating the struggle of the client and suggesting areas for growth and change. By maintaining awareness of the need to both validate and promote change, therapists are able to intervene in ways that maximize the possibility of clients openly engaging in therapy and willingly considering new options. Statements that first validate how painful or hard something is and then gently suggest acting in a desired direction or trying out a different way of responding (like willingness or mindfulness) are most likely to be effective. The goal is for the client to feel as though the therapist is standing with him or her, not in opposition.

Cultivating the Therapeutic Stance

Research is clearly needed to guide recommendations for the optimal training of acceptance-based behavioral therapists. Specific guidelines for therapists/teachers vary significantly from approach to approach. The Center for Mindfulness at the University of Massachusetts Medical School provides very specific guidelines for MBSR instructors (*www.umassmed.edu/Content.aspx?id=41322&linkidentifier=id&itemid=41322*). Instructors who wish to be certified in this approach must minimally have professional experience and a graduate degree in the field of health care, education, and/or social change; daily meditation practice and a commitment to the integration of mindfulness into daily life; regular participation in silent, teacher-led meditation retreats of 5–10 days; and experience with mindful body-centered disciplines such as Hatha yoga. Furthermore, they must attend MBSR training programs and teach a number of classes before the certification process is complete.

To our knowledge, there is not a formal set of qualifications for therapists who wish to incorporate MBCT into their clinical practice, but it does require that therapists maintain their own active mindfulness practice (Segal et al., 2002). Similarly, a voluntary self-assessment of core competencies for ACT therapists has been developed that emphasizes the importance of therapists understanding that they are "in the same boat" as their clients and that they need to be willing to hold contradictory or difficult emotions without needing impulsively to resolve them (*www.contextualpsychology.org/complete_the_act_core_competency_self_assessment*).

From our personal experiences as therapists, supervisors, and trainers, we strongly believe that acceptance-based behavioral therapists benefit from reading multiple sources on the theory and research underlying mindfulness, acceptance-based, and behavioral approaches to treatment. Participating in training, supervision, and/or peer consultation may also be extremely beneficial. Finally, we encourage therapists to engage in a range of acceptance and mindfulness practices outside of the therapeutic context. While we do not think extensive meditation practice is a requirement to be an effective therapist, we believe some form of mindfulness practice is necessary.

Benefits to Cultivating the Therapeutic Stance

We encourage some form of mindfulness practice for therapists prior to and within sessions for a number of reasons. First, mindfulness practice allows us to become aware of our own thoughts, feelings, and sensations as we engage in the therapy process. We may be affected by some personal event in our life, such as worrying about our children or thinking about a conflict with our partner. We might be bored or sleepy during a session on a busy day or with an emotionally disengaged client. We might be saddened by a client's poignant description of a loss or frightened by the disclosure of an assault. We might find our client's expression of emotions painful or struggle with thoughts of our incompetence as a therapist.

This compassionate awareness of our experiences fosters our ability to empathize with our clients' struggles and to provide genuine validation and feedback. Regular mindfulness practice can strengthen our capacity for genuine and sustained attention to clients, decreasing the probability that we will "tune out" or become restless or bored in session with an emotionally disengaged client (Fulton, 2005). A mindful, accepting stance allows us to remain engaged in the therapeutic process even when painful emotions emerge in our clients and in ourselves. In our experience, when we are being mindful it is easier to notice our urge to alleviate distress in our clients and in ourselves and to be able to override that urge and behave in accordance with our long-term values as therapists. Finally, this stance allows us to model the essence of the treatment to our clients and to draw from our experience in providing examples that help make the concepts more accessible and personal.

Modeling the Treatment

We often use an adapted version of the "two-mountain metaphor" (Hayes, Batten, et al., 1999) drawn from ACT to illustrate to our clients the universality of their struggles and to acknowledge that we are not immune to these forces.

> "As your therapist, I will sometimes offer some observations about your struggle and make some suggestions about possible options in response to those struggles. It may seem as if I am on the top of a mountain, with the mountain representing the barriers you face as you work toward obtaining a life that is fulfilling and satisfying. It may seem that from my perch on the mountain I can more clearly see the things that contribute to your struggle, as I have already succeeded with the climb, but that is not my view of therapy. I believe that the struggles you are experiencing are common to all human beings and that therapists are not immune to those struggles. In fact, therapists are just like other human beings in that we all have our own mountain with our own struggles and obstacles. As your therapist, I may at times be able to offer some perspective on your struggle because I have some distance and a unique perspective from my perch over here on my own mountain."

We encourage therapists to consistently disclose examples when it is therapeutically appropriate of the thoughts and feelings they experience in difficult situations. For instance, a therapist might disclose her thoughts of inadequacy that are elicited by an invitation to present at a scientific conference or describe his urge to withdraw from a situation of conflict. We have found these disclosures particularly useful when a client is uncomfortable reporting on his or her own internal experiences. For example, a female client who presented with MDD and highly valued her role as a parent was initially unwilling to explore the ways in which her problems might have been interfering with her relationship to her children. Her therapist disclosed that being an available, connected parent was a value for her as well but admitted that when she was feeling significant pressure at work she noticed herself being more critical toward and detached from her children. Following the therapist's honest disclosure about herself, the client was willing to provide examples of times that she was feeling sad and worthless and that she withdrew from her children. While these types of disclosures can be powerful, they should be carefully chosen and guided by the intention of providing a model of the universality of these struggles.

We also recommend therapists use language in session that reflects a mindful, cognitively defused stance. For example, therapists should use precise, nonpathological terms when discussing the client's experience and encourage clients to use the same form of language. The interchange below illustrates this concept.

CLIENT: I had plans to go out to dinner with my friends on Friday night, but I couldn't because of my depression.

THERAPIST: I understand that you have been diagnosed with major depressive disorder and that sometimes you use the word "depression" as shorthand for many different thoughts, emotions, and physical sensations that you are experiencing. In order for us both to really understand your moment-to-moment experience, I am going to ask you to try to be more specific when talking about your experiences. Is it OK with you if we try that? (*Client nods.*) So, what emotions did you notice were present on Friday night?

CLIENT: I felt depressed.

THERAPIST: Would you say that you were feeling sadness?

CLIENT: Yes, I definitely felt sad.

THERAPIST: Any other emotions?

CLIENT: No, just sad.

THERAPIST: How did you feel physically? Did you notice anything going on in your body?

CLIENT: My body felt very heavy, like I was a block of lead.

THERAPIST: How about any thoughts? Did you notice yourself thinking or saying anything to yourself?

CLIENT: Just the usual. I felt useless, like a loser.

THERAPIST: So you had the thought "I am useless. I am a loser."

CLIENT: That's right.

THERAPIST: Often emotions are linked with what we call "action tendencies." In other words, certain emotions urge us to behave in certain ways. Like when we feel anxious, we have the urge to run away or fight whatever is making us scared. Did you notice some sort of behavioral urge that arose when you felt sad?

CLIENT: Sure. I felt like going back to bed. I just wanted to avoid my friends, jump back into bed, and pull the covers over my head.

THERAPIST: OK, one last thing. What did you choose to do?

CLIENT: I stayed in bed. I didn't answer the phone when my friend called.

THERAPIST: OK, so let me see if I understand what your experience was like on Friday night. You noticed feelings of sadness, your body felt heavy, you had the thought that you were useless, and you felt the urge to go back to bed and avoid your friends. In the end, you chose to go back to bed rather than to go to dinner. Does that capture your experience?

CLIENT: Yup.

THERAPIST: If you are willing, I am going to ask you to try and talk about your experience in that very specific way, rather than using the shortcut term "depression." Is that ok with you?

CLIENT: OK, I can try. But it is not how I am used to talking.

THERAPIST: I completely understand that. I am going to ask you to try a lot of new things that might seem strange and different at first.

In response to a client who stated, "I self-medicated my PTSD flashback," the therapist might explore the elements of that statement, encouraging the client to notice that he had experienced an image of a painful past event, along with feelings of sadness and fear, and that he had noticed thoughts such as "I cannot cope with this," felt an urge to drink, and opted to drink a pint of whiskey with the hope that the painful images, thoughts, and feelings would go away.

Sometimes, the modeling takes a more subtle form with less intervention, such as in the following exchange.

CLIENT: Wednesday was a terrible day. I woke up knowing that it was a "fat" day.

THERAPIST: So, as soon as you woke up you noticed the thought "I feel fat today"?

CLIENT: That's right. I couldn't stand the thought of putting on my jeans and going to class. I knew I had to go to the gym and work out for an extra session.

THERAPIST: So, you noticed the urge to go to the gym and skip class. It sounds like it felt very powerful.

CLIENT: I was just disgusted with myself. I had to go to the gym.

THERAPIST: Those emotions can be so intense and powerful. It sounds like you really felt an urge to exercise.

Similarly, we encourage therapists to use the concept of valued action to commit to the work that is required of them. In other words, agreeing to be a therapist involves committing to preparing for sessions, following up with clients on all of the out-of-session work that was agreed on, being willing to experience the clients' and your own discomfort, keeping adequate notes, and preparing for and using supervision or peer consultation effectively.

INTRODUCING THE CLIENT TO TREATMENT

Once a thorough assessment has been completed and the therapist has developed an individualized treatment plan informed by an acceptance-based behavioral conceptualization of the client's presenting issues, a feedback session devoted to presenting this plan, obtaining the client's informed consent and setting the stage for therapy can be useful. This session can be challenging in that many topics are covered briefly, by necessity. Therefore, the therapist should expect that the issues discussed during this session may need to be revisited repeatedly throughout treatment. Included in this session are a very brief conceptualization of the client's presenting problem, an overview of the plan for treatment, a discussion of alternative treatments that the client could consider, the development of shared goals for treatment and a plan to assess progress toward those goals, and the development of expectations about the roles of the therapist and the client in therapy.

Conceptualization of Presenting Problem

Although both the conceptualization and the treatment plan have been developed through a collaborative process with the client over several sessions (as discussed in Chapter 3), reiterating this information in a systematic way during the feedback session may facilitate the client's observation of the costs associated with experiential avoidance and the limited utility of attempts at internal control. As discussed in Chapter 2, we typically assess the nature and extent of the client's presenting problems and associated features, pertinent historical influences, attitudes toward internal experiences (e.g., emotions, physical sensations), mindfulness, common coping strategies, past treatment, and, most important, current quality of life. During the feedback session, our conceptualization integrates this information, validates the client's experience, provides a rationale for the treatment model, and sets the stage for change.

Overview of the Plan for Treatment

ABBT approaches underscore the importance of experiential rather than verbal learning. For example, although one can hear or read about mindfulness, the experience of observing and noticing events as they unfold is necessary in order to really understand the concept. Similarly, in ACT, therapists are warned that clients' efforts to prematurely "make sense" of the concepts of acceptance and defusion can sometimes reflect experiential avoidance. Although ABBT is a treatment best experienced rather than explained, therapists need to provide enough information about the rationale and methods to be used in treatment to allow clients to make an informed choice when agreeing to a treatment plan. We have found it useful during the feedback session to touch on the three main components of treatment and to describe how each method directly addressed the client's presenting problems.

Altering One's Relationship with Internal Experiences

As discussed in Chapter 1, an acceptance-based behavioral conceptualization of psychopathology assumes that our responses to internal experiences significantly affect our functioning. Our tendency to become fused with our thoughts, feelings, and sensations; to respond fearfully to a range of internal experiences; to judge painful experiences as negative and stigmatizing; to feel as if these experiences are holding us back; and to attempt repeatedly to avoid and escape these experiences can cause significant psychological distress and negatively affect our functioning. Therefore, a major goal of treatment is to change the relationship clients have with their internal experience. We tell clients that we will examine the function of their emotions and teach them some methods to observe their internal experiences with curiosity and compassion and to notice the transience of each thought, feeling, and sensation. We also describe how increasing awareness and altering the quality of this awareness will enhance their ability to make choices regarding their actions and the way they want to live their lives. We explain that one goal of treatment is to help clients pursue valued activities without having to get rid of or in any way control their internal experiences.

Decreasing Experiential Avoidance and Increasing Choice and Flexibility

As discussed earlier, throughout the assessment and case formulation phases, significant effort is made to highlight the ways in which attempts at experiential avoidance have been ineffective and interfered with the client's life. In ACT, this process is described as "drawing out the system," and it involves determining what the client wants, the methods he or she has used to try and get it, and an accurate assessment of the "workability" of each approach. During the introductory session, we explicitly convey our impression, based on general clinical knowledge and our specific understanding of the client's past struggles, that experiential avoidance has not been effective and that our treatment recommendation involves the development of a more accepting stance toward internal experiences.

At this early stage in treatment, many clients are receptive to the idea of acceptance, even though they may struggle with applying the concept as treatment progresses, but it is also not uncommon for clients to be less enthusiastic about this treatment goal and to maintain that experiential control is both a possible and a desirable goal for treatment. Clients might express a variety of responses ranging from skepticism to outright rejection. From a clinical standpoint, we expect and welcome this reaction as it fits with our conceptualization of psychological struggle. If a client is experiencing a mixed reaction to our model of treatment, our goal is to determine his or her willingness to explore more carefully the "workability" and costs of experiential avoidance and control efforts and to consider trying some different ways of responding. If a client feels strongly that he or she would rather pursue a course of treatment aimed at internal control, we might recommend an alternative treatment (discussed in more detail below). Clients may need to experience more fully the futility of experiential control before they can commit to trying a different approach.

Increasing Engagement in Valued Activities

In addition to targeting experiential avoidance, ABBTs aim to decrease behavioral avoidance. During the introductory session, we reflect the ways in which the client's life has become limited and restricted through experiential avoidance and recommend that treatment involve a commitment to pursuing activities consistent with the client's values. While all psychological treatments are implicitly aimed at increasing quality of life, traditional cognitive-behavioral approaches can sometimes overemphasize symptom reduction or elimination as the primary goal of treatment. In contrast, an acceptance-based approach explicitly focuses on increasing behavior in valued domains.

While most clients hope that treatment will change their life in some way, not every client expects its focus to be behavior change. Clients may come to treatment to gain insight, or to receive support for a condition they think is chronic and incurable. Changing internal experiences such as reducing anxiety, feeling self-confident, increasing self-esteem or feeling happy might be a client's focus for treatment. Therefore, it is important to convey explicitly that this model of treatment emphasizes behavior change in the service of increasing the client's quality of life.

Discussion of Alternative Treatments

Hayes, Strosahl, and Wilson (1999) underscore the importance of describing alternative forms of therapy to ensure that the client gives a fully informed consent to treatment with ABBT. We absolutely agree, particularly when there is compelling empirical support for an alternative approach, such as behavioral activation for MDD or panic control treatment for panic disorder. There is, of course, much debate and controversy in the field about developing lists of empirically supported treatments and recommending them as first-line treatments for several disorders. As scientist-practitioners, we feel strongly that an evidence-based approach to treatment is critical. However, acceptability is also an important criterion on which to judge the effectiveness of different treatment approaches. We often encounter clients with PTSD or panic disorder who undoubtedly would benefit from exposure therapy but are unwilling to engage in this form of treatment. In those cases, these highly effective treatments can be (and have been) effectively integrated with an acceptance-based approach, as noted below and discussed more fully in Chapter 10.

In our own practice, we often describe the differences between traditional cognitively oriented therapies and ABBT to our clients. Specifically, from a traditional cognitive perspective, psychopathology is assumed to arise from the presence of irrational thoughts. Thus, a traditional cognitive therapist might work to uncover the cognitive distortions underlying a client's social anxiety, systematically challenge the veracity of the thoughts, and encourage the client to develop a more rational approach to social situations. We also acknowledge the similarities between the two approaches. Both underscore the importance of increasing awareness of internal experiences, describing experiences using multiple channels of responding (e.g., thoughts, sensations, emotions), and increasing proactive behavior. (The theoretical and clinical differences and similarities between acceptance-based behavioral approaches and other CBTs are discussed in more detail in Orsillo, Roemer, & Holowka, 2005; Orsillo et al., 2004; and Chapter 10, this volume.) We have found acknowledgment of these similarities and differences to be particularly important when working with clients who have previously received CT with mixed results. For instance, if we were to treat a client who had already completed a trial of CT for MDD, we might have this discussion.

"It sounds as if you had mixed results from your last therapy experience. You mentioned that you feel like you learned a lot about the relationship between your mood and your behavior through self-monitoring. You used to think that depression was something that hung over you for weeks, but you learned that your mood fluctuates depending on different situations. It also sounds like you got some benefit from pleasant event scheduling, although when you were feeling very sad and lethargic, you did not follow through on the assignments.

"From what you told me, sometimes cognitive restructuring was very helpful to you. Taking some time to stop and notice what you were thinking and feeling seemed helpful. Viewing thoughts as just thoughts made them seem less scary. At times you were able to come up with a different interpretation of an event or talk yourself out of thinking a certain way, but other times those methods were not effective.

"Does that sound right?

"Well, my recommendation for treatment will involve continuing many of those strategies, while changing some and adding others. Specifically, I definitely would like us to continue to think about the ways in which you spend your time and to schedule some activities each week. I also want to spend a bit more time exploring what you really want to be doing with your time and particularly how you would like to spend the time you have in your relationships, at work and at play. I would like to work together to increase the time you spend doing what really matters to you.

"I also think it makes good sense to continue observing your thoughts, feelings, sensations, and behaviors. If you are willing, I would like to show you a slightly different way of noticing those experiences that involves developing compassion toward them. If you are willing, we will practice some mindfulness skills to see how we might change the relationship you have with your internal experiences.

"One thing that might be different between your last therapy and this therapy is the idea of trying to change your irrational thoughts. I agree with your experience that sometimes that method seems to work, although other times it doesn't. There is actually some evidence to show that the more you try and change thoughts, the more distressing they become and the more they stick around. So, if you are willing, we might put that strategy on hold for some time and try something a bit different."

It is also important to note that, as discussed in Chapter 10, many of the most common applications of ABBT already involve the integration of acceptance with other well-established approaches to therapy. For example, MBCT integrates acceptance with CT, a more established approach to addressing depression, and there have been acceptance-enhanced applications of panic control treatment (Levitt & Karekla, 2005). Often, acceptance-based approaches can be used to increase a client's willingness to engage in the required elements of these other evidence-based approaches to treatment.

It can also be useful to contrast ABBT with less structured supportive or humanistic approaches to psychotherapy. Our approach to therapy integrates a client-centered stance with more directive behavioral strategies. Thus, it is important that clients understand that, while this approach to therapy aims to validate their experiences and to facilitate their growth in desired domains, it is also structured and organized, with explicit expectations that the client engage in active practice of a number of skills outside of therapy.

Finally, we have found it useful to contrast ABBT with mindfulness-based practice outside of the therapeutic context (e.g., yoga or meditation classes, Zen Buddhism). Sometimes clients have had experience with Eastern meditative practices and expect that therapy will follow a similar path. Depending on the client's experience with specific forms of mindfulness, this may or may not be the case. Similarly, the work our clients do in therapy is often mirrored and bolstered by their practice of mindfulness in other contexts; we have had clients use yoga or meditation very effectively in conjunction with and following our treatment. On the other hand, sometimes these practices do not coincide well with the work of therapy. For instance, we treated one client with GAD who had developed a ritualized approach to meditation. He felt as if he had to complete a sequence of meditations in order to prepare for the day and felt highly anxious if something interfered with this routine. Through therapy, the client came to realize that meditation itself had become another strategy aimed at controlling his anxiety. Another client with a history of meditation practice regularly engaged in meditation as a way to avoid conflict-laden interactions with his wife. In therapy, mindfulness was introduced as a strategy that could facilitate his ability to approach his wife and communicate with her compassionately.

Occasionally, we encounter clients who are wary about the spiritual connotations of mindfulness and concerned that the inclusion of mindfulness practice in treatment suggests a spiritual focus to therapy that they do not desire. We carefully choose our language when describing ABBT and clarify that the mindfulness practices we incorporate into therapy are removed from the context of the Eastern spiritual traditions that inform them. We think it is important to distinguish the use of mindfulness in the context of psychotherapy from personally or spiritually based mindfulness practice. A huge array of mindfulness-based practices is available and may be pursued for a wide range of purposes. Clients who present for psychotherapy are pursuing a specific type of assistance. We are not meditation teachers or spiritual counselors. We draw strategies from these traditions but use them for psychologically related and articulated purposes, specifically to help clients more actively engage in their lives in ways that are meaningful to them.

Defining the Roles of Therapist and Client

A number of client-related variables, including cultural factors, past therapy experience, and interpersonal style, can dramatically influence the expectations clients have about the nature of their role in psychotherapy. Clients may expect therapists to be relatively silent observers, active advisors, or supportive friends. Therefore, we have found that it can be very useful explicitly to share our own assumptions about the role of the therapist and the client in our approach to therapy, as well as to assess clients' expectations.

Traditional cognitive-behavioral approaches underscore the importance of collaborative identification of problem areas, goals, and markers of progress in the client–therapist relationship. Similarly, the establishment of a collaborative relationship between client and therapist is essential in ABBT. While the overarching general theory of ABBT suggests that avoidance is negatively impacting the client's life and offers several clinical methods for addressing this avoidance, it is the client's personal concerns and values that ultimately dictate the course of therapy. We assume that the client is the expert on him- or herself, but we also acknowledge that fusion, avoidance, and rule-governed behavior may at times obscure the client's ability to accurately observe his or her own experience and to be aware of the contingencies guiding his or her behavior. Therefore, although we expect that clients initially may be confused about some of the concepts we discuss or disagree that certain strategies might be useful to them, we ask them to be open to the possibility that making radical changes in the way they view their internal experiences and choose their responses may be helpful. In other words, we ultimately defer to the clients' view of the utility of certain approaches or strategies in enhancing quality of life, but we ask that they consider taking some time to observe their behavior closely and to try some new methods of responding before they reach a conclusion. To describe this relationship to a client who is struggling with an anxiety disorder, we might say:

> "Here are my views on each of our roles in therapy and how we can best work together. As a therapist, I have some knowledge of general principles of anxiety and worry, the ways in which they can limit people's lives, and methods to help people struggling with anxiety to lead more satisfying and fulfilling lives. But my knowledge is general, and you are the expert on your personal experience and how these general principles do or don't apply to you. So, I will do my best to present all of this information to you, to share thoughts and ideas I have, and to offer my support, understanding, and guidance, but I believe that you are the only expert on you. Only you can say what is really important to you and how you would like to live the rest of your life. You are the only one who can honestly observe your own experience to see if the things we talk about together that might be causing your struggles really are and to judge if the changes we come up with enhance your life. If we are to work together, I would like to ask you to consider some of the suggestions I make to you based on my general knowledge to see if they fit your experience. I am also going to ask you to try out some new ways of responding that initially may not seem logical or useful to you. Your experience with these new approaches will help us determine whether they are helpful to you or not. I would like you to commit to considering some new approaches, and I will commit to listening to and honoring your experiences with these approaches."

To summarize the issues we raise in this chapter, we provide below a comprehensive example demonstrating the type of information we might try and convey to a client with social anxiety disorder during an initial session. Although we have provided this information as a monologue to represent all of the points we would try to touch on, in clinical practice it would be a discussion peppered with the client's questions and reactions.

> "Based on everything you have shared with me so far about your struggles with anxiety and the previous ways you have tried to improve your life, I have some thoughts about what might be getting in your way and how we might be able to work together to make some changes. It sounds as if the physical sensations (e.g., palpitations, arousal), thoughts ("I am a loser"), and behavioral urges (to escape or avoid) you experience when you are in or imagining a socially threatening situation are increasingly distressing to you. On some of the questionnaires you completed, you noted that overall you are somewhat fearful of your emotions and that you prefer to avoid situations that are likely to evoke strong emotions. You also described the ways in which your family is uncomfortable with your expressions of anxiety and how from an early age you were encouraged to appear strong and competent in all social interactions.
>
> "You have been trying to get rid of your anxiety for as long as you can remember, and you believe that you cannot really live a meaningful and rewarding life unless you are able to learn a strategy to get your anxiety under control. In the

past, you have tried relaxation strategies, distraction tactics, medication, and self-talk directed at changing your thoughts and feelings. While you had some success with these approaches, you haven't experienced the significant improvement that you were hoping to achieve. Sometimes your control efforts seem to work in the moment, but the anxious thoughts and feelings always return. Also, you described some situations during which you felt it was critically important to control your anxiety, but you were unable to do so. You also tried having a few glasses of wine before each social interaction to put yourself at ease, and, while you find that somewhat helpful, you have developed some concerns about relying on alcohol to get through social situations. You don't really have any close, satisfying friendships, and you would like to feel less anxious so that you could start dating and develop some intimate connections. You also worry that you might be holding yourself back at work because you refuse promotions that will involve presentations or any significant social contact.

"You have given a great deal of thought to your problems, and it seems to you that the best way out of this struggle is to learn how to control your internal experiences more successfully. On the other hand, it sounds like your experiences have told you that this approach may not be the answer. So, while you are feeling somewhat hopeful about therapy, deep down you are also concerned that you might not be able to make the significant life changes that you are hoping for.

"Does that sound right to you? Have I left anything out that you think is important for us to consider?

"Everything you have shared with me makes perfect sense and fits with the knowledge I have about anxiety and how it interferes in people's lives. I understand why you think that gaining complete control of those anxious thoughts and feelings is the most important thing you could do for yourself. That belief is communicated to us in many ways in our society, but there is actually a growing body of research to support what your experience has already told you. Specifically, some research has found that the more we try and suppress thoughts or feelings, the stronger and more distressing they become. Also, the kinds of active problem-solving efforts you make to try to suppress your thoughts and feelings (like drinking wine and keeping others at arm's length) seem to be taking you even further from living the sort of life you really want for yourself.

"If we work together, I would ask that you consider a different approach from the one you have been trying for so long. My suggestion would be that we start by really exploring the specific ways you would like your life to be different, particularly the ways in which your struggles related to anxiety have prevented you from living life the way you wish it could be. It sounds like you have a general idea of what you want but that in some ways you haven't really thought about how you would like your life to be better, as most of your goals seem unattainable to you.

"Once we really know some of the specific ways in which you would like your life to be different after therapy, I will ask you to consider some new ways of responding to your thoughts, feelings, and sensations. Up until now, your habit has been to notice them and quickly turn away in the hope that they will disappear. You have labeled them as dangerous and a sign of weakness, and you have done all you can to make them disappear. I am going to suggest a different way of responding that involves compassionately observing yourself and that may open up more options for you. While I don't think it is possible for anyone to escape feeling anxiety or any other of the full range of human emotions, we could work toward decreasing the hold that anxiety has on your life. Specifically, this approach to therapy would focus on improving the quality of your life through encouraging you to pursue activities that really matter to you while teaching you mindfulness and some other skills to help you develop a more accepting stance toward your emotions and thoughts. Learning to relate to thoughts and emotions in a different way typically decreases the intensity and frequency of distress.

"I know you have been in therapy in the past and you have tried a lot of things to improve your life. I want to be clear that this approach to therapy involves a significant commitment on your part. As you noted, you have developed habitual ways to respond to anxiety and anxiety-eliciting situations. In order to break those habits and develop new ones, you will need to devote a significant amount of time outside of session practicing the new methods you learn in therapy. If we work together, I will ask you to make a commitment to clearing some time in your life to focus on yourself and the changes you would like to make in your life.

"I also want to let you know that I may ask you to do some things in therapy that will bring up strong emotions and painful thoughts. Of course, you always have the choice whether or not to try the things I suggest, but I want you to know that taking risks will be required to make the meaningful changes you are hoping for. You should also know we will be working together to develop skills that might make taking risks less frightening than it has been in the past.

"This approach to therapy is somewhat new, and, while there are some very promising findings from research, we are still in the early stages of testing this approach. As we have discussed, cognitive-behavioral therapy is another approach to treating social anxiety that has shown some significant progress. I know that you have already tried CBT with mixed results and you are looking for an alternative. If we decide to work together, I will monitor your progress closely, and we will check in periodically to see if any change in your treatment plan is indicated. You should also let me know at any time if you are concerned with your progress in therapy.

"All I have done today is given you a very broad overview of the work I think we could do together. I would like to hear your reactions, and I am happy to answer any questions you might have. I also want to tell you that it is perfectly normal to have some doubts and concerns about any approach to treatment. You don't need to be certain that this approach will work for you. It is really hard to know until you get started with the work, so I welcome you to bring any worries or concerns you have with you. If we decide to go forward, all I ask is that you consider keeping an open mind as you try some new approaches for a limited amount of time. Then we can check in and see if you want to continue them."

FIVE

Offering the Client an Acceptance-Based Behavioral Model of Human Functioning

Psychoeducational elements are standard in cognitive-behavioral approaches to psychotherapy. There is some range across the ABBTs in their formal inclusion of and emphasis on psychoeducation, but they all emphasize developing a shared conceptualization and understanding of an acceptance-based model. DBT includes four psychoeducational skills–based modules in which key elements of treatment are introduced, described, explained, illustrated, and discussed in group settings. MBSR and MBCT are both presented in an educational format, although they also emphasize the primacy of practice and personal experience. The developers of ACT (Hayes, Strosahl, & Wilson, 1999) caution against overexplanation of the tenets of therapy, emphasizing the need for clients to experience concepts rather than rationally understand them so that they are guided by their contingency-based learning, rather than rule-governed principles that can become rigid and inflexible.

Within this context, we see presentation and understanding of the model as necessary but not sufficient elements of ABBTs. Transparency is an important element of these (and other cognitive and behavioral) approaches, with therapists clearly conveying the underlying model of therapy and the rationale for interventions so that clients can continue the work on their own between sessions and following termination of therapy. Although experiential understanding and enactment of new behavioral patterns (in order to alter habitual, overlearned responses) are considered central change mechanisms, intellectual understanding is thought to set the stage for these behavioral changes, providing clients with a rationale and motivation for making difficult changes in their lives and encountering temporary increases in distress as a result. This understanding is also thought to help clients self-administer treatment following termination when new contexts and challenges arise in their lives. Thus, we spend considerable time early in treatment presenting, illustrating, and helping clients observe basic elements of a shared conceptualization of their difficulties and methods to promote change. In this chapter, we review those elements that relate to a shared understanding of clients' presenting problems, types of learning, the function of emotions, and the problems with efforts at experiential control. In the three subsequent chapters, we discuss mindfulness/acceptance and valued action in more detail.

METHODS OF PRESENTING INFORMATION

Our method for providing psychoeducation is drawn from many empirically supported behavioral and cognitive approaches to treatment, as well as from the psychoeducational elements of other acceptance-based behavioral therapies. As described in Chapter 4, we emphasize psychoeducational elements primarily in the early sessions of treatment. After an initial mindfulness practice and review of between-session tasks from the preceding week, we share an agenda for the session with the client, highlighting the new concepts that will be presented and the old concepts that will be revisited. We typically introduce a new concept with an experiential exercise so that the client immediately engages with the topic at an experiential level rather than a solely intellectual one. For instance, prior to discussing the cycle of anxiety with an anxious client, we would have the client imagine a recent anxiety-provoking situation and notice her responses. We would then use these observations in our discussion of the factors that elicit and prolong anxious responses. Her reactivity to her own anxiety, along with failed efforts of experiential control, would illustrate important aspects of the cycle of anxiety.

We also typically provide handouts for newly presented topics. Clients review the handout while we discuss the concept, giving them an organizational scheme for the information. We give our clients three-ring binders to keep all of their handouts, so they have references to remind them of elements of treatment. The binders also provide clients with a record of the key elements of therapy that they can return to following termination if they find themselves experiencing heightened distress or experiential avoidance. (As we describe in Chapter 10, we also develop summaries with clients to help guide them through future lapses that are also placed in their binder.) We include examples of the handouts we commonly use throughout this book (other very useful examples are presented in Eifert & Forsyth, 2005; Hayes & Smith, 2005; Hayes, Strosahl, & Wilson, 1999; Linehan, 1993b; Segal et al., 2002). We adapt handouts to meet the needs of specific clients depending on their presenting problems, education level, language abilities, and other relevant factors.

Clients are encouraged to respond to the material with any questions, and the relationship between the general material and their own experience is explored through discussion and demonstration. Although concerns and refutations should be responded to at this point, clients are generally encouraged to consider exploring new concepts between sessions regardless of their initial skepticism. They are reminded of our initial discussion regarding the likelihood that some of these ideas may not seem accurate because of the rigid habits they have developed over time and are asked to consider and closely observe each concept that is raised in therapy before coming to any conclusions about the accuracy or applicability of a particular idea. The stance that we ask clients to take toward therapy is similar to a more general stance we hope them to cultivate. Rather than accepting what they know to be true based on past experience, what "should" be true, or what we suggest may be useful in therapy, we ask clients to bring "beginner's mind," or a fresh, fully aware curiosity, to life experiences in the hope that they may see something new in their old patterns of responding. At the same time, their concerns are validated, and the possibility that a specific concept may not apply fully to their experience is certainly considered. Therapists need to remember to be open to altering models and incorporating specifics of clients' experience or background that may slightly or significantly alter a conceptual model. Models are always considered hypotheses that are tested through clients' experiences and observations; these understandings are, therefore, revisited throughout therapy and altered based on clients' experiences as they try out new ways of responding in different contexts.

A critical aspect of presenting and sharing these general models is the development of relevant between-session exercises that help clients observe or apply specific concepts in their daily lives. We design and expand self-monitoring exercises in which clients either stop at several prescribed points during the day (e.g., morning, noon, dinnertime, and before bed) or before or after significant emotional events (e.g., panic attacks, social anxiety–provoking incidents, depressive reactions, urges to drink) and note contextual cues, emotional responses, reactions to these reactions, and/or actions taken (depending on the point in therapy). We include examples of monitoring forms we might use at different times in treatment with different clients throughout this chapter after we discuss the relevant concepts. These forms should be adapted to meet the needs of specific clients. The basic principle of monitoring is to promote self-observation that will illustrate concepts developed in therapy and to build on this observation by adding new elements to observe throughout treatment (while still trying to keep monitoring relatively straightforward and simple). Many therapy books contain other examples of useful monitoring forms (e.g., Hayes, Strosahl, & Wilson, 1999; Linehan, 1993b; Segal et al., 2002).

In addition to self-monitoring between sessions, clients might be asked to practice specific exercises (for instance, mindfulness exercises, described in more detail in the following chapter) or engage in particular actions. During the later part of therapy, actions that are consistent with the client's values are chosen and he or she is asked to attempt these actions between sessions and notice what occurs and what gets in the way (see Chapter 8 for more detail). Practice creates examples of alternative responses that provide information that can alter clients' understanding of potential responses and their consequences as well as function as skills-building efforts that weaken old habits of responding and strengthen new habitual responses.

SHARING THE MODEL OF HUMAN FUNCTIONING AND CHALLENGES

Chapters 6 and 7 describe the psychoeducational elements directly addressing mindfulness- and acceptance-based strategies as well as valued action/behavioral strategies that we commonly use. Here, we provide some examples of how a general model of human functioning and challenges can be presented within an acceptance-based behavioral perspective (drawing from the model described in Chapter 1 but emphasizing how to share these concepts with a client). These explanations combine traditional cognitive-behavioral formulations with acceptance-based elements.

General Model of Learned Responses

We find a basic behavioral model of learned responding (both by association and by consequences) extremely helpful with clients who present with a broad range of psychological difficulties. For instance, we might say something like the following in presenting the model (although we would typically break it up more and use a lot of personal examples from what the client has told us so far):

"Human beings naturally learn from past experiences. We learn to associate things that have occurred together in the past—for instance, we might come to associate threat or comfort with a particular sound, smell, or situation. We also come to expect certain consequences for our actions (such as rejection for expressing feelings or showing weakness). It's good that we're able to learn this way and that we can learn quickly and without giving it a lot of thought. This is how we can rapidly avoid threats and how we are able to function in our usual environments.

"On the other hand, we can also overlearn certain responses and associations. Sometimes we learn a response or association so well and so strongly that we have it all the time, even when it isn't useful anymore. This is particularly likely as we're growing up, when it's most important that we learn how to adapt to our environment well. Our responses might become so rigid and automatic that we have them all the time, even when they aren't helpful in a particular situation. [Here, we would usually provide a direct example from the client or a hypothetical example that relates to his or her presenting concerns, such as anxiety, sadness, or fear of rejection.]

"Sometimes responses we have can be useful immediately but get in the way of our lives over the long term. For example, we might learn to walk away from conflicts, which feels better in the short term but leaves these issues unresolved. These habits can be particularly hard to unlearn because they have desirable consequences at first, and we tend to learn from what happens first.

"Another hard thing about the way we learn is that it usually happens outside of our awareness, so it's more of an instinct than something we reason through. This makes it hard to change overlearned habits just by thinking about how we'd rather act. Have you noticed this? We've found that the most helpful way to learn new habits is to try them out rather than just understand them better. On the other hand, we can learn problematic responses just from what people have told us. For instance, when growing up we may get messages that it's important to be emotionally strong and independent. If we have learned the message well, we may not easily notice that our efforts to be independent are actually making us lonely. One of the things we're going to do in treatment, then, is try to start noticing more what's working and what isn't. This awareness will also help with finding times to change these habits and try something new. Changing habits is really hard though, so it will take patience and time!"

We find that sharing this type of model can be quite therapeutic for clients in and of itself. It immediately begins to address some of the judgments and negative reactions they have to their own responses by cultivating an attitude of compassion and understanding toward those difficulties. It also quickly establishes that *we* view their difficulties with compassion and understanding (see Gilbert, 2005, for a book-length review of the role of compassion in psychological well-being and therapy). This type of learning model is also useful because it suggests that new responses can also be learned, as described more fully below.

We draw from clients' particular histories and presenting concerns to provide specific examples of how problematic responses can be learned. For instance, Janine described habitually agreeing with others rather than stating her own needs in order to avoid being criticized or rejected. She reported that her mother often withdrew from her and criticized her when they had disagreements. The therapist observed that she very accurately learned at an early age to expect criticism and withdrawal after disagreeing with others and that her habit of acquiescence was a natural outgrowth of that learning. The therapist also took developmental considerations into account, highlighting how important it was for Janine to learn to minimize rejection from her mother as a child because attachment is a primary need of children. While validating Janine's early experience, the therapist asked her to consider that now, as an adult, she had other resources and could perhaps expand her behavioral repertoire and assert her own opinions and needs in relationships. In addition, they explored together the range of current contexts in which Janine's concerns might no longer be warranted. While encouraging Janine's willingness to develop new patterns of interaction, the therapist also acknowledged that, at times, people will be critical and rejecting following disagreements and that this does feel distressing. The goal was to help Janine to reach her own decisions, balancing the risks involved with potentially being hurt while trying to develop more intimate relationships with the safety of avoiding pain by distancing herself from others.

As discussed in Chapter 3, we always present specific examples as hypotheses and note that we do not really know how various habits have been established. The original cause of a particular behavior does not need to be established in order to alter it effectively; maintaining factors need to be identified to make these kinds of changes. The historical perspective is helpful primarily because it provides clients with an understanding of their own responses that reduces blame and stigma and promotes care and understanding (although in some cases it may interfere with treatment, as mentioned in Chapter 3). This type of validation is thought to provide an optimal context for behavior change.

Although our model differs in some ways from traditional cognitive models (in that we do not suggest that thoughts or beliefs are causes of emotional responses and that these thoughts must be changed in order to change emotional responses), we do note that thoughts and appraisals of situations are internal learned responses and may influence other modes of responding (emotional, behavioral). We draw from ACT and its basis in relational frame theory to describe how, through bidirectional learning, our words and thoughts come to take on the same psychological properties as the phenomena they represent, leading us to have the same reactions to them that we would have to external stimuli (such as fear and avoidance). We describe the model of experiential avoidance presented in Chapter 1, using clients' experiences, responses, and behaviors to illustrate it. Exercises from ACT like "trying not to think about a chocolate cake" help demonstrate how challenging it can be to try to avoid or eliminate a thought or image and how these efforts may paradoxically increase the prevalence of the target thought.

We ask clients to spend a few minutes thinking of anything except eating a piece of chocolate cake. Inevitably, clients report that thoughts of just that arose, often quite persistently.

Within the context of a typical learning model of psychological difficulties, we particularly emphasize the role that learned reactions to our internal experiences and associated efforts to avoid these internal experiences play in developing and maintaining difficulties. As discussed in Chapter 1, different clients have different methods of avoidance. Some engage in problematic behaviors (e.g., arguments, compulsive rituals) to avoid internal experiences that they react to and judge. Others refrain from desired behaviors (such as pursuing a relationship, meeting new people, or going out in public) to avoid unwanted internal experiences. Others engage in obsessions, worry, or rumination because these cognitive activities serve an experientially avoidant function. While the specifics of these presentations are important, the overarching role of experiential reactivity and avoidance is a particular focus of treatment and often helps explain associations among apparently disparate comorbid presentations.

As part of psychoeducation, we often share research findings with clients in a simplified, accessible way. For instance, we describe how studies have shown that when individuals try not to think of something (like a white bear), they actually report thinking about it more subsequently (Wegner, 1994). With our anxious clients, we like to illustrate the human ability to learn fearful associations without being aware of the initial pairing of a stimulus with a threat. For instance, LeDoux (1996) describes a female patient with anterograde amnesia whose doctor poked her with a pin while shaking her hand. The next time they met, the patient did not remember her doctor but would not shake his hand, demonstrating her learned fear. These examples can help clients see their difficulties as understandable and worthy of compassion.

We pay particular attention to methods that will help increase clients' understanding of their own responses. Seeing these responses more clearly is one aspect of changing the client's relationship to them. Thus, we have clients monitor multiple components of their responding (cognitive, emotional, somatic, behavioral) so that they begin to see each part of what they have been calling "distress," "anxiety," "binge eating," and so on. We also have them imaginally recall a significant episode of their presenting problem, describing the thoughts, feelings, and sensations they notice so that they can begin to see how each element leads into and feeds other elements of their response. This process helps us build a collaborative understanding of how difficulties have been unfolding and begin to target opportunities for new habits to be developed and new responses to be tried.

Addressing Specifics of Clients' Presenting Problems

Along with presenting and developing a general model of human functioning and difficulties, it is important for therapists to specifically address the clients' presenting problems. Behavioral, cognitive, and acceptance-based models of specific disorders can be found in multiple sources (e.g., Barlow, 2008; Hayes & Strosahl, 2004; Orsillo & Roemer, 2005) and presented to clients. We provide Handout 5.1 (p. 106) to clients with GAD, showing them an acceptance-based behavioral model for understanding anxiety, worry, and avoidance that draws heavily on Borkovec and colleagues' (2004) model of GAD and incorporates acceptance-based elements.

With a client with GAD, we typically present some version of Mowrer's (1960) two-factor model of fear. We explain how fearful associations are learned through pairings and how these associations can generalize to other, related cues and even be the source of new learning experiences (for instance, when a learned fearful response to driving occurs so strongly that fear becomes associated with all of the cues in a new driving context, such as the place one is going). The tendency to avoid feared cues is described and illustrated from the client's own experience. We explain that this avoidance precludes learning new, nonfearful associations with the feared cues, thus maintaining the fearful response. We also highlight the way that individuals often come to feel distressed by their own responses, leading to a similar process of learned distress, avoidance, and maintenance of distress with internal cues. Again, we highlight the functionality of this system—it is evolutionarily adaptive that we learn fear and anxiety and that we stay away from the things we fear—and the ways it can become rigid, habitual, and no longer adaptive. We also describe the ways that anxiety influences our attention to and processing of information (with bias toward detecting threat and interpreting ambiguous information as threatening), highlighting research findings in this area. This discussion sets the stage for clients to begin to observe their anxious responses, both in and outside of the session, with a little bit of distance and perspective. It provides a premise for seeing responses and appraisals as just reactions and appraisals, not necessarily accurate reflections of reality. After presenting this information, we might use a monitoring form like Anxiety Awareness (Form 5.1, p. 111). The filled-out version (Figure 5.1) gives an example of a client with anxiety in social situations, who has been asked to notice both the context and the nature of her anxiety (what sensations and thoughts seem to characterize the experience she labels "anxiety"). This exercise is meant to help her turn toward her feared internal experiences as they arise rather than trying to avoid them. Monitoring helps the client observe the cycle of anxiety and begin to decenter from her fused experience of anxiety by observing and dismantling its components.

With a client who presents with MDD, we would give information about the bidirectional relationship between activity and mood, meaning that feelings of sadness can lead one to withdraw and be inactive, which can maintain and exacerbate feelings of sadness and apathy. Although inactivity feels consistent with the very real sadness and anhedonia that individuals are experiencing, it often worsens the problem. We would also describe the bidirectional relationship between mood and cognitive abilities, describing how depressed mood can slow thinking, lead to a heightened ability to recall sad events and a diminished ability to recall pleasant events, and result in a bias toward negative interpretation. We would also discuss how disruptions in routine have been found to have significant mood effects, highlighting again the effect of behavior on mood. Using information from the client's self-observations and reports, we would collaboratively develop a model of how mood, cognition, and behavior may be interacting to affect the client's experience, setting the stage for the client's enhanced observation of these patterns as they unfold.

We provide similar specific details for clients with other presenting problems (e.g., the impact of extreme dieting on metabolism and hunger, the addictive properties of substances) in order to help them more fully understand the various factors that may account for some of their difficulties. Thus, we blend a more general model of human functioning with symptom-specific information to develop a comprehensive working model of clients' difficulties.

ANXIETY AWARENESS

We would like you to begin to notice the nature and context of the anxiety you experience in social situations. Therefore, we would like you to try to observe more closely when you experience this anxiety and what that experience of anxiety is like. When you notice you are experiencing sensations of anxiety before or during a social situation, please take a moment to write down what you observe and the situation you are in. For instance, you might notice a tightening in your chest and your palms sweating, and the situation that triggers this might be having lunch with your partner's family, or you might notice thoughts about someone thinking badly of you when you are speaking up in class.

Date/Time	Experience of Anxiety	Situation
3/14 1 p.m.	Heart racing, can't think straight	Class presentation
3/14 7 p.m.	Tight chest, palms sweating, blushing	Dalia brought three guys over and introduced me to them
3/15 2 p.m.	Everyone can see what an idiot I am!	Called on in class, didn't know answer
3/15 3 p.m.	Can't stop thinking about class, not concentrating, heart racing	Bumped into someone in the hall
3/15 6 p.m.	Heart racing, tight chest	Ordering food in a restaurant

FIGURE 5.1. Example of a completed Anxiety Awareness form.

Model of Psychotherapy

It is helpful to clearly review a model of treatment with clients, both in session and in handout form, so that the rationale for between-session tasks and within-session activities is transparent. We provide Handout 5.2 (p. 108) within the context of our current GAD treatment study. It draws from the conceptual of model of worry presented in Chapter 1, noting that worry serves an experientially avoidant function, and provides clients with a clear, concise rationale for what will follow in therapy as well as something to look back at in order to keep the main tenets of treatment in mind. We adapt this model in our clinical work with clients with various presenting problems, either explicitly providing a model or more informally presenting the central aims of therapy and their underlying rationale. As discussed previously, this typically includes (1) helping clients change their relationship to their internal experiences, (2) reducing experiential avoidance and increasing choice and flexibility, and (3) increasing intended, mindful, valued action. An acceptance-based behavioral model of treatment builds on the model of presenting problems that has been collaboratively developed with the client, highlighting the habitual nature of problematic responses and the ways that new responses can be learned through increased awareness and repeated practice. We emphasize the challenges inherent in changing overlearned patterns of responding in order to help clients patiently practice while they continue to habitually engage in old patterns of responding. We also predict that enhanced awareness of patterns of responding and reductions in experientially avoidant behaviors will likely lead to a temporary increase in distress as clients become more aware of their own responses, as discussed in the previous chapter.

Function and Regulation of Emotion

We have found it very helpful to review the nature and function of emotions with clients, who often present for treatment with a desire to reduce their negative emotions and increase their positive emotions as well as with an undifferentiated sense of their own emotional experience (i.e., an experience of "distress" or "upset" without a clear sense of specific cues and emotions and their correlates). Drawing from DBT (Linehan, 1993b), Greenberg's (2002) emotion-focused therapy, and Mennin's (2006) emotion regulation therapy, we spend time exploring the nature of clients' emotional experiences (as described above) and the function that even unpleasant emotions serve.

We have found it helpful to review this information early in treatment, after developing a model of the client's presenting problem and our proposed treatment approach and after a brief introduction and demonstration of mindfulness (as described in the next chapter). We suggest to clients that, although people often want to control their emotional experiences, these efforts are not always successful because emotions serve a useful function. We begin by asking them what purpose they think their emotions serve, then ask specifically about "unpleasant" emotions and times they have experienced them when they might have been useful. We then give clients a handout on the function of emotions (Handout 5.3, p. 109) and review it with them in detail, providing examples.

In reviewing the top part of the handout, it is helpful to provide examples of each function, using either the client's experiences or the therapist's. Therapists can illustrate how our emotional reactions can tell us when there is a potential threat present (anxiety or fear), when our needs are not being met (anger), or when we are losing something we value (sadness). Emphasis should be placed on the communication function of emotional expressions. Clients can be asked for examples of times that the emotional expression on a loved one's face helped them understand the significance of a concern and really attend to what the person was telling them. Although people are often given the message that it is important to control emotional expressions, clients can usually readily think of times that their or someone else's clear communication of emotions helped generate change. Additionally, we discuss how advertisements and commercials aim to elicit specific emotions to increase the probability that consumers will remember the product being promoted.

Clients can also be asked for examples of times when their emotional response helped them perform an important action, illustrating the ways that emotions can organize us for effective action in certain contexts. For example, excitement and fear about an upcoming competition can motivate an athlete to maintain a challenging and time-consuming practice schedule. When we discuss this function of emotion, we acknowledge how emotions are associated with specific action tendencies. For instance, when we are afraid, we are prepared to fight, flee from a dangerous situation, or freeze in the hope that a threat will pass. Anger prepares us to fight or defend ourselves from a potential threat. We underscore that, although emotions can prepare us physiologically for action and increase the probability that we will choose a particular behavior, our actions are not caused by emotional responses. As discussed later, a major component of treatment involves distinguishing emotional and behavioral responding.

Finally, we ask clients to imagine having no emotional responses (sometimes we use examples from science fiction, such as Data from *Star Trek: The Next Generation*, who was often puzzled by the human experience of emotion but yearned to have it) in order to see how emotions deepen their lives. With some clients, it can be useful to acknowledge the often uncomfortable paradox of being human and feeling the full range of emotions. For instance, it is impossible to feel the joy and love associated with close relationships without also experiencing the pain of separation. One cannot feel the exhilaration of taking a risk or responding to a personal challenge without also experiencing some fear of what is new or potentially threatening. It is important to demonstrate how emotional states that we often label as "positive" and "negative" are intimately connected.

Similar to other approaches in describing emotion to clients, we use the metaphor of a hot stove to illustrate the informational aspect of our emotional responses as well as the complexity of effectively responding to them. We highlight the main points of the metaphor in Handout 5.3 but present it in full to the client in a manner similar to the following example.

> "Frequently, we wish to avoid negative emotions, which seems like a natural and adaptive human response. If there is any way we can turn off emotional pain (such as drinking or using drugs, distracting ourselves, or avoiding a task that we really need to attend to), we try it. This makes perfect sense, and unfortunately we can run into problems when we ignore our basic biological programming. Think of emotional pain as being similar to physical pain. Most people would agree that physical pain is unpleasant and should be avoided at all costs. Now imagine that

you put your hand on a hot stove. You would obviously be strongly motivated to try and avoid the associated pain, so what could you do?

"You could take a really, really strong pain reliever and keep your hand on the stove. You could distract yourself from focusing on the pain (like women do during childbirth or some cultures do when they attempt to walk on hot coals). You could tell yourself that the pain is not really there (what we sometimes refer to as denial).

"What would happen if you successfully engaged in these avoidance/distraction techniques? Your hand would be severely burned. What you obviously need to do is remove your hand from the stove.

"But removing your hand is not enough to ensure that you never get burnt again. If you remove it without paying sufficient attention to the process, you could risk repeating the same mistake. In order to respond adaptively, you need to:

1. Be aware that you are experiencing the pain.
2. Be aware of what kind of pain you are experiencing.
3. Be aware that the stove is what is causing the pain.
4. Be ready to take action.

"If you don't take each of these steps, you may stop the pain for the moment but run into other difficulties later. For instance, if you burn your hand on a pan on the stove, you may blame the pan for your pain and avoid pans when the stove is really what caused the pain. You might try to remove pain from your life by throwing out the stove or never cooking again, but then your attempts to avoid pain would have become more important to you than your need to feed and care for yourself.

"Let's see how this metaphor fits with an emotional example. Imagine you are experiencing sadness and disappointment because your current job is not fulfilling. Those feelings are uncomfortable, so you naturally want to get rid of them. You might start staying out late at night spending time with friends and hanging out at bars so you don't notice that you're feeling sad. You might start finding reasons to miss work or daydreaming when you're at work. All these things reduce the pain of the sadness, but none of them resolves the problem, and they may create new problems as you start sleeping less and doing worse at work. Instead of getting rid of the pain, you need first to notice that you are experiencing pain, recognize that pain is sadness and disappointment, and realize that it comes from your work situation. Then you can take the final step and engage in action to resolve the situation, such as looking for a new job or new challenges in your current job.

Emotional pain can be more complicated than physical pain because sometimes we want to override the response associated with an emotional signal. For instance, we might experience anxiety in response to a potential threat, such as meeting a new person. Even if we correctly identify the source of our emotional pain as exposure to the new person, we may not want to avoid him or her. If we value connectedness, it may be more in line with our values to approach this person, even though it may increase our emotional pain in the moment. In this case, after we do the first three steps (become aware of the pain, identify the type of pain, identify the source of pain), we might choose an action in accordance with our values rather than one that eliminates the pain."

Of course, awareness and identification of emotional responses is a complex, challenging process. We have adapted the concept of "clean" and "dirty" emotions from ACT, combined with Greenberg and Safran's (1987) construct of primary and secondary emotions, to explore with clients the ways that sometimes emotions are *clear*, while other times (perhaps much more often) they are *muddy*. Clear emotions are directly related in both content and intensity to the situation at hand. For instance, when a car is heading toward us as we cross the street, we experience fear in direct relation to that event, and that fear motivates us to hurry across the street and avoid being hit. Many factors, however, can lead us to experience emotional reactions that are either more intense than the present context warrants or are unrelated to the present context. These factors are listed on the bottom of Handout 5.3, and we review them with clients, providing personal illustrations of the ways that all human beings can have muddied emotional responses. Physiological dysregulation, such as lack of sleep or poor nutrition, can make us emotionally vulnerable, leading us to have more intense emotional responses than a given context warrants. I (Roemer) share with clients that, at the beginning of a day when I haven't slept well, I remind myself that I shouldn't take action on any emotional reactions I have during the day but wait to see if the situation remains emotionally evocative after I have had more rest. A mental focus on the past or the future can also affect our emotional responses in the moment. Excessive worry about the future may worsen the impact of present events, leading to anxious responses due to presumed associations with imagined catastrophic future events. Similarly, current events may remind us of past emotional situations, leading to a more intense response in the moment due to feelings related to a previous context. For instance, if we fight with our partner in the morning and our anger remains unresolved, we may have a strong response to a mildly critical remark by a coworker that reminds us of something our partner said. Also, often we respond to people and contexts in the present that remind us of painful experiences in our past. As already discussed, our reactions to our own emotional responses, including our efforts to control or eliminate them, may amplify and exacerbate them, leading to muddy emotions that do not provide clear information. Relatedly, feeling defined by or entangled with our emotions makes them muddier, more intense, and more pervasive. Each of these factors results in an emotional signal that is not tied to its true source, so there is no clear indication of how to respond appropriately. Mindfulness- and acceptance-based responses help one clarify emotional responses and choose appropriate actions. In addition, these modes of responding facilitate chosen, intended action in response to emotional signals, allowing clients sometimes to choose actions that run counter to emotional action tendencies but are consistent with what matters to them.

This latter distinction between reacting to emotional stimuli and acting in response to emotions has been identified as an important aspect of emotion regulation and adaptive functioning by many clinical scholars (e.g., Barlow, Allen, & Choate, 2004; Germer, Siegel, & Fulton, 2005; Greenberg & Safran, 1987; Linehan, 1993a, 1993b). One client referred to our approach to treatment as "pause therapy" in that we help clients pause between their emotional reaction and their behavioral action so that their actions can be informed but not dictated by their emotional responses. Extensive observation, application, and practice help clients develop this response set, but increasing their understanding of their emotions and the reasons that emotions should be attended to but not followed blindly is an important first step.

Finally, in our discussion of the function and regulation of emotion, we address the complex ways that emotions relate to valued actions. Emotional responses can provide us important information about what matters to us. We may be trying to live a life that is influenced by what is important to someone else (e.g., a parent or partner) rather than following our own valued path. Our continued emotional experience of discontent is an important cue that this is happening, and our examination of this response may help us determine the path we truly want to follow. On the other hand, sometimes our muddied emotions interfere with the path we want to follow, such as when we respond to our overlearned fear of rejection by avoiding intimacy rather than pursuing a valued intimate relationship. Repeated, mindful attention to contexts, consequences, and our own responses will help us identify each of these situations and adjust our actions accordingly.

After presenting this information, we typically expand clients' self-monitoring so that they begin noticing their emotional responses. For instance, a client whom we're treating for GAD might fill out the Mindful Worry form in Figure 5.2, in which he is asked to begin to observe his emotional responses when he notices he is worrying. This gives him an opportunity to see the way his worry arises in different emotional contexts and may, in fact, be functioning to distract him from his emotional experience. A blank version of the Mindful Worry form is provided in Form 5.2 (p. 112).

The Problem of Control Efforts

Acceptance-based behavioral approaches emphasize and illustrate the problems inherent in rigid efforts at experiential control. In our own work, we like to address this issue after we have reviewed the function of emotions because the utility of emotional response is one reason that excessive control efforts can be problematic. Drawing from ACT, we present clients with a handout that outlines the problem of trying to live a meaningful life while simultaneously trying to limit negative internal experiences. Handout 5.4 (p. 110) highlights the choices that individuals have in trying to negotiate this dilemma.

We find it useful to present this issue after clients have begun to explore what matters to them (their values) and the ways that their presenting problems and experiential avoidance have gotten in the way of their actions in these domains (described in more detail in Chapter 7). This context helps prepare clients to examine the way that their desire to avoid experiencing negative internal experience is at odds with their desire to live a fulfilling life (although they may still hope that there is a way to do both). We find it useful to thoroughly review the first two response options on the handout with our clients. First, a client might choose to restrict her life in order to avoid distress, but it is unlikely that limiting her life will actually protect her from unpleasant internal experiences, and this course of action will lead to other negative internal experiences associated with constriction. For instance, she might not pursue an intimate relationship in order to avoid the distress associated with potential rejection, but other instances of apparent rejection may still occur, and she may experience other distressing reactions such as loneliness or envy because her life is restricted.

MINDFUL WORRY

Please continue to notice the nature and triggers of your worry as you have been doing. When you notice you are worrying, please take a moment to write down what you are worrying about and the situation you are in. For instance, the topic of the worry may be finances, and the situation that triggers this worry may be having lunch with your partner's family, or the topic of the worry may be your safety and well-being, and the situation may be driving. Also note any particular emotions you experienced when you were worried. For instance, you might notice that you feel anxious, sad, or angry while you are worrying.

Date/Time	Topic	Situation	Emotion
6/22 11 p.m.	Dealing with issues at work tomorrow	Trying to sleep	Sad about S leaving
6/23 8 a.m.	How I'll be able to concentrate at work	Getting ready for work	Nervous, frustrated
6/23 8:30 a.m.	Being late to work	On the subway	Tense, anxious, still sad about S
6/23 4 p.m.	People's reactions to what I'm saying	Meeting	Embarrassed
6/23 11 p.m.	Not being able to fall asleep	Trying to sleep	Agitated, anxious

FIGURE 5.2. Example of a completed Mindful Worry form.

A second option is the choice that individuals often make, although typically not with full awareness, to continue engaging in their lives but attempt to control their negative thoughts and feelings. For example, a client may be trying to develop friendships and build a career while simultaneously trying to avoid feelings of anxiety or self-doubting thoughts. He may have a long history of failed coping strategies aimed at managing his emotions and thoughts and present to treatment hopeful that therapy will motivate him to step up his efforts and finally overcome his difficulties. A number of experiential exercises can help illustrate the problem with this approach. For instance, we use the following adaptation of the polygraph metaphor from ACT with our anxious clients:

> "Sometimes people feel like they could control their anxiety or worry if they were only more highly motivated to do so. Let me give you an example in which you would have the ultimate motivation to control your anxiety, but it might still be impossible. Imagine that I hook you up to a machine that could tell with 100% accuracy whether or not you were experiencing feelings of anxiety, and I tell you that your job in this situation is to stay relaxed. If you get the least bit anxious, the machine will sense it. Your motivation to control your anxiety would be extremely high because if the machine senses any anxiety, it will explode (likely causing you serious injury). What would happen in this situation?"

We also use examples from ACT that illustrate the difficulties of controlling positive emotional experiences. For example, could you feel love for someone if you were paid 10 million dollars? Clients are quick to note that they could *act* like they were in love, but they would not be able genuinely to experience love, even when they were highly motivated to do so. Many clients can relate to the example of a man or woman who might break up with a "great guy" who was handsome and kind and on the surface a perfect match for him or her simply because he or she could not make him- or herself love him. We highlight the ways that this difficulty controlling our internal experience is very different from the effect of control efforts on our actions. For instance, if someone told us to clap our hands or there would be some negative consequence, we would be able to do so, even if we felt like it was silly and really did not want to do it.

Some clients can readily provide examples of times that their experiential control efforts have failed, but many will recount incidents when they were able to reduce or even eliminate their emotional reactions. As with all new information, we encourage clients to consider what we are suggesting and then actively to test different hypotheses, attempting to control an emotional response and mindfully observing the consequences versus allowing an emotion and similarly seeing what unfolds. It is important to avoid general debates about these concepts with clients. Early in treatment, clients may not have an accurate sense of the efficacy of the strategies they use. For instance, a client who avoids opening up to others in order to prevent himself from getting hurt may think that strategy is working because he strongly believes it should, despite evidence that he experiences pain even while using this strategy. Furthermore, it is critical for therapists to be open to hearing clients' specific experiences with different strategies and not assume that general principles are true for everyone. Self-monitoring and extensive observation and discussion of specific situations and experiences that the client encounters provide the best opportunity for discovering what works for a particular client.

During the psychoeducational component of therapy, we find it useful to acknowledge that, while control efforts do result in a lessening of our distress, particularly in the short term, often these effects do not last long. Moreover, control efforts are least likely to work when we most want them to. For instance, we may be able to use breathing to lessen the anxiety we feel when fielding a hostile question from an undergraduate in a class, but trying to reduce anxiety in a similar way before a particularly important and well-attended public presentation is effective less often and, in fact, will likely increase our anxiety. Also, habitual efforts to avoid distress can lead to restricted awareness of our emotional responses and limited attention to the present moment, both of which can interfere with our ability to respond adaptively to different contexts.

A common point of confusion regarding control efforts should be addressed here. Sometimes statements regarding difficulty controlling internal experiences seem to suggest that any efforts to alter internal experience will have paradoxical effects and that we are unable to regulate our internal experiences at all; however, we have all had successful experiences modulating the intensity of our emotional responses. Sometimes breathing deeply, shifting our attention, or seeking emotional support leads to reductions in our distress. Similarly, practices of mindfulness and acceptance are likely to reduce the muddiness of our emotional experience, limiting the amplification associated with rigid control efforts, and will, therefore, likely reduce distress at times (although being fully present with our experience may sometimes result in heightened distress and emotional pain). No strategy can completely eliminate negative internal experiences, which are a natural part of being human. Furthermore, the extent to which we desire to eliminate these experiences seems to be directly related to the paradoxical effects of these efforts. Therefore, even when we engage in strategies that may reduce arousal or distress, it seems to be important that we hold these strategies lightly rather than requiring that they effectively comfort us before we engage with our lives. Thus, the problem is focusing exclusively or predominantly on efforts to eliminate negative internal experiences, not attempting to lessen them occasionally. When the latter attempts are engaged in flexibly, with an openness to whatever emotional consequences occur, they are adaptive rather than problematic.

Drawing from ACT, we also share with clients that control efforts are ubiquitous because it seems as though other people are able to control their internal experiences. People rarely share their distressing reactions, and we are often given messages that suggest we can control our internal experiences ("Cheer up!", "Don't cry"), so we grow up believing it is possible to exert this kind of control and that there is something wrong with us if we are not able to do it as well as everyone else.

Control efforts are also successful in many other areas of our lives. If we need to clean our house, we just do so, regardless of how we feel about it. We can make ourselves go virtually anywhere and do virtually anything (if our skill level permits it), so it makes sense that we would try to will ourselves to think and feel certain things and not think and feel other things. Our experience tells us, however, that these efforts are not successful and bring with them problems of their own, particularly when we engage in them rigidly without awareness and intention. In fact, some experimental evidence suggests that trying to suppress our thoughts actually leads us to view those thoughts as more anxiety-provoking (Roemer & Borkovec, 1994), suggesting that these control efforts increase the negative subjective quality of the target content, further perpetuating the cycle.

After fully exploring the problems inherent in this option with our clients, we introduce a third option, which we will spend the rest of therapy investigating. In this option, clients choose to engage in their lives in meaningful ways while being willing to experience whatever internal reactions arise. This willingness is cultivated through mindfulness- and acceptance-based strategies described in the next chapter, and it is in service of the valued domains detailed in the chapter after that.

We then have clients begin to monitor their efforts to control throughout the week. A client with alcohol problems who had been monitoring her urges and the emotions she experienced during them would now be asked also to monitor her engagement in control efforts in these contexts (see Figure 5.3; a blank version is provided in Form 5.3, p. 113). This monitoring would help her begin to see the frequency with which she tries to control her internal experience and the effects of these efforts. As therapy progresses, we typically diminish the emphasis on specific presenting problems and ask clients to monitor the unfolding of their responses to emotionally significant contexts in general (directions may be altered to help clients identify these contexts based on their specific presenting problems). In the filled-in Mindful Monitoring form (Figure 5.4), a client documents his initial responses to a particular situation, how he responded to them (for instance, with avoidance or judgment or, conversely, with mindfulness or acceptance), and the actions he then chose to take (for instance, avoiding the situation or taking an action that was valued regardless of his emotional reaction). This process helps the client begin to see how certain reactions and actions may initially feel helpful but actually prolong distress, while others can facilitate functioning even if they do not feel natural or desirable in the moment. A blank version of the Mindful Monitoring form is provided in Form 5.4 (p. 114).

CHALLENGES IN PRESENTING MODELS

Compliance in Between-Session Tasks

One of the most common challenges in the methods described above comes from whether or not clients engage in between-session tasks. Clients often have an especially difficult time engaging in self-monitoring, which is a particularly effective way of illustrating numerous psychoeducational concepts. We predict these challenges and attempt to address many of the potential obstacles to complying with these tasks in therapy. Clients may not see the point of them, so therapists need to take time to make the rationale clear and to address any questions clients have about how these tasks relate to the goals of therapy. This means that therapists themselves need to be clear about this connection and sure that they are assigning useful tasks. Immediate review of self-monitoring in subsequent sessions and using the material from self-monitoring within the course of sessions help illustrate its relevance to clients. Particular attention to the observations that emerge from these tasks also helps reinforce completion of the task. Relatedly, therapists should be quick to alter assignments that are not seeming particularly helpful and should take client feedback regarding the burden versus the utility of self-monitoring seriously. They may, however, simply ask the client to stick with it for another week or two due to the belief it will become useful over time. Often, self-monitoring assignments become so rote for therapists that they fail to really engage with a client's individual experience of them and adapt them accordingly.

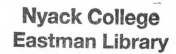

URGE AWARENESS

Please continue to notice the nature and triggers of your urges to drink as you have been doing. When you notice an urge, please take a moment to write down the nature of the urge and the situation you are in. For instance, you might notice a thought about an alcoholic beverage, accompanied by salivation, and the situation might be a phone conversation with your mother. Also note any particular emotions you experienced immediately prior to or during this urge. In addition, write down any efforts you made at controlling your emotional experience (e.g., trying to distract yourself from feeling anxious or sad).

Date/Time	Urge	Situation	Emotion	Efforts to Control?
11/1 5 p.m.	Imagining a cold beer	Got home from work	Frustrated from the day, tired, sad	Just wanted to feel better. Told myself to get over it and be strong
11/1 11 p.m.	Can't stop thinking about a drink, taste it in my mouth	Fighting with M	Angry, scared	Trying not to show anger or fear, want so much to stop feeling this way, hate feeling like this
11/2 8 p.m.	Imagine holding a drink, sipping it, the feeling that goes with it	Serious conversation with M	Scared, sad	Noticed wanting the feeling to go away. Tried to let the feeling be there instead. It actually helped a little!
11/3 1 p.m.	Saw liquor store, felt strong urge to walk in and buy bottle	Coming back from lunch	Angry at self for urge	Tried to push away urge, anger. Felt worse. Then tried to practice acceptance. It helped briefly but still felt angry about the urge. Will I ever be free of them?
11/2 3 p.m.	Strong urge to leave work and drink, can taste liquor	Just got out of meeting that went badly	Feel embarrassed, anxious about job	Wanted feelings to go away. Wanted to give up. Still trying to get earlier urge out of my head. Tried to notice the feelings and allow them. That seemed better.

FIGURE 5.3. Example of a completed Urge Awareness form.

MINDFUL MONITORING

Use the space below to jot down anything you notice regarding your thoughts, feelings, or reactions throughout the week. This can include situations that cue distress, the emotional signals you notice, the thoughts or worries you have, and the ways you respond to your thoughts, worries, or distress.

Date/Time	Situation	First reactions (thoughts, feelings, sensations)	Second reactions (efforts to control, muddy emotions, willingness, acceptance)	Actions/Responses
7/14 3 p.m.	Picking up S at school	I know I'm going to be late, feel tense, the teacher thinks I'm not responsible	Feel bad that my anxiety still comes up so easily and strongly, wish it were different	Rush to get there, keep my head down once I do so I don't look at the teacher, feel worse
7/14 9 p.m.	Trying to unwind with D	Keep thinking about things I need to do, worrying about money, feel uneasy	Remember to practice mindfulness, allow these thoughts and feelings, breathe	Focus on what D is saying, tell him that I'm feeling tense but also glad to be spending time with him
7/16 12 p.m.	Reading my HS newsletter	Pit in stomach, feel like other people are more successful, sad, ashamed	Tell myself I'm being stupid, shouldn't care what other people think	Throw out the newsletter, feel worse
7/16 6 p.m.	Dinner with D	Irritable, snapping at D, feel like a loser and bad about myself	Tried to notice the feelings and thoughts, kept trying to push them away but came back to just noticing them	Remembered my value of spending time with D, focused on that, felt my mood lighten a little
7/18 12 p.m.	In my room	Just had an argument with S. Feel like a jerk. Angry, frustrated	Noticed how fast my mind was going, how tight my body felt. Breathed, paused.	Went back in to talk to S more calmly, expressing my feelings and also understanding. Felt good!

FIGURE 5.4. Example of a completed Mindful Monitoring form (later in treatment).

Related difficulties include clients filling out all the forms but in a cursory way or putting words in each column but not really following the directions. In these cases, it can be useful to have the client give fewer examples but do so thoughtfully, going through each of the columns so that the process of self-monitoring is done in a meaningful way. We often tell clients that we would prefer a few examples provided thoughtfully, with awareness and intentionality, than a long list of nonreflective entries.

We also make a point of predicting to clients that self-monitoring can increase their distress initially. Often, clients have been ignoring the extent of their own distress or the degree to which they have disengaged from parts of their lives so that monitoring this distress or disengagement more closely can feel discouraging. We suggest to clients that we often need to experience the discomfort of seeing the extent of a problem before we can make meaningful changes and that this distress is an important aspect of change. Here, again, research can be helpful. Recent process studies have shown that change in psychotherapy is nonlinear, with spikes in symptoms (associated with exposure) predicting subsequent therapeutic gains (Hayes, Laurenceau, Feldman, Strauss, & Cardaciotto, 2007). We have found the "path up the mountain" metaphor from ACT a helpful illustration of this phenomenon:

> "Suppose you are taking a hike in the mountains. You know how mountain trails are constructed, especially if the slopes are steep. They wind back and forth; often they have 'switchbacks,' which make you literally walk back and forth, and sometimes a trail will even drop back to below a level you had reached earlier. If I asked you at a number of points on such a trail to evaluate how well you are accomplishing your goal of reaching the mountaintop, I would hear a different story every time. If you were in switchback mode, you would probably tell me that things weren't going well, that you were never going to reach the top. If you were in a stretch of open territory where you could see the mountaintop and the path leading up to it, you would probably tell me things were going very well. Now, imagine that we are across the valley with binoculars, looking at people hiking on this trail. If we were asked how they were doing, we would have a positive progress report every time. We would be able to see that the overall direction of the trail, not what it looks like at a given moment, is the key to progress. We would see that following this crazy, winding trail is exactly what leads to the top."[1]

This perspective can keep clients from responding negatively to their own increase in distress and either prematurely terminating therapy or refraining from self-monitoring. It can also provide a behavioral example of choosing *not* to engage in experiential avoidance and instead continuing with a task despite the distress associated with it because of a broader goal of increasing understanding in service of change. Therapists and clients may need to return to this issue repeatedly as clients express their concerns about self-monitoring assignments.

Often, clients describe pragmatic obstacles to self-monitoring, such as overscheduled lives with multiple demands. Also, some clients may have strong negative reactions to writing, fear evaluation of their writing, or respond poorly to the concept of

---

[1] From Hayes, Strosahl, and Wilson (1999, p. 222). Copyright 1999 by The Guilford Press. Reprinted by permission.

"homework." We do not use the word "homework" for this reason. Instead, we refer to "between-session exercises" or "practices." We clearly conceptualize these exercises as in service of the client, not the therapist. (This explanation is more complicated in the context of a therapy trial, where we need to acknowledge that some assessments are for research purposes in addition to clinical purposes, although all assessments also serve a clinical function.) We also adapt assignments so that they fit into clients' lives more effectively. For instance, some clients prefer to keep a journal of their observations rather than using forms. Others use small notebooks they can carry with them. We encourage clients who have concerns about writing or evaluation to use their own shorthand or notes and simply share their observations with us each session. If the task of writing down self-monitoring is so aversive that it is interfering with clients' ability to observe themselves, we experiment with self-monitoring without any record keeping, sometimes using imaginal recall when reviewing observations in sessions. Our main goal is to work with clients so that they become more aware of all their responses in the moment; all choices about between-session assignments are made in service of this goal. Record keeping seems to be a particularly effective way to move toward this goal with many clients, but if it is becoming a hindrance rather than a help, we drop it or have clients take a break from it. If we see that clients are integrating the concepts into their lives, we are less concerned about compliance in self-monitoring, but if we feel that clients are still struggling with aspects of the treatment, we encourage them to take up some form of self-monitoring again, focused specifically on apparently troublesome areas. As therapy progresses, we explicitly encourage clients to bring some of their newly developed skills, such as mindfulness and willingness, to completion of these tasks.

Interestingly, with some of our clients with GAD, we found that overcompliance was an issue. Some clients would record every observation so diligently that it seemed they were spending more time recording their lives than engaging in them. For these clients, we began to reduce self-monitoring assignments and invite clients intentionally not to complete some assignments so that they can experience flexibility in this behavior and observe their reactions to not fully completing a form. A similar approach may be needed with some clients with obsessive–compulsive disorder.

Issues of compliance with between-session exercises also provide an excellent opportunity for work within the therapeutic relationship. Often, clients report concerns about what the therapist might think if they do not complete an assignment, providing an opportunity for in-session exploration of interpersonal patterns that emerge for them around expectations and potential conflict. Paying attention to these patterns and sharing observations of clients' responses and hypotheses about patterns while listening to clients' responses and adjusting accordingly can help clients have a corrective emotional experience in this type of interpersonal context. Clients often exhibit significant behavioral changes when they do not comply with an assignment and are able to tell the therapist without avoiding a session, becoming preemptively angry or following some other characteristic pattern. Conversely, clients may expand their behavioral repertoires by noticing the way that they have retreated from expectancies and not complied with assignments when they *do* want to pursue the therapy for themselves and, therefore, begin to do exercises for themselves rather than for the therapist. This process is strengthened to the degree that therapists are able to remain mindful of their intention to help clients take a path of their own choosing rather than a path determined by their therapists.

Therapists should keep in mind that studies have yet to determine exactly how much compliance is necessary for therapeutic effects to occur. Although daily self-monitoring seems preferable, it may be that some clients can increase awareness without this frequency. Furthermore, if some clients simply will not or cannot self-monitor that frequently, it makes more sense to adjust to what they are able to do and proceed from there. Again, attention to the function of the assignment is important—efforts should be made to enhance clients' awareness of their responses through whatever means are possible. We saw a client with GAD who very rarely completed self-monitoring or formal practice assignments, yet she came to sessions with reports of observations from the week, expanded on concepts presented in-session with her own metaphors, and seemed to be truly engaging with the concepts of therapy. I (Roemer) made a decision to scale back her assignments and de-emphasize self-monitoring forms in order to focus more on the aspects of treatment in which she was engaging. This client responded to therapy according to symptom-based assessments at both posttreatment and 3-month follow-up and recently contacted us (3 years after completion of her therapy) to report on how helpful she found the therapy. She particularly wanted us to know that the therapy had helped her even though she had not done the between-session assignments.

It is important to develop an understanding of the cultural and situational constraints that may impact compliance (this issue is discussed in more depth in Chapter 11). Clients who are living with economic disadvantages may have real constraints on their time that make it difficult to focus on tasks between sessions. Working with clients to develop an individualized, feasible plan for completing tasks can help keep them engaged in treatment. Modifications also need to be made for clients for whom English is a second language. We saw one client who was able to do more homework if she spoke into a tape recorder rather than writing her assignments down.

Avoiding Overintellectualization and Detached Teaching Styles

Another challenge in presenting these concepts is maintaining a focus on experiential rather than intellectual understanding, an issue that is particularly highlighted in the context of ACT. Although therapists present concepts in words and talk about them rationally, ultimately clients are asked to rely on their own experience to see what works for them. As stated earlier, although an educational element can help set the stage for experiential learning, therapy is not a process of convincing clients of certain ideas or principles. Nonetheless, it can be easy to slip into an intellectual debate about any of these ideas. When we present a concept, we discuss clients' reactions to it briefly and ask clients to use the next couple of weeks to see whether it fits or not and what its limitations are with regard to their specific experience. Usually, clients will begin to see how something like experiential avoidance plays a role in their lives, with at least some contexts in which their experiential control efforts add to their suffering becoming evident. If this does not occur, we explore other possible models with them while continuing to attend to whether some subtle avoidance is taking place.

A related concern in psychoeducation is that sessions can become too educationally focused, interfering with the development of a therapeutic relationship and experiential presence. While therapists are presenting handouts and concepts, they need to be sure that they remain experientially present and connected to clients. Using examples from both therapists' and clients' lives helps maintain this personal connection. Experiential exercises also help bring clients fully into the room, and clients sharing reactions to these exercises helps therapists empathically connect to them. Taking time at the beginning of a session to review self-monitoring forms and weekly events also helps establish and strengthen the therapeutic relationship. Shared mindfulness practice at the very beginning of a session also enhances this shared presence and connection. While all of these strategies help with this challenge, therapists must continue to attend to this concern, checking in with clients and actively cultivating a meaningful therapeutic connection in the midst of presenting these concepts. Sometimes this will require postponing or truncating presentation of material; these choices should be made based on careful observation and reflection regarding what will most benefit clients and help them move forward. Shared mindfulness practice, as described in the next chapter, also facilitates deepening experience and the therapeutic relationship.

MODEL OF FEAR AND ANXIETY

This handout contains a lot of information about how we think about anxiety and worry. Please read it over and note any reactions or questions you have. We will go over it in detail in the next session and we will continue to talk about it throughout your treatment.

Anxiety and Fear Are Natural Responses That Help Us Deal with Threat

Anxiety and fear are natural, helpful reactions that help us stay safe. We feel fear when we are in a situation that we think is dangerous. We get anxious when we think about or imagine something threatening might happen in the future. Anxiety and fear are made up of thoughts, feelings, physical sensations, and behaviors. When we are anxious or afraid, we see threat easily and think about the worst possible thing that could happen, feel tension and arousal in our bodies, and try to escape or avoid the things we fear. All of these responses are helpful in telling us that a threat is present, and helping us to stay safe. They get us ready to fight or escape from a dangerous situation or to freeze (or not respond at all) in the hope that the danger will pass. Because these reactions have been so important to our survival as humans, they happen quickly, without much thought or effort on our part, anytime we see a possible threat. We can feel scared and tense without even knowing what is causing the reaction. We can also automatically avoid situations that seem dangerous without even realizing it. All of these reactions can really help us stay safe, especially when we are faced with physical danger.

Sometimes We Ignore Survival Reactions and Choose to Face a Threat

While fighting or running away may be the best reactions to physical danger, they do not always work as well with other types of threats. For example, it is natural and adaptive to want to be liked by others. Even animals are sensitive to possible rejection. They try and get along with others in their pack because it increases their chances of survival. But sometimes trying to avoid being rejected by others actually causes *more* problems. For example, if you are anxious about giving a presentation at work because people might not think you did a good job, you might decide to call in sick and avoid it. But calling in sick will not make the work situation safer in the same way that running away from a tiger would. Also, you may feel that doing a presentation is really important to you and you might want to do it even if you are afraid. Or, you might be afraid to say "I love you" to someone for the first time because you are not sure he or she feels the same way. But you may decide that you want to take that risk because you really value having a close relationship. One of the tricky things about being human is that taking steps toward the things we care about (relationships, jobs, personal goals) usually requires that we take some risks. It is natural that taking a risk will make us feel vulnerable, insecure, or anxious. So, despite the fact that our survival system tells us to avoid doing things that we are afraid of, sometimes we have to if we want to live a more rewarding life.

(continued)

Our Ability to Think Complicates the Survival System

Our survival system can also be thrown off by our memories and imagination. We can feel just as scared remembering something scary that happened *before* or imagining something threatening that *could* happen as we would if we were in actual, physical danger. We get the same threat signal in response to events in our mind as we do to physical threats in our environment. We can remember all kinds of past events and imagine all sorts of future dangers. So, we are often preparing for and reacting to dangerous situations that have already passed or that may never happen. This means we get more danger signals than we should and that they are often very confusing.

Worries are one type of thought that can definitely increase our anxiety and make our lives more difficult. If we are worried that something bad might happen, we might avoid doing things that could be fun and rewarding. For example, we might avoid starting a new relationship because we are afraid of being rejected. Or we might feel like we have to spend a lot of time doing things that we hope will prevent something bad from happening. For example, someone might keep calling her or his children to make sure they are safe when they are with the afternoon babysitter even if it is not necessary and may cause extra stress and frustration.

Our ability to think and imagine can leave us in an almost constant state of fear and anxiety.

Anxiety and Fear Can Take Us Away from What Is Really Happening in Our Lives and Get in the Way of Our Enjoyment

One of the most troubling things about being constantly afraid and anxious is that it can really take a toll on our quality of life. Thoughts about frightening things that happened in the past and worries about things that could happen in the future distract us from what is happening in the present. For example, if during a job interview you are worried about what could happen if the interviewer doesn't like you or if you do not get hired, you might find it hard to actually listen to the interviewer and respond. Or, if you are thinking about something stressful that happened at work while eating dinner with your family, you are less likely to enjoy their company. As we mentioned before, people sometimes avoid doing certain things or taking risks because they are afraid of becoming even more anxious. This can make it seem like we don't have a lot of choices in life because we have to spend most of our time and energy making sure bad things don't happen. Anxiety and worry can take up a lot of time and energy and make people feel busy, tired, and as if they are on automatic pilot, going through the motions, watching life rather than fully engaging in it. We believe that the effect that anxiety and worry has on people's lives is actually more troubling than the experiences of worry and anxiety themselves.

TREATMENT MODEL FOR AN
ACCEPTANCE-BASED BEHAVIORAL THERAPY FOR GAD
Increase Awareness
Increase Choice and Flexibility
Increase Mindful Action

GAD interferes with awareness.

- Anxiety narrows our attention so that our focus is on threat.
- Worry focuses us on the future so that we often miss what is happening in the present.
- This cycle happens outside of awareness, so it is hard to change.
- Awareness of thoughts, feelings, and sensations can be critical, negative, or "entangled," making these responses more intense.

In this treatment you will:

- Become more aware of your internal responses to events, and you will feel more present in your life by:
  - Monitoring your experiences during the week.
  - Trying some awareness exercises in and between treatment sessions.
- Learn to develop a different kind of relationship to your internal responses.

GAD can create inflexibility.

- Anxious responding is automatic and rigid.
- The most natural response to threat is to avoid/escape/freeze.

In this treatment you will:

- Become aware of different possible responses to events that bring up anxiety or distress.
- Break the automatic relationship between thoughts ("something bad will happen if I try this," "I can't do this") and behavior.
- Learn to choose actions rather than automatically avoid situations.

GAD can cause you to feel like you are on automatic pilot, stuck, and/or a spectator in your own life.

- Worry is about what might happen next, and it takes people away from what is happening now.
- Worry can make it seem like you have no choices and must behave in certain ways.
- Worry can be so exhausting it can leave no time for doing things that make your life fulfilling.

In this treatment you will:

- Identify the important directions in your life that worry has prevented you from pursuing.
- Take action to live a meaningful and satisfying life.
- Develop practical solutions to problems that increase worry.

THE FUNCTION OF EMOTIONS

Why do we have emotions?

- Emotions give us important information.
- Emotions communicate to others.
- Emotions organize us and prepare us for action (often *quickly*).
- Emotions deepen our experience of life.

Hot-stove analogy: In order to respond effectively to the hot stove, you need to:

- Be aware that you are experiencing the pain.
- Be aware of what kind of pain you are experiencing.
- Be aware that the stove is what is causing the pain.
- Be ready to take action.

"Clear" and "muddy" emotions (why it can be hard to know what our emotions are telling us):

- Emotions can be clear (linked in intensity and type to an event) or they can be muddy.
- How do emotions become muddied?
    - When we are not taking care of ourselves (e.g., overtired, not enough down time, poor eating patterns).
    - When they are reactions to imagined future events (rather than actual current events).
    - When our reactions to a current event are added to "leftover" reactions.
        - Unrelated recent events (e.g., a fight with my friend at work muddies my emotional reaction to my child's tantrum that evening).
        - Related events (e.g., my emotional response to my boss giving me critical feedback is muddied by my experiences with overly critical parents).
    - When we have reactions to our initial emotional responses.
        - We have emotional reactions to our emotions.
        - We view having emotions as bad or problematic.
        - We try and change how we feel or prevent an emotion from happening.
    - When we feel defined by our emotions.
        - When it is difficult to see emotions as natural human responses that come and go.
        - When we start to feel entangled and stuck in our emotions.

THE PROBLEM

- We want to avoid negative thoughts and feelings.
- We want a meaningful life.
- A meaningful life brings us into situations that will stir up negative thoughts and feelings.

Possible responses

1. **Limit life by making choices about relationships, work, and self-care that are driven by the desire to avoid painful thoughts and experiences.**
   - You can successfully avoid some difficult situations, but it is impossible to completely avoid fear, sadness, vulnerability, and critical thoughts about yourself.
   - Making the choice not to pursue some things you care about also brings difficult and painful thoughts and feelings.

2. **Attempt to live a meaningful life and to control your responses and reactions.**
   - Total control over one's thoughts, feelings, and bodily reactions is not possible, and control attempts often make those reactions worse.
   - It is hard to let go of control attempts because:
     - Sometimes they seem to work.
     - Other people seem to control their internal experiences.
     - Control works so well in other parts of life.

3. **Live a meaningful life and be willing to experience the thoughts and feelings that come up along the way.**
   - Perhaps a change of focus is needed.
     - Give up the tug-of-war with negative thoughts and feelings.
     - Think about what you would like to do to make your life more fulfilling to you and take some action.
   - Mindfulness techniques can be helpful if you choose a willingness stance.

ANXIETY AWARENESS

We would like you to begin to notice the nature and context of the anxiety you experience in social situations. Therefore, we would like you to try to observe more closely when you experience this anxiety and what that experience of anxiety is like. When you notice you are experiencing sensations of anxiety before or during a social situation, please take a moment to write down what you observe and the situation you are in. For instance, you might notice a tightening in your chest and your palms sweating, and the situation that triggers this might be having lunch with your partner's family, or you might notice thoughts about someone thinking badly of you when you are speaking up in class.

Date/Time	Experience of Anxiety	Situation

MINDFUL WORRY

Please continue to notice the nature and triggers of your worry as you have been doing. When you notice you are worrying, please take a moment to write down what you are worrying about and the situation you are in. For instance, the topic of the worry may be finances, and the situation that triggers this worry may be having lunch with your partner's family, or the topic of the worry may be your safety and well-being, and the situation may be driving. Also note any particular emotions you experienced when you were worried. For instance, you might notice that you feel anxious, sad, or angry while you are worrying.

Date/Time	Topic	Situation	Emotion

URGE AWARENESS

Please continue to notice the nature and triggers of your urges to drink as you have been doing. When you notice an urge, please take a moment to write down the nature of the urge and the situation you are in. For instance, you might notice a thought about an alcoholic beverage, accompanied by salivation, and the situation might be a phone conversation with your mother. Also note any particular emotions you experienced immediately prior to or during this urge. In addition, write down any efforts you made at controlling your emotional experience (e.g., trying to distract yourself from feeling anxious or sad).

Date/Time	Urge	Situation	Emotion	Efforts to Control?

MINDFUL MONITORING

Use the space below to jot down anything you notice regarding your thoughts, feelings, or reactions throughout the week. This can include situations that cue distress, the emotional signals you notice, the thoughts or worries you have, and the ways you respond to your thoughts, worries, or distress.

Date/Time	Situation	First reactions (thoughts, feelings, sensations)	Second reactions (efforts to control, muddy emotions, willingness, acceptance)	Actions/Responses

SIX

Mindfulness- and Acceptance-Based Strategies

Cultivating an accepting, nonjudgmental, nonreactive, open awareness of one's internal experiences is a central element of ABBTs. Although cultivation of this kind of relationship to internal reactions may be a common factor across a wide range of psychotherapies (Germer et al., 2005; Martin, 1997), an explicit emphasis on this cultivation is a defining characteristic of acceptance-based behavioral approaches. In this chapter, we review the ways that this stance is understood, cultivated, practiced, and strengthened in ABBTs.

THE NATURE OF ACCEPTANCE

A conceptual model that emphasizes the problematic nature of reactivity toward, judgment of, and avoidance of one's responses suggests that learning a new way of responding to internal reactions may be therapeutic. If reactivity and avoidance are characteristics of a detrimental response to internal experiences, then openness and acceptance are likely to be more beneficial. "Acceptance," in this context, refers to allowing what is to be rather than wishing or attempting to make it otherwise, but it does not necessarily mean liking things as they are. We can notice our anxiety and that we wish we were not anxious without actively trying to fend off or avoid our anxiety in ways that are problematic. Acceptance refers to a recognition that thoughts, feelings, and sensations will inevitably arise (and inevitably fall) and that judging, fighting, or avoiding them is not very useful. Thus, rather than exhibiting a narrowed attentional focus toward experiences, characterized by judgment, evaluation, and control efforts, we can work toward cultivating an open, compassionate stance, noticing whatever occurs. This stance can help us move from seeing our internal responses as obstacles to doing what matters to seeing them as occurrences along the road toward wherever we want to go (as discussed more fully in the next chapter).

Although acceptance is often mistaken for resignation, or a passive response to events or experiences, Sanderson and Linehan (1999; cited in Robins, Schmidt, & Linehan, 2004) note that the Middle English root for accept is *kap*, meaning to take, seize, or catch, suggesting a much more active response. Acceptance is actively entering into the reality of what is rather than attaching to how we wish it to be or how much we like the way it is.

Acceptance is a continually evolving process. We can accept our sensations of anxiety, or we can judge them, notice we are judging them, and accept those judgments as inevitable and human. We might judge our judgments and only be able to introduce acceptance at this third level, or we might find that we cultivate acceptance but continually slip into judgment and avoidance. Each time we notice difficulties, we have a new opportunity to practice a more open, accepting stance. It is the noticing and cultivation of a different response that is important, not how often it is needed or how long it lasts. Thus, we encourage clients to see the practice of acceptance as lifelong. Although we may find it easier to be accepting at times, and we may find we remember more readily to cultivate acceptance due to our consistent practice, new opportunities and challenges will continually present themselves. And, when our practice has diminished or been forgotten, we still have the opportunity to pick it up again so that it is never lost.

CULTIVATING ACCEPTANCE THROUGH MINDFULNESS-BASED PRACTICE: AN OVERVIEW

Many of the ABBTs use mindfulness-based practices in order to cultivate this accepting stance.[1] These approaches vary in terms of the prominence and extent of mindfulness practices in the treatment. MBSR and MBCT teach clients mindfulness meditation (in a form called the body scan) and yoga and have them practice for at least 45 minutes each night. DBT includes a psychoeducational module on mindfulness skills and uses these skills throughout the other modules and treatment, opting for brief mindfulness practices rather than formal sitting meditation due to concerns that individuals with borderline personality disorder might have difficulty with extensive sitting (Linehan, 1993b). (Segal and colleagues, 2002, suggest that meditation might be problematic for individuals in a depressive episode; they advocate its use with individuals who have recovered from repeated episodes.) ACT uses numerous exercises to illustrate and cultivate acceptance experientially, including several mindfulness-like practices. We draw from DBT in combining mindfulness with traditional behavioral skills training approaches. Consistent with behavioral approaches, we teach multiple methods to cultivate this skill so that clients can use the methods that work best for them (e.g., Borkovec et al., 2004). We find that it is important to balance providing clients with multiple practices in order to enhance flexibility with helping clients achieve a consistent practice that they are able to maintain. Multiple methods can make it more difficult to develop a strong practice in which a single method is used consistently, allowing for habit formation and new discoveries to emerge in a constant context. On the other hand, multiple methods can

---

[1]As Hayes and Shenk (2004) note, one point of confusion in the literature has been whether the term *mindfulness* refers to a process (such as the self-regulation of attention toward immediate experience, with that attention having the quality of openness, curiosity, and acceptance; Bishop et al., 2004) or to practices, such as meditation, that are thought to evoke that process. We use the term *mindfulness* to refer to the process and *mindfulness-based practices* to refer to those practices that have traditionally been used to evoke this process. We also discuss nontraditional mindfulness practices here that we believe similarly evoke the process of mindfulness.

help clients find practices that fit them best and not rigidly attach to a single method of practice. Thus, we work to help our clients develop some type of flexible consistency over time, first introducing multiple methods and then encouraging regular practice of a handful of preferred methods.

As noted in the preceding chapter, mindfulness and acceptance can be described and discussed, but they need to be experienced. In-session exercises and between-session practice help clients develop these skills and notice the effects of this way of responding, providing experiential evidence that can support efforts at continued practice. An emphasis is placed on both formal practice, which involves setting aside a specified period of time to engage in some type of mindfulness practice (usually one in which clients have already engaged during session), and informal practice, which involves applying mindfulness to everyday activities. Formal practice helps cultivate these skills, while informal practice is a critical application of these skills to living. (This approach is similar to the methods contained in applied relaxation, where relaxation is taught in formal, initially lengthy practice but is intended to be applied in anxious situations; e.g., Bernstein, Borkovec, & Hazlett-Stevens, 2000.) No research is available regarding the optimal amount of between-session practice. While MBSR and MBCT, as mentioned, advocate 45 minutes of daily formal meditation, we have tended to use shorter periods with clients unless they choose on their own to engage in more extensive practice. MBSR and MBCT also include a day-long meditation retreat, which has not been part of our approach to treatment. Although extensive formal practice may be optimally beneficial, we have preferred to incorporate a great deal of flexibility so that clients can find modes and dosages of practice that they can adhere to and use effectively. We encourage clients who are interested in more extensive formal practice to seek outside contexts that support this practice (e.g., meditation centers, sanghas, yoga studios) rather than incorporating these methods formally into our treatment. We suspect that different approaches work well with different clients, although research is not yet available to guide clinicians in making these choices.[2] We suggest careful assessment of clients' responses to specific practices, encouragement to try out practice for a sufficient period of time (e.g., 2 weeks of conscientious effort), assessment of reactions and effects, and adjustment of practice accordingly.

In our experience, consistency and quality of practice is perhaps more important than quantity. We have clients self-monitor their mindfulness practice using the Mindfulness Practice form (Form 6.1, p. 141), including both assigned specific formal or informal practice, based on the content of the day's session (described more fully below) and other practices in which they engage. We purposely made this monitoring form minimally detailed to facilitate clients completing it and focusing on the practice rather than the form. With clients who are struggling with practice, we might develop a more detailed form for them to use for a period of time to help them bring their attention to their practice.

We have also found that it is helpful to present a progression of mindfulness practices, starting with easier foci of awareness and gradually expanding to more challenging practice such as awareness of thoughts and cultivating compassion. This is similar to traditional Buddhist practices, which often begin with a focus on the breath in order

---

[2]For example, clinicians working with clients with serious mental illness have shared with us their observation that very brief practices are necessary with these clients due to challenges in maintaining focus. In this case, a minute or two of mindfulness practice may be the best way to give clients an experience of decentering and defusion. More frequent, briefer practices may be desirable.

to develop attentional abilities before cultivating a more expanded mindful awareness. Interestingly, Patel (2006) has suggested that, when working with anxious clients, it may be beneficial to reverse match the order of exercises to their dominant mode of anxiety presentation (cognitive vs. somatic). Thus, with a client with OCD who had a particularly somatic presentation of anxiety, she began with sitting meditation focused on thoughts and progressed to yoga and then a body scan; with someone with a more cognitive presentation, she would have reversed the order, focusing on the body first. Optimal progression of exercises is an area in need of further study. For now, clinicians should attend to the ways that specific exercises interact with clients' symptomatic presentation and either adapt exercises accordingly or adjust their order in order to optimize client response. As with the selection of behavioral exercises, therapists should try to maximize the likelihood that clients will complete and learn from the exercises by minimizing potential obstacles. Careful attention should be paid to their responses in order to adjust exercises to be optimally performed and experienced. It is important to distinguish between selecting or altering exercises in order to enhance clients' learning and making choices that serve the function of experiential avoidance. The goal is *not* to ensure that clients do not experience distress in these exercises. In fact, the mindful, nonjudgmental, nonavoidant experience of distressing thoughts and feelings is a central goal of this aspect of treatment. As with exposure exercises, it is important that clients are willing and able to remain in contact with these responses rather than avoiding them. Thus, choices regarding the order of exercises are based in part on developing a graduated exposure hierarchy so that clients are more likely to remain fully engaged in each exercise rather than prematurely terminating or distracting during the exercise.

We have developed a standard progression of exercises (adapted from MBSR, MBCT, ACT, DBT, and other sources) that we typically use with all clients for the first several sessions. We have found this progression matches well with most clients, particularly when we alter breathing focus instructions in order to minimize anxious responding to an attentional focus on the breath (again, to maximize engagement in the exercise, not to promote experiential avoidance). We introduce most exercises in session, where we do them with clients at the beginning of a session and then discuss their reactions/experiences. Clients then practice the exercises during the week and report further on their observations and reactions. Once clients have made their way through the full progression, we return to exercises that represent particular challenges or develop new, individually tailored exercises to meet clients' specific needs. We also have clients select the exercises they want to focus on for a particular week or that they want to make part of their regular practice so that they begin to develop their own mindfulness practices, which they will continue after the end of treatment (as discussed more fully in Chapter 9).

Acceptance-based and other behavioral approaches emphasize the importance of eliciting clients' reactions to any exercises. Therapists ask clients what each exercise was like for them, what they noticed, and what they reacted to. This feedback helps therapists develop a better sense of clients' unique experiences and helps tailor future exercises so that the language used in instruction corresponds to the language the client uses to describe his experience. The feedback also informs therapists of any potentially problematic reactions. In acceptance-based exercises, therapists need to listen carefully for indications that clients are using the exercises as a way to control or avoid distressing emotions or are beginning to attach to a particular reaction to exercises and become distressed if they have another one. Therapists can then remind clients of the importance of being open to *any* experiences rather than trying to cultivate only one kind of response (although, of course, it is natural to have an initial response of wanting to feel calm or happy and to want to experience that again).

For instance, one client responded to an initial mindfulness of breath exercise by describing how she felt calmer during it than she had in years. The therapist was careful to validate this experience and share the client's excitement about it, while also noting that sometimes mindfulness does not feel calming and that it is important to practice being open to distressing experiences as well. Another client initially had a lot of challenging responses to mindfulness exercises but was able to remain engaged in the practice. Over time, he began to find a sense of peace and tranquility when he practiced and was disappointed when this sense did not come during an exercise. The therapist validated this experience, noting how natural it is to want that kind of tranquility, but she reminded the client of his experiences early in therapy and asked if he could remain open to a range of experiences in his practice, including wishing he felt otherwise.

Therapists should practice delivering mindfulness practice instructions in an optimal, slow, paced style. Practicing mindfulness prior to session helps cultivate a calm, slow voice that helps listeners follow instructions and bring awareness to their experience. (Although Segal and colleagues [2002] suggest speaking in a matter-of-fact voice rather than changing one's tone.) Pausing frequently during instruction allows clients to really engage the practice rather than solely listening to the therapist. We always tell our supervisees to speak *much* more slowly than feels natural; it is very rare that we have heard a clinician guide a practice speaking too slowly. We also follow Segal and colleagues' (2002) suggestion of using "-ing" verbs (e.g., "noticing," "bringing awareness to") to highlight the continual process of mindfulness.

SPECIFIC INSTRUCTION AND PRACTICE IN MINDFULNESS- AND OTHER ACCEPTANCE-BASED PRACTICES

Introduction of Mindfulness: Mindfulness of Breath, Eating, and Sensations

We begin (typically in the first couple of sessions) by presenting both the experience and the concept of mindfulness. With anxious clients, we like to introduce the traditional behavioral technique of diaphragmatic breathing adapted to emphasize mindfulness. We begin by having clients simply observe their breath, noticing whatever arises. Often, they will notice a tightness in their chests, shortness of breath, and so on, or that anxious thoughts arise as they bring their attention to their breath. We respond to all of these observations as natural parts of the process. We then ask clients to gently shift their breath so that it starts lower down, in their diaphragm, and observe the effects of this shift.[3] We discuss their observations, noting any judgments or efforts at control

---

[3]This type of instruction is not typical of mindfulness- and acceptance-based strategies. We are adapting relaxation instructions (Bernstein et al., 2000) with demonstrated efficacy, particularly with clients with GAD, so that they can potentially benefit from this activation of the parasympathetic nervous system while noticing their own responses and practicing a nonjudgmental response to them. We predict that they may actually experience increased anxiety or have difficulty following the instructions; in all cases, they are asked to practice allowing whatever is to be, while gently altering their breath. We feel this instruction in gentle change helps clients with high levels of anxious arousal or tension to engage more fully in awareness of breath (which otherwise can generate such heightened judgment and anxiety sensitivity that they have difficulty complying with instructions).

or avoidance that arise. We ask clients to practice this awareness and gentle altering of their breath informally throughout the week, providing them with some practice noticing their habitual responses and the effects of a slight change in these responses. Sometimes clients become concerned with doing this exercise "right." We encourage them to practice in whatever way they can and to notice what emerges. If they cannot bring their breath into their abdomen, then noticing that and continuing to breathe is the practice. If they forget to notice their breath, then their practice might be periodically noticing that they are not noticing their breath. Any practice is useful and something we can work with.

We also provide clients with Handout 6.1, What Is Mindfulness? (pp. 137–138), which we ask them to review between sessions and review in depth with them the following week. Over the same period, we also like to assign the following initial formal mindfulness exercise, adapted from MBSR, to give clients more experience with mindfulness that can inform later discussion.

Initial Formal (Mindfulness) Breathing Exercise

1. Assume a comfortable posture lying on your back or sitting. If you are sitting, keep the spine straight and let your shoulders drop.
2. Close your eyes if it feels comfortable.
3. Bring your attention to your belly, feeling it rise or expand gently on the inbreath and fall or recede on the outbreath.
4. Keep[ing] the focus on your breathing, practice "being with" each inbreath for its full duration and with each outbreath for its full duration, as if you were riding the waves of your own breathing.
5. Every time you notice that your mind has wandered off the breath, notice what it was that took you away and then gently bring your attention back to your belly and the feeling of the breath coming in and out.
6. If your mind wanders away from the breath a thousand times, then your "job" is simply to bring it back to the breath every time, no matter what it becomes preoccupied with.
7. Practice this exercise for fifteen minutes at a convenient time every day, whether you feel like it or not, for one week and see how it feels to incorporate a disciplined [mindfulness] practice into your life. Be aware of how it feels to spend time each day just being with your breath without having to *do* anything.[4]

We often begin early sessions with a mindfulness of breath exercise that builds on this first practice. We provide gentle verbal guidance that encourages clients to draw attention to their breath and to deepen it. For instance, we might say something like:

"Noticing the way you are sitting in the chair . . . Noticing where your body is touching the chair . . . Now beginning to bring your attention to your breath . . . Noticing how the air enters your body, where it travels, and how it leaves your body . . . Noticing the parts of your body that move as you are breathing . . . Now, placing

---

[4]From Kabat-Zinn (1990, p. 58). Copyright 1990 by Jon Kabat-Zinn. Reprinted by permission of Dell Publishing, a division of Random House, Inc.

your hand on your abdomen and noticing whether it moves as you are breathing ... Gently deepening your breath so that you are breathing from your abdomen ... Noticing your abdomen, chest, and shoulders expand as you inhale ... Continuing to deepen and slow your breath ... Paying attention to the sensations you experience ... Just continuing to focus on your breath for the next several moments. ..."[5]

The ellipses indicate places where the therapist can insert a substantial pause to allow the client to follow instructions and fully experience the practice. This exercise is a somewhat nontraditional mindfulness exercise because there is a gentle emphasis on change rather than on simply observing what is. In our experience, this emphasis helps counteract the potential for increased distress among individuals who may react negatively to their initial awareness of their own breath and prematurely terminate the exercise. Nonetheless, it is important to emphasize that anxiety and distress may arise throughout the exercise and that it, too, can be noticed without judgment. If clients become overly focused on trying to shift to diaphragmatic breathing, therapists may want to drop that portion of the script and simply emphasize a focus on the breath. In postexercise discussions with clients, we pay particular attention to any aspects of the script that seemed to interfere with their experience, as well as their own descriptions of their process, so that we can tailor what we say in the future to the client. Although we use scripts to guide these exercises, we do not read these scripts in session, and we encourage therapists to develop their own instruction delivered without a script so that it sounds natural.

We also like to use another mindfulness exercise early in treatment in which clients are instructed to eat an object (often a raisin) mindfully, bringing "beginner's mind" to the activity (Segal et al., 2002). Clients are guided through very slowly eating a familiar object as if they had never seen it before. They begin by looking at the object carefully from all angles and then move on to touching it and smelling it. They then place the object in their mouth, noticing their responses and the urge to chew or swallow. Finally, they slowly chew and swallow the object, attending to all their sensations, thoughts, and reactions as they do so. After the exercise, we take time to review clients' experiences of this exercise, which typically evolves into a discussion of how different it would be to do daily tasks (like washing the dishes, eating, brushing our teeth) with this type of awareness and "beginner's mind."

After clients have engaged in one or two mindfulness tasks so that they have an experience of mindfulness, we go on to a more formal introduction of the concept. We emphasize the experiential nature of mindfulness, noting that, although we can try to talk about what it is, it is really learned through repeated practice and observation. Therefore, as noted in the previous chapter, we are careful not to engage in extensive discussion of the concept but introduce a few skills that we (and other acceptance-based therapists) see as central to the therapeutic use of mindfulness. We give clients Handout 6.2, Skills of Mindfulness (p. 139), and discuss its major points, as well as Handout 6.1.

Nonjudgmental observation is a particularly important skill and difficult to cultivate. Our clients often report that they are already extremely aware of their inter-

---

[5]There are numerous excellent references for mindfulness/meditation scripts from which clinicians may want to draw or adapt specific practices. See the resources list at the end of this volume for those we have found particularly helpful in our clinical work (and personal practices).

nal experiences and would like to be less aware. We validate that perception and ask whether they find that their awareness is characterized by compassion and understanding or by criticism and judgment. They are quick to note that the latter type of awareness is far more common. We suggest that it may be this aspect of their awareness that is problematic and that a more compassionate or kindly awareness might have very different consequences for them. Imagining how we might respond to a friend if he or she were to share the types of thoughts, emotions, or reactions we're having with us often shows that we are more able to be compassionate toward another than ourselves. Often, clients find this perspective helps them imagine a more compassionate response to their own experiences. We share with clients that this is a particularly hard attitude to cultivate and that we will be working together extensively on strengthening their ability to respond compassionately to their own experience. We find that a judgmental response to internal experiences is often so overlearned that it takes extensive practice and direct attention to alter it. Clients sometimes express their belief that their own judgmental responses motivate them to strive and do more. In response to this assumption, early in treatment, we ask clients if they are willing to try out a different way of responding to see if this belief is accurate. We might share our own experience of finding that we can actually do more when we are kinder to ourselves, while our own harsh judgments can interfere with our ability to act as we would like to. We are careful not to try to convince clients that this is true or even particularly to attach to this truth for ourselves; instead, we encourage clients to notice for themselves whether this stance has been working for them and consider if another stance might work.

The concept of beginner's mind can be linked to the raisin exercise so that clients have an experiential example of seeing something as if for the first time rather than allowing their past experiences or expectations to cloud their current experiences. We use the example of having a discussion with a partner that we have had many times before, noting how easy it is to respond to what we expect her to say rather than what she has said and how different it would be to really hear each comment as if for the first time. By intentionally bringing beginner's mind to these kinds of situations, we can be more open to what is actually happening in the moment and can have an expanded experience rather than one dictated by our reactions and expectations. We encourage clients to practice approaching various daily experiences with beginner's mind.

During this discussion, it is important to assess clients' reactions to the idea of mindfulness. Clients may have their own experiences with different kinds of mindfulness practice, or they may have preconceived notions of what mindfulness is. We elicit their responses and address any concerns they may have. Sometimes clients express concerns about the connection between mindfulness and Buddhism and its potential inconsistency with their own religious traditions and beliefs. In response, we discuss the role of mindfulness or awareness in different religious traditions and our use of mindfulness within a secular rather than a religious context. When clients have a background with mindfulness-based practices, we ask them to draw from their past experiences but to attend to ways that their past use of mindfulness may differ from our intended use (as discussed in Chapter 4).

Early on and throughout treatment, we emphasize that mindfulness, like acceptance, is a process. Returning to our awareness is the action of mindfulness; it is irrelevant how many times our attention wanders and important only that we return. We sometimes quote the traditional Zen saying "fall down seven times, get up eight" to illustrate this concept. Similarly, we return to compassion repeatedly rather than reaching a steady state of compassion that never wavers. For each moment of judgment, we have the opportunity to practice nonjudgment. Thus, each apparent failure at mindfulness is simply an opportunity to practice again. We also emphasize the importance of both formal and informal practice, providing a handout that details various types of informal practice for clients to try (Handout 6.3, p. 140).

In early sessions, we use several other mindfulness/awareness exercises that emphasize awareness of senses and sensations. With our clients with GAD, we use a modified version of progressive muscle relaxation (PMR; Bernstein et al., 2000) in which we emphasize drawing attention to the sensations associated with both tensing and releasing each muscle group and allowing whatever response occurs to occur. Similar to our use of diaphragmatic breathing, this mindfulness exercise is somewhat unusual because it includes an action that may actively change the client's experience (tensing and releasing muscles typically leads to more relaxed muscles); however, we find integration of this empirically supported treatment for GAD helps our clients broaden their experience (by introducing a more relaxed response into what is typically a rigid style of tension) while also allowing whatever arises. We are careful not to suggest that the exercise will result in relaxation and encourage clients to notice whatever occurs, including thoughts and sensations associated with anxiety that are likely to occur along with relaxation responses. We have these clients practice PMR at home between sessions, gradually reducing the number of muscle groups so that it becomes briefer and eventually an applied exercise.

We have also found that mindfulness of sounds (Segal et al., 2002) is another helpful exercise that helps clients cultivate beginner's mind and develop their mindfulness skills. After bringing clients to an awareness of their body, we encourage them to bring their awareness to their ears and allow it to expand to any sounds as they arise. We suggest that they notice sounds as they arise, both near and far, obvious and subtle, and also notice silence. We encourage them to be aware of sounds as sensations rather than of their meanings or implications and to notice when their awareness shifts away from sounds or they begin to think about sounds rather than hearing them.

This exercise often illustrates for clients and for therapists how challenging it is *not* to label our observations. We put names and judgments on our experiences almost at the same instant that they register. This exercise helps us see that automatic process and begin to extend the time between noticing and judging so that we can start to observe without judging and more clearly see our judgments as separate from our experiences.

Another useful beginning exercise with a wide range of clients that can also be used later in treatment, when clients have more practice with mindfulness, is "3-minute breathing space," also from Segal and colleagues (2002). We begin by asking clients to take:

> "a very definite posture . . . relaxed, dignified, back erect, but not stiff, letting our bodies express a sense of being present and awake.
>
> "Now, closing your eyes, if that feels comfortable for you, the first step is being aware of what is going through your mind; what thoughts are around? Here, again, as best you can, just noting the thoughts as mental events . . . So we note them, and then noting the feelings that are around at the moment . . . in particular, turning toward any sense of discomfort or unpleasant feelings. So rather than trying to

push them away or shutting them out, just acknowledging them, perhaps saying, 'Ah, there you are, that's how it is right now.' And similarly with sensations in the body . . . Are there sensations of tension, of holding, or whatever? And again, awareness of them, simply noting them. OK, that's how it is right now.

"So, [you've] got a sense of what is going on right now. We've stepped out of automatic pilot. The second step is to collect our awareness by focusing on a single object—the movements of the breath. So focusing attention down there in the movements of the abdomen, the rise and fall of the breath . . . spending a minute or so focusing on the movement of the abdominal wall . . . moment by moment, breath by breath, as best we can. So that you know when the breath is moving in, and you know when the breath is moving out. Just binding your awareness to the pattern of movement down there . . . gathering yourself, using the anchor of the breath to really be in the present.

"And now as a third step, having gathered ourselves to some extent, we allow our awareness to expand. As well as being aware of the breath, we also include a sense of the body as a whole. So that we get this more spacious awareness . . . A sense of the body as a whole, including any tightness or sensations related to holding in the shoulders, neck, back, or face . . . following the breath as if your whole body is breathing. Holding it all in this slightly softer . . . more spacious awareness.

"And then, when you are ready, just allowing your eyes to open."[6]

This exercise begins to introduce flexibility of attention, with clients first noticing all of their experience, then focusing on their breath to ground themselves, and then expanding back out to their full experience. This allows beginning practice in noticing thoughts and reactions without attaching to them, which will be cultivated more fully in later exercises. Sometimes clients find this exercise challenging, especially if they have found focus on the breath or on the body to be relaxing in some way, which can present an opportunity to address the ways that mindfulness includes all of our experiences, including those that are less pleasant. The brevity of the practice can also be difficult, with clients reporting frustration at not having longer to settle down. Again, this can provide an opportunity to practice with frustration and to begin to develop a briefer, more portable mindfulness response. With practice and acceptance of the frustration that may arise, the 3-minute breathing space can become an excellent, brief mindfulness practice that clients can use continually, even after treatment, to reconnect to the central principles of mindfulness. We encourage our clients to practice it daily, and for some it becomes a regular part of their daily routines that continues beyond treatment.

Mindfulness of Emotions and Thoughts and Defusion Exercises

Once clients have begun to develop an ability to gently shift their attention toward their sensations and senses, we begin expanding their practice to the challenge of noticing and allowing thoughts and feelings, bringing curiosity and compassion to these experiences. Similarly to DBT, we link mindful awareness of emotion to our discussion of the function of emotion (described in the preceding chapter) so that clients understand the

---

[6]From Segal, Williams, and Teasdale (2002, p. 174). Copyright 2002 by The Guilford Press. Reprinted by permission.

utility of noticing and understanding rather than avoiding their internal experiences. We frequently use an exercise that allows clients to recall an emotional event in their recent experience and practice an expansive awareness of their emotional responses to this event. Initially, we have clients choose a moderately distressing experience to maximize the likelihood that they will be able to remain aware of their emotions throughout the exercise. After continued practice, we begin to use the exercise with highly emotional, very recent events, and we encourage clients to practice on their own as these events occur in their lives.

The therapist and client select an event before the exercise. The therapist then guides the client into awareness of herself in the room, gently bringing awareness to the way she is sitting in the chair, how her breath moves through her body, and so on. The client is then instructed:

> "Now bringing [the emotional event] into your awareness . . . Imagining yourself back in that situation . . . Noticing what you can see, the sounds you hear . . . Noticing the sensations in your body . . . Noticing any thoughts running through your mind . . . and now noticing how you are feeling . . . Just noticing each feeling as it arises . . . not trying to alter or change your experience . . . Noticing any desire to alter or change what you are feeling and gently letting go of that effort . . . Expanding to allow your full experience . . . Noticing what the feelings are like . . . Noticing if the feelings change in any way. . . . "

Clients can also practice mindfulness of emotions using the Letting Go of Emotional Suffering handout from DBT (Linehan, 1993b). This handout instructs clients to *observe* their emotion by noting its presence, stepping back, and getting unstuck from the emotion. They can then *experience* it (1) as a wave, coming and going; (2) trying not to block the emotion; (3) not trying to suppress the emotion; (4) not trying to get rid of the emotion; (5) not trying to push it away; (6) not trying to keep the emotion around; (7) not holding on to the emotion; and (8) not amplifying it. They are instructed to *remember* to not necessarily act on emotion and to remember times they have felt different. Finally, they can *practice* loving their emotion by not judging it, practicing willingness, and radically accepting it.

Often, clients report that bringing mindfulness to their experience in session allows them to notice more complex emotions than they had initially noticed during the situation. For instance, Sondra reported a high level of anxiety and worry when her daughter won an opportunity to go on a trip for a sports competition, fearing for her daughter's safety and well-being. She noticed during this exercise that, in addition to fear, she felt pride in her daughter and happiness at her success. Although awareness of these feelings did not eliminate the fear, it provided a context in which the fear did not have to guide her behaviors as strongly and reminded her why she might want her daughter to go on the trip despite her fear. Sometimes, clients simply notice that their emotional responses come and go, which helps lessen the intensity of their responses, that their emotions are very strong and very distressing but not "intolerable" because, in fact, they are able to tolerate them. This experience weakens the learned avoidance response to emotional experience, opening up the possibility of staying with emotional responses rather than trying to eliminate them regardless of the costs involved (such as restrictions in life or subsequent increases in distress).

We have also found that Rumi's poem "The Guest House," translated by Coleman Barks and also used by Segal and colleagues (2002), can help clients imagine a different way of responding to their emotional experiences. We use it as a mindfulness exercise, first guiding clients to be aware of themselves in the room, their sensations, and their breath and then asking them just to listen openly as we slowly read the poem:

> This being human is a guest house.
> Every morning a new arrival.
>
> A joy, a depression, a meanness,
> Some momentary awareness comes
> as an unexpected visitor.
>
> Welcome and entertain them all!
> Even if they're a crowd of sorrows,
> who violently sweep your house
> empty of its furniture,
>
> still treat each guest honorably.
> He may be clearing you out
> for some new delight.
>
> The dark thought, the shame, the malice,
> meet them at the door laughing,
> and invite them in.
>
> Be grateful for whoever comes,
> because each has been sent
> as a guide from beyond.[7]

Clients often find this imagery particularly helpful in cultivating a compassionate response to their emotions. The poem is another, more experiential approach to the psychoeducation about the function of emotion described in the preceding chapter. Often, clients will report that when they found themselves experiencing anxiety or sadness or anger and initially wishing it away, they recalled the poem and imagined themselves welcoming the emotions rather than trying to banish them. This kind of alteration in habitual responding allows clients to experience the transience of their emotional response, weakening the threatening associations they have with their negative emotions and strengthening their ability to refrain from futile efforts to eliminate these responses.

We draw from ACT, DBT, and MBCT in our choice of exercises that specifically emphasize noticing thoughts without getting caught up in them. We have adapted the clouds exercise from DBT to help clients practice this kind of detached or decentered awareness of the thoughts that arise for them.

"Close your eyes . . . First focusing on your breathing, just noticing your breath as you take it in, it travels through your body and then back out of your body. Notic-

---

[7]Copyright 1995 by Coleman Barks. Reprinted by permission.

ing how your body feels . . . Now picturing yourself lying someplace outside where you can see the sky. You can picture any place that feels comfortable and vivid to you—lying on a raft in a pond, on a blanket in a field, on the deck of a house, any place where you have a clear, full view of the sky. Now imagining yourself, comfortably lying, your body sinking into whatever you're lying on, as you gaze at the sky. Noticing the sky and the clouds that hang in the sky, moving across it. Seeing how the clouds are part of the sky, but they are not the whole sky. The sky exists behind the clouds. Imagining that your thoughts and feelings are the clouds in the sky, while your mind is the sky itself. Seeing your thoughts and feelings gently drifting across the sky . . . As you notice thoughts and feelings, placing them in the clouds and noticing them as they pass across the sky . . . Noticing yourself as you become distracted, or immersed in the clouds, losing sight of the sky . . . Noticing how the clouds can be very light and wispy or dark and menacing . . . Noticing how even when the clouds cover the sky, the sky exists behind them . . . Noticing moments when your thoughts and feelings feel separate from you . . . and moments when they feel the same as you . . . Picturing the sky behind the clouds and the clouds drifting across the sky . . . Practicing putting your thoughts and feelings onto the clouds . . . Noticing the different shapes they take . . . the different consistency of the clouds they are on . . . When you find yourself on the clouds, slowly shifting your attention back to the sky behind the clouds and practicing putting your thoughts and emotions on the clouds. . . . " [Leave the client time to do the exercise in silence, then gently guide awareness back to the room, present sensations, how he or she is sitting in the chair, and invite the client to open his or her eyes when ready.]

A similar exercise from ACT, "leaves on a stream," can also be used for this purpose (Hayes, Strosahl, & Wilson, 1999). Segal and colleagues' (2002) mindfulness of sounds and thoughts is also a nice exercise that expands the previous practice of mindfulness of sounds to mindfulness of thoughts. Eifert and Forsyth (2005) also present an exercise on acceptance of thoughts and feelings that could be used to practice awareness and acceptance of a wide range of internal experiences.

Often, clients find these exercises the most challenging so far (we find this true as well and share that fact with them). They provide an excellent context for emphasizing the process of mindfulness—the aim is repeatedly to draw our attention back, to notice our thoughts again. We cannot continually maintain this type of awareness; instead, we hope to develop our ability to remember to practice this awareness so that at difficult times it is easier for us to remind ourselves to see our thoughts as thoughts and our feelings as feelings. Practicing formally this way helps us develop this skill. Clients can practice these exercises during the week and begin to notice how sometimes achieving this awareness is easier than others, some thoughts grab them more than others, and, while the process may get easier over time, it never gets easy. Gradually, clients can begin to apply this practice informally, seeing if, when a challenging situation arises, they can notice thoughts as they arise, seeing them as thoughts and not attaching to them as truths.

We find defusion techniques drawn from ACT are also very helpful to draw awareness to thoughts as thoughts. For instance, we adopt the strategy with our clients of labeling our internal experiences as internal experiences. Thus, rather than saying, "My partner is angry at me," or "I am never going to be ready for this presentation," we would encourage our clients to practice saying (even to themselves), "I am having the thought that my partner is angry at me," or "I am having the thought that I will never be ready for this presentation." This slight change in construction can help increase awareness that thoughts are just thoughts, rather than statements of things as they are (which is how we often experience them). This stylistic convention can, therefore, enhance clients' sense of decentering or defusion from their thoughts. We think of it as a mini-mindfulness exercise because it really draws attention to the nature of thoughts, enhancing awareness.

Cultivating Self-Compassion

As we noted above, cultivating compassion toward one's experience is one of the most challenging aspects of these interventions. We talk about this directly with clients, high-lighting the ways that we may learn not to be compassionate toward ourselves (e.g., parents or other role models may model a lack of compassion, we may mistakenly learn to associate compassion with letting ourselves off the hook or being lazy and giving up). We invite clients to notice the effects of their noncompassionate responses to themselves and the effects of others' noncompassionate responses to them. We also remind them of the function of emotions and the humanness of a range of internal experiences as a foundation for cultivating compassion for these experiences.

Perhaps the most powerful mode of cultivating self-compassion in therapy is through the therapist's compassionate response to clients' reports of their experiences. Rogers (1961) long ago noted the therapeutic impact of empathic concern, and our clinical experience certainly echoes his observations. Throughout treatment, our clients share the internal experiences that they judge most negatively in themselves, and we consistently respond to these reports in the way that we experience them: as natural aspects of human experience. We also communicate our compassion toward and accep-tance of their responses by *not* trying to eliminate their experiences; this shows that we do not see their responses as dangerous or bad, even though we understand that they feel that way. Clients working with us and with the therapists we have supervised fre-quently report beginning to hear their therapist's compassionate words in their head as a first step toward cultivating their own compassionate response to their experiences. Therapists' own mindfulness practices can help them cultivate this compassion toward and attunement to clients' emotional experiences (Fulton, 2005), and specific exercises can be used to cultivate empathy toward clients (see Morgan & Morgan, 2005).

We have also collected a set of mindfulness exercises that we use with clients who are having a particularly difficult time cultivating self-compassion. Williams, Teasdale, Segal, and Kabat-Zinn (2007) describe a brief breathing space exercise aimed at soften-ing one's reaction toward one's own pain and distress that we often use with some adaptations (e.g., expanding the emphasis on bodily sensations to include all internal situations). We have clients begin by focusing on their breath and then expanding to their full body. Then we ask them to bring to mind a current difficulty in their lives and continue as follows.

"Now, once you are focusing on some troubling thought or situation—some worry or intense feeling—allow yourself to take some time to tune into any physical sen-sations in the body that the difficulty evokes. See[ing] if you are able to notice and approach any sensations that are arising in your body, becoming mindful of those physical sensations, deliberately [but gently] directing your focus of attention to the region of the body where the sensations are the strongest in the gesture of an embrace, a welcoming. This gesture might include breathing into that part of the body on the in-breath and breathing out from that region on the out-breath, exploring the sensations, watching their intensity shift up and down from one moment to the next.

"[. . .]Seeing if you can bring to this attention an even deeper attitude of compassion and openness to whatever sensations, [thoughts, or emotions] you are experiencing, however unpleasant, by saying to yourself from time to time: 'It's okay. Whatever it is, it's already here. Let me open to it.' Then just stay with the awareness of these [internal] sensations, breathing with them, accepting them, letting them be, allowing them to be just as they are. It may be helpful to repeat, 'It's here right now. Whatever it is, it's already here. Let me open to it.' Soften[ing] and open[ing] to the sensations you become aware of, letting go of any tensing and bracing. Remember that by saying 'It's already here' or 'It's okay,' you are not judging the original situation or saying that everything's fine, but simply helping your awareness, right now, to remain open to the sensations in the body. If you like, you can also experiment with holding in awareness both the sensations of the body and the feeling of the breath moving in and out, as you breathe with the sensations moment by moment.

"And when you notice that the bodily sensations are no longer pulling your attention to the same degree, simply return 100% to the breath and continue with that as the primary object of attention."[8]

Clients can begin by softening in response to distressing sensations and then gradually soften and open up to distressing thoughts and feelings as well. Practicing this daily in a formal manner (for instance, with any distressing reactions the client wakes up with) can help strengthen the response so that clients can apply it during a distressing experience, breathing and opening up to their experience rather than trying to avoid it or judge it.

We often adapt the "accepting yourself on faith" exercise from ACT (Hayes, Strosahl, & Wilson, 1999) to help clients practice with a broader compassionate response to counter the overriding sense of self-criticism that clients have often developed from past experiences. We ask clients to consider the ways they repeatedly analyze themselves and find themselves not good enough. We ask them to consider an alternative—that being acceptable is a choice, a leap of faith, rather than something to constantly test and evaluate. In this exercise, we ask if they are willing to take this leap, to see themselves as worthy and whole just as they are, in this moment and each moment.

Other exercises used in mindfulness-based approaches draw from traditional Buddhist practice (see Germer, 2005, for a review) to cultivate compassion. The Tibetan practice of Tonglen, which involves breathing in (and opening ourselves up to) our own or others' pain and suffering and breathing out relief (Brach, 2003; Chodron, 2001) can be used to cultivate a nonavoidant, open response to any occurrence of pain or suffer-

---

[8]From Williams, Teasdale, Segal, and Kabat-Zinn (2007, pp. 151–152). Copyright 2007 by The Guilford Press. Reprinted by permission.

ing. Continued practice with any suffering that arises can help clients develop a sense of their ability to hold pain and suffering rather than needing to turn away from it. Loving-kindness meditation or *metta* (e.g., Kabat-Zinn, 1994) can be used to cultivate a warm, caring response to oneself and then direct that loving-kindness out toward other people. Practicing compassion toward other people can be helpful in the context of interpersonal difficulties clients are having and can help clients develop more skillful, effective ways of resolving conflicts.

Bringing It All Together: Developing a Sense of the Transience of Experience and Definitions of Self

We use several exercises with clients that bring the multiple aspects of mindfulness (awareness of the breath, sensations, thoughts, feelings) together, highlighting the over-all transience of human experience. The "observer self" exercise from ACT systematically takes clients through each aspect of their experience, noticing the ways that no specific sensation, feeling, or thought is constant or defines them. This exercise highlights the ways that some aspect of us exists beyond the experiences we have in a given moment and labels it the observer self.

Kabat-Zinn (1994) describes several meditation exercises that similarly evoke an experience of the transient nature of our experience. We often use an adapted version of the mountain meditation exercise, and many of our clients find it extremely useful in cultivating this perspective. After guiding clients to bring their awareness to themselves in the room, their sensations, and their breath, we would introduce the following meditation:

The Mountain Meditation

"Pictur[ing] the most beautiful mountain you know or know of or can imagine, one whose form speaks personally to you. Focus[ing] on the image or the feeling of the mountain in your mind's eye, noticing its overall shape, the lofty peak, the base rooted in the rock of the earth's crust, the steep or gently sloping sides. Not[ing] as well how massive it is, how unmoving, how beautiful whether seen from afar or up close . . .

"Perhaps your mountain has snow at the top and trees on the lower slopes. Perhaps it has one prominent peak, perhaps a series of peaks or a high plateau. However it appears, just sit[ting] and breath[ing] with the image of this mountain, observing it, noting its qualities. When you feel ready, see[ing] if you can bring the mountain into your own body so that your body sitting here and the mountain of the mind's eye become one. Your head becomes the lofty peak; your shoulders and arms the sides of the mountain; your buttocks and legs the solid base rooted to your cushion on the floor or to your chair. Experienc[ing] in your body the sense of uplift, the . . . elevated quality of the mountain deep in your own spine. Invit[ing] yourself to become a breathing mountain, unwavering in your stillness, completely what you are—beyond words and thought, a centered, rooted, unmoving presence.

"Now, as well you know, throughout the day as the sun travels the sky, the mountain just sits. Light and shadow and colors are changing virtually moment to moment in the mountain's adamantine stillness. Even the untrained eye can see changes by the hour . . . As the light changes, as night follows day and day night, the mountain just sits, simply being itself. It remains still as the seasons flow into one another and as the weather changes moment by moment and day by day. Calmness abiding all change.

"In summer, there is no snow on the mountain, except perhaps for the very top or in crags shielded from direct sunlight. In the fall, the mountain may display a coat of brilliant fire colors; in winter, a blanket of snow and ice. In any season, it may at times find itself enshrouded in clouds or fog, or pelted by freezing rain. The tourists who come to visit may be disappointed if they can't see the mountain clearly, but it's all the same to the mountain—seen or unseen, in sun or clouds, broiling or frigid, it just sits, being itself. At times visited by violent storms, buffeted by snow and rain and winds of unthinkable magnitude, through it all the mountain sits. Spring comes, the birds sing in the trees once again, leaves return to the trees which lost them, flowers bloom in the high meadows and on the slopes, streams overflow with waters of melting snow. Through it all, the mountain continues to sit, unmoved by the weather, by what happens on the surface, by the world of appearances.

"As we sit holding this image in our minds, we can embody the same unwavering stillness and rootedness in the face of everything that changes in our own lives over seconds, hours, and years. In our lives and in our [mindfulness] practice, we experience constantly the changing nature of mind and body and of the outer world. We experience periods of light and dark, vivid color and drab dullness. We experience storms of varying intensity and violence, in the outer world and in our own lives and minds. Buffeted by high winds, by cold and rain, we endure periods of darkness and pain as well as savoring moments of joy and uplift. Even our appearance changes constantly, just like the mountain's, experiencing a weather and a weathering of its own.

"By becoming the mountain in [this exercise], we can link up with its strength and stability and adopt them for our own. We can use its energies to support our efforts to encounter each moment with mindfulness, equanimity, and clarity. It may help to see that our thoughts and feelings, our preoccupations, our emotional storms and crises, even the things that happen *to* us are more like the weather on the mountain. We tend to take it personally but its strongest characteristic is impersonal. The weather of our own lives is not to be ignored or denied. It is to be encountered, honored, felt, known for what it is, and held in high awareness since it can kill us. In holding it this way, we come to know a deeper silence and stillness and wisdom than we may have thought possible, right within the storms. Mountains have this to teach us, and more, if we come to listen."[9]

Kabat-Zinn (1994) also provides instruction for a standing and lying-down meditation (tree meditation and lake meditation) with similar themes that we sometimes use with our clients. These meditations often allow clients to develop a vivid image that they can recall in difficult situations to remind them at an experiential level of the transience of their experience and their ability to transcend whatever distressing responses emerge

---

[9]From Kabat-Zinn (1994, pp. 136–139). Copyright 1994 by Jon Kabat-Zinn. Reprinted by permission of Hyperion. All rights reserved.

for them. We introduce this broad range of exercises because we have found that clients respond to different practices and different images and are then able to bring them more fully into their lives. Some clients will really connect to the clouds exercise and will often liken their strong, compelling emotional and cognitive responses to very cloudy skies, reminding themselves of the sky that exists behind the clouds even if they cannot see it. Other clients will evoke the image of a mountain when they are distressed, finding that sense of stillness inside themselves in the midst of disruptions on their surface and continuing to act in their lives in part due to that sense of stillness and transcendence.

One aspect of these practices that can be very clinically useful is their illustration of how clients are not their thoughts, reactions, feelings, or sensations. The observer self exercise and mountain meditation both evoke a sense of some kind of transcendent observer of these experiences who is distinct from the content-driven self with which clients so often identify. This sense allows clients to disentangle from ideas of themselves that have developed over their lifetimes, such as "I am a nervous wreck," "I am unassertive," or "I always fail at things." Experiencing these evaluations as thoughts that rise and fall and are no more constant than the weather or the seasons can help clients open themselves up to acting in ways that are inconsistent with these definitions of self. For instance, a client can have the thought that she is unassertive while she clearly communicates her needs to someone.[10] The repeated experience of separateness from these formerly defining thoughts and feelings increases clients' behavioral flexibility and reduces their motivation to avoid these thoughts and feelings (because nondefining thoughts and feelings are less threatening than defining ones).

Noticing the Wisdom of Experience and the Limits of Language

Other defusion strategies can be drawn from ACT. Therapists can talk to clients about the ways that language fails to capture the complexity of experience. For instance, we talk about how we do not tell babies how to walk—they have to experience it, take risks, have accidents, and try something new to learn. Similarly, reading a book doesn't teach one how to play tennis or drive a car—language leaves a great deal out, and direct experience is often needed for learning.

We also encourage therapists to adopt certain language conventions and encourage clients to do the same to cultivate a different relationship to their internal experiences. As we noted above, thoughts, feelings, memories, and sensations are labeled as such. Similarly, to break the fusion between internal experiences and behavior, clients are urged to move away from using thoughts and feelings as reasons for action or inaction. While it is socially acceptable to say, "I wanted to keep my appointment, but I was too depressed," or "I couldn't ask her out on a date because I was too anxious," those statements are typically not entirely accurate. While reasons for inaction and avoidance can sound like facts, they may actually reflect judgments and/or choices that are often hidden or difficult to see. One can physically attend an appointment while being depressed or ask someone on a date while feeling anxious. Our reasoning happens so quickly

---

[10]Within Buddhist traditions, these experiences gradually lead to an awareness that all definitions of self are insufficient, leading to a perception of no-self. While transcending limited definitions of oneself falls within the psychological domain, the broader implications of transcending any sense of self fall within a more spiritual domain and are not a part of our treatment approach. Instead, we direct clients who begin to raise these types of questions to Buddhist sources and resources for exploration of these issues.

and others take us at our word, so we do not even notice the assumption inherent in that kind of reasoning (i.e., that we cannot do something if we will be anxious doing it). Thus, we ask clients to consider whether replacing the "but" in these sorts of statements with "and" might be a more accurate way of conveying the relationship between internal experiences and behavior. Combining these two language conventions, a client might be encouraged to say, "I wanted to keep my appointment" *and* "I noticed some sad feelings" *and* "I noticed an urge to avoid the appointment." Loosening the relationship between our words and our experience allows us to be guided more effectively by our experience rather than limited by our language.

OBSTACLES IN CULTIVATING MINDFULNESS AND ACCEPTANCE

Mindfulness as a Way to Avoid Distress

Clients often find the practice of mindfulness pleasant or relaxing and can begin to engage in it to alleviate their distress. It is important to notice and discuss this process, both validating the inevitability of enjoying that consequence and highlighting the cost of clinging to that outcome. We encourage clients to be present to whatever emerges from their practice, to notice when they begin to judge an outcome as more or less desirable, and to gently let go of that judgment and return to the experience itself. Clients will usually notice variability in their responses to their practice, providing an opportunity to observe the effects of wishing for one outcome when another occurs. This situation can help clients see how their desires to reduce their distress can, in fact, escalate it. Clients should practice noticing any distress that occurs, observing their understandable desire for their distress to subside, and choosing instead to acknowledge their experience, perhaps "invite" it to "sit next to" them, and continue with their practice.

If clients repeatedly experience mindfulness practice as pleasant, we invite them to practice mindfulness in more distressing contexts in order to ensure that they also have experiences during the course of therapy in which mindfulness is difficult or challenging rather than have these experiences emerge as obstacles following termination. Mindful emotion practice provides an excellent opportunity to practice with distressing responses, as does informal mindful practice in challenging emotional contexts that arise during their lives. Also, when clients begin to engage in valued actions (as described in the next chapters), they often find that they experience increased distress and emotional arousal, leading to more challenging mindfulness practice.

Sometimes clients engage in mindfulness practice that serves an experientially avoidant function by emphasizing concentration over mindfulness. Although ABBTs may use concentration forms of mindfulness initially to help clients develop their attention abilities (such as focusing on the breath), clients are encouraged over time to broaden their attention so that they are aware of whatever arises rather than using a concentrative focus (such as the breath, an image, or a mantra) as a way to avoid any distressing content that occurs. We often talk to clients about expanding awareness to include whatever arises or adding new content to what is already present; thus, clients can notice their breath *and* the anxious thought that just arose rather than using the breath to avoid the thought. Clients' own experiences will usually show them the futility of the latter approach, as the anxious thought usually comes right back, during life if not during practice. We remind clients that we are trying to cultivate a way for them to be engaged in their lives, not a way for them to get a brief respite from their lives.

Experiential Avoidance

Conversely, sometimes clients have been so actively avoiding their own pain and suffering that they immediately find mindfulness practice and an acceptance stance very distressing and begin to avoid it. Clients who have restricted their lives significantly without noticing may feel saddened when they begin to attend to their experience more openly. They may find the thoughts and feelings that arise during practice and during their daily lives upsetting and look for reasons to avoid practice and awareness. Therapists can respond empathically to these experiences; if it were easy to open up to our experiences, we would all do it naturally, and clearly we do not. It is human to want to stay away from pain and distress, but clients can look at their own experiences to see whether these efforts to shut out or stay away from pain have been helpful. We find the tug-of-war metaphor from ACT can be helpful to illustrate the way that the struggle actually keeps distress present. We ask clients to imagine their distress (sadness, anxiety, anger, pain, etc.) is a monster and that they are engaged in a tug-of-war with it, with a large pit between them. The distress monster is trying to pull them toward the pit, which is a deep abyss that they do not want to fall into, so they pull with all their might, using both hands and planting their feet. The harder they pull, the harder the monster pulls back. It seems like the only thing they can do to avoid falling into the pit is keep pulling. Yet there is another option—they could drop the rope. The monster would still be there, but they would no longer be moving toward the pit, and they would be able to do other things with their hands and feet rather than struggling with the monster. Mindfulness practice can be one example of "dropping the rope." We find that clients often take to this metaphor and actually imagine themselves dropping a rope as they make a choice *not* to struggle with their pain either during their formal practice or, most important, as they live their lives. As clients begin to practice "dropping the rope" or allowing their emotional experience and find that their internal experiences may not dissipate but do not intensify in the same ways, it often becomes easier for them to continue to practice.

Mindfulness Requires Too Much Time

We have found that it can be difficult for clients to see the value of mindfulness practice, particularly early in treatment, so sometimes we have to work to enhance their motivation to practice. We find that revisiting our model for why mindfulness practice may be beneficial can be helpful in these cases. While validating doubts clients may have about the potential usefulness of this practice, therapists can ask them to commit to trying some of the prescribed exercises and watching to see whether or not they seem beneficial. For instance, the following exchange might take place:

> CLIENT: I just couldn't set aside any time for the practice this week. I have too much else going on.
>
> THERAPIST: I know how challenging it can be to find extra time. Can you give me an example of a particular day and what happened when you tried to practice?

CLIENT: Well, the day after I saw you, I thought I would wake up in the morning and do the breathing for a few minutes. I got up, and I went to the corner of my room where I was planning to set up my practice. But then I started thinking about everything I had to do that day, and I just didn't see how sitting and doing nothing would help at all.

THERAPIST: I see. So, part of what happened is that it didn't feel like practicing would be useful for you, given everything you have going on. Is that right?

CLIENT: Yeah, I guess so. I mean I understand what you said about how doing this would help me to see my emotions differently, but when I have so many things on my plate, I just don't feel like I can indulge myself in this kind of thing. People are counting on me to do things for them.

THERAPIST: I really understand that reaction. I find that myself when I'm trying to set aside time to practice. It's so incredibly hard to feel like sitting and not doing anything will do anything other than give us less time to do all the things we need to. And it can feel selfish. Yet, in my experience, when I force myself to take a little time and do these kinds of exercises, I actually find that I am able to do the other things I need to do more efficiently and with less distress than if I don't, and I'm able to be with other people and meet their needs better. But it's really hard to trust that, particularly at the beginning. So, in a way, I'm asking you if you can take a leap of faith and just do these practices, even if they feel like a waste of time, for a couple of weeks. I promise if, after a few weeks of practicing, you haven't seen anything about them that seemed useful, we can move on to trying other things. But I really think that practicing noticing your experience and your breath is going to help you feel less overwhelmed by the rest of your life over time. Do you think it's worth trying it out, given how bad you have been feeling?

CLIENT: Well, when you say it like that, I guess it's worth trying something instead of not trying at all.

THERAPIST: Great. Now, just to really help you get started, what about trying to practice for only 5 minutes a day this coming week?

CLIENT: Really? Is that enough time?

THERAPIST: The main thing is to start to develop this new habit. And it's a hard habit to develop. It's much better to practice for 5 minutes regularly than to set your goals so high that you don't do it at all. So, let's make it easier for you to feel like it's worth the sacrifice to start out. Then maybe we can increase the time if you find it useful.

CLIENT: OK, I can definitely do 5 minutes.

THERAPIST: OK. Now, remember, you're still probably going to feel like it's a waste of time. And you might still feel that after you practice. Practice might be boring or anxiety-provoking, or you might feel bad at it and think, 'Why did she tell me to do this?' Do you think you can stick with it even if all of those things happen?

CLIENT: Yeah, I can do anything for 5 minutes. I'll remember what we said and just do it anyway.

In this example, the therapist used several strategies to help the client make this initial commitment. First, she validated the feeling that mindfulness practice is a waste of time. She shared her own genuine experiences of feeling the same way. She acknowledged that practicing initially really involves a leap of faith. She also addressed the client's concern that practicing is selfish by describing her own experience of feeling more connected to and responsive to others when she practices. This is something that clients often notice on their own later in therapy, but it can be helpful to suggest the possibility before they have had the chance to experience it themselves. Finally, she reduced the assigned practice so that it would seem particularly manageable for the client. We wouldn't necessarily do all of these in a single exchange, but they are all ways to address clients' concerns about practice being a poor use of their time.

In our experience, even early, brief mindfulness practices increase many clients' awareness of how rarely they attend to the present and how they may be missing out on living their lives as a result. Detailed discussion of practice experiences will help identify any effects that emerge and highlight them for the client to reinforce continued practice. Furthermore, clients often have at least some experience of mindfulness deepening their experience of life after some degree of practice, so a commitment to practice for a few weeks is usually enough to engage them in more consistent and sustained mindfulness practice. When practice lapses later on, as it often does, clients typically have their own experience and observations to draw from regarding how regular practice improves their lives.

Evolving Challenges of Acceptance

We have found that, while some clients experience challenges with acceptance and mindfulness when the concepts are first introduced, others seem to take to the ideas immediately and develop difficulties later in treatment. For instance, one client initially opened himself up to his emotional experiences, engaged fully in mindfulness exercises, and expressed a strong commitment to practicing acceptance in his life. When he began identifying the areas of life that mattered to him and taking actions in valued directions, however, he reverted to a more avoidant emotional style and began questioning the value of accepting his responses. Altering habitual patterns of restricting one's life can be unsettling and distressing, opening up fears and responses that clients have been successfully avoiding for years. It is important to validate clients' understandable reluctance to accept these reactions and their impulse to avoid or reduce this distress in any manner that seems available to them. We find it helpful to reiterate the treatment model, using examples of clients' own observations from earlier in treatment to help them reconnect to the experiences that support this model. This approach can help clients continue their practice in the face of increased distress and have new experiences that support its usefulness to their lives. We often predict for clients that mindfulness and acceptance may become more challenging as they begin to engage their lives more fully, suggesting that they may feel more pain initially as they expand their lives, but their practice of mindfulness can help them notice this distress as it arises, see it as transient thoughts and feelings, and open up fully to the experience (rather than trying to push it away), thus lessening the potentially disruptive nature of this distress.

WHAT IS MINDFULNESS?

In this treatment, we will talk about the role of *awareness* as a first step to helping us make changes in our lives. In particular, we will focus on a special kind of awareness called *mindfulness*. The term *mindfulness* comes from Eastern spiritual and religious traditions (like Zen Buddhism), but psychology has begun to recognize that, removed from the spiritual and religious context, it may be used to improve physical and emotional well-being. Although many of the ideas we suggest here will be consistent with Eastern philosophies and traditions, we will not be focusing on the religious or spiritual parts of mindfulness, and we believe this approach can be useful no matter what your religious or spiritual preference.

Mindfulness is nonjudgmental (or compassionate), present-moment awareness of what is going on inside of us and around us. We often live our lives focused on something other than what is happening in the moment—worrying about the future, ruminating about the past, focusing on what is coming next rather than what is right in front of us. It is useful that we can do a number of things without paying attention to them. We can walk without thinking about walking, which allows us to talk to the person we're walking with without having to think, "Now I should lift up this foot." However, this ability to do things automatically, without awareness, also allows us to lose touch with what is happening right in front of us. We can develop habits (such as avoiding conflict) that we aren't aware of and that may not be in line with our broader goals.

Sometimes we do pay close attention to what we are thinking and feeling, and we become very critical of our thoughts and feelings and either try to change them or to distract ourselves because judgmental awareness can be very painful. For example, we might notice while we are talking to someone new that our voice is wavering, or we aren't speaking clearly, and think, "I'm such an idiot! What is wrong with me? If I don't calm down, this person will never like me!"

Being mindful falls between these two extremes. We pay attention to what is happening inside and around us, we acknowledge events and experiences as what they are, and we allow things we cannot control to be as they are while we focus our attention on the task at hand. For example, when talking to someone new we might notice those same changes in our voice, take a moment to reflect, "This is how it is now. There go my thoughts again," and gently bring our attention back to the person and our conversation. This second part of mindfulness—letting go of the need to critically judge and change our inner experience—is particularly tricky. In fact, often being mindful involves practicing being nonjudgmental about our tendency to be judgmental!

We think that being mindful is a personal experience that can bring some flexibility to your life, and we will work together to find the best ways to apply this approach.

Here are a few points about mindfulness:

• *Mindfulness is a process.* We do not *achieve* a final and total state of mindfulness. It is a way of being in one moment that comes and goes. Mindfulness is losing our focus 100 times and returning to it 101 times.

• *Mindfulness is a habit.* Just like we have learned to go on automatic pilot by practicing it over and over, we can learn mindfulness through practice. The more we practice, the easier it can be to have moments of mindfulness.

(continued)

• *Mindfulness activities come in many different forms.* People engage in formal mindful practices like meditation, yoga, and tai chi. These practices can take hours or even days. People can also be mindful for a moment—attending to their breath at any point during the course of their day and noticing their experience. All forms of mindful practice can be beneficial. We will focus most on briefer, daily practice within treatment, but you may find that you also want to seek other, more formal modes of mindful practice outside of therapy or once therapy ends.

• *Mindfulness brings us more fully into our lives.* Sometimes, especially early in treatment, we will practice mindfulness in ways that seem very relaxing and removed from the stressors of our daily lives, but the ultimate goal is to use mindfulness to keep us more fully in our lives and to improve our overall life satisfaction. Mindfulness can allow us to pause and ready ourselves for some event (e.g., focusing on our breathing for a moment *before* we answer the phone) and bring us more fully into an event (e.g., being present and focused in the moment when we are interacting with someone rather than thinking about what they may be thinking or worrying about what might be coming next).

SKILLS OF MINDFULNESS

These aspects of mindfulness require practice and cultivation. We can all continue to attend to these elements and develop them further throughout our lives. Keep them in mind as you develop your own practice and watch how they emerge, fade, and reemerge.

Awareness

- Learning to focus one's attention rather than having it be in many places at once
- Becoming aware of thoughts, emotions, and bodily sensations as well as sights, sounds, smells, and tastes

Nonjudgmental Observation

- Developing a sense of compassion toward one's internal experience
- Becoming aware of the constant judgments we make about our experiences
- Stepping back and noticing experiences without labeling them as "good" or "bad"

Staying in the Moment

- Observing the here and now rather than focusing on the past and future
- Practicing patience with the present moment rather than rushing to whatever is next
- Participating in experiences as they occur

Beginner's Mind

- Observing things as they really are rather than letting what we think we "know" to be true cloud our experience
- Becoming open to new possibilities

PRACTICING MINDFULNESS

Mindfulness skills can be practiced both formally, during scheduled meditation, and informally, during your everyday activities. Below is a list of activities that may be practiced mindfully. While doing these activities, practice the skills of mindfulness covered in session.

- Notice internal and external events, trying to focus your attention on the things happening around you and the thoughts, feelings, sensations, and images that come up and noticing when your attention wanders.
- Practice patience with the present moment, staying in this moment and noticing the urge to rush ahead to the next thing.
- Try to notice judgments of your experience and of yourself. Try to be compassionate in your awareness of your internal experience, practicing having your thoughts and feelings without labeling them as "good" or "bad."
- Notice the urge to judge things based on past experiences. Attempt to bring beginner's mind to the experience, observing things as they are rather than as you think they will be.
- Notice the urge to hold on to certain feelings (e.g., happiness, relaxation) and the urge to push other feelings away (e.g., sadness, anxiety). Practice letting go of this struggle, just allowing thoughts and feelings to come and go as they will.

You can practice mindfulness while you do just about anything. Here are some suggested activities to try mindfully:

Eating	Driving
Breathing	Cooking
Sitting	Listening to music
Walking	Examining an object
Washing dishes	Hugging someone
Taking a shower	Working
Talking on the phone	Listening to a friend

MINDFULNESS PRACTICE

Please complete a row of this monitoring sheet at the end of each day.

This week, please practice the following mindfulness exercise:

We would like you to note how often you practice mindfulness. We are interested in both *formal* activities that may be used to promote mindfulness (e.g., yoga, meditation, etc.) and any other activities that you performed in a mindful way (*informal*). For instance, although it is not usually done this way, it is possible to wash dishes in a mindful manner, attending to the experience fully (for instance, the feel of the hot water, the smell of the dish soap, etc.). Other *informal* activities that you can perform mindfully might include breathing, playing with your kids, or driving your car. So, at the end of the day, please note in the columns how many times you did each type of activity. You don't have to write the type of activity. If you notice anything related to your practice of mindfulness that you want to remember, feel free to jot down these thoughts in the comments section.

Date	Assigned Activity	Formal Mindfulness Activities	Informal Mindfulness Activities	Comments

SEVEN

Setting the Stage for Behavioral Change

The ultimate goal of ABBT is to expand the behavioral repertoire of the client such that the quality and vitality of the client's life is enhanced. Clients often develop restricted behavioral repertoires in an attempt to limit their exposure to situations and activities that elicit painful and negatively evaluated internal events. Furthermore, because we are able to *imagine* potentially threatening or painful future events, clients can also develop a defensive and ineffective way of responding to what *could happen* that often gets in the way of responding to what is *actually happening*. ABBT is aimed at moving the client from a place where action is dictated by what one must do or not do to avoid stress/anxiety to a place of choice and valued action. It involves encouraging clients to attempt and repeatedly practice new responses such as approach behaviors and mindful engagement in activities as they unfold. Practicing new responses opens up the possibility of behavioral choice and allows clients to be more flexible in choosing from a range of possible options.

Improving the quality of a client's life is a universal goal shared by all theoretical orientations to psychotherapy, but it is often considered secondary to other goals such as insight or symptom reduction. In traditional CBT approaches, behavioral change is often most notable as a marker of symptom reduction. For example, the relative success of a course of treatment for MDD might be partially indicated by the extent to which the client engages in daily pleasant events. A positive outcome of exposure therapy for anxiety disorders includes regular engagement in situations that were previously feared or avoided. Finally, the development and employment of a previously missing skill set is often the focus of behavior therapy. In contrast, although acceptance-based behavioral approaches are often associated with symptom reduction and the development of new skills, the overarching goal of living a valued life is an explicit focus of therapy.

In this chapter, we provide a broad overview of the concept of valuing, a component of ACT that can be incredibly powerful in evoking meaningful behavioral change (Hayes, Strosahl, & Wilson, 1999; Wilson & Murrell, 2004). In therapy, we feel it is important to engage clients experientially with their values prior to defining those values, so we begin this domain with assessment and a series of between-session writing assignments related to values (described later in this chapter), before we discuss the characteristics of values in session. In the current chapter, however, we define the characteristics of values first (using examples of how we present this material to clients) to enable the reader to develop a deeper sense of this construct. Next, we describe our assessment process and present a progression of clinical methods that can be used to encourage clients to reconnect with and define their values and to observe obstacles to their ability to consistently engage in valued behavior. Throughout this chapter, we also discuss some obstacles to behavioral change that we often encounter and offer some suggestions to consider when responding to these issues. The work described in this chapter sets the stage for the remainder of therapy, in which acceptance and mindfulness techniques are integrated with values and commitment work in the service of significantly impacting the client's behavior and quality of life.

AN INTRODUCTION TO THE CONCEPT OF VALUES

Values are "chosen qualities of action that can be insinuated in behavior but not possessed like an object" (Hayes, 2004, p. 22) and reflect what it is a client wants his or her life to stand for. For example, one might value developing and maintaining intimate relationships, engaging in challenging and fulfilling work, and living a healthy lifestyle. Valued actions are specific activities that clients engage in (or avoid) that are consistent with their personally held values, such as asking a friend to lunch, heading up a new project at work, or participating in a yoga class.

Given the various uses of the word "values," we have found it useful to clarify that we use the term to represent what personally matters to our clients and that it does not have any moral or religious connotations for us. We use a number of psychoeducational methods, experiential exercises, and between-session assignments to help clients connect with the concept of values and bring values into their lives. Specifically, we try to communicate several core characteristics of values in our clinical work.

Values versus Goals

Values are distinguished in several ways from the more traditional CBT concept of goals. Although goals can sometimes be quite useful in directing behavior, they also have some characteristics that can limit their utility in promoting a healthy and fulfilling lifestyle. For instance, goals are future-focused and inherently favor where *someone should be* over where he or she currently is. While these properties can make goals motivating, they can also engender feelings of discontent and hopelessness and promote nonacceptance of the present moment. In contrast, values are present-centered and encourage ongoing participation and engagement in meaningful activities.

Valuing is conceptualized as process or direction (e.g., caring about one's physical health and well-being), whereas a goal is an end point or outcome (e.g., losing 10 pounds). Although one can often meet or achieve a particular goal, values can never be fully satisfied or permanently obtained. Despite their different functions, goals and values are often interrelated: values can be thought of as the glue between goals. For example, one might have the goal of going out on a date, which may be driven by a closely held value of developing, nurturing, and maintaining intimate relationships.

Whereas the goal can be met, valuing is an ongoing process that can direct behavior before a relationship is initiated and continue to inform and cultivate a deeper, more intimate relationship as it unfolds.

In our own clinical work, we ask clients to consider and discuss both their positive and negative experiences with goals. Clients can often appreciate times when goals have kept their behavior on track and connect with ways in which goals have been associated with procrastination and disappointment. We often use Handout 7.1 (p. 162) to summarize many of the points described above. We also use the following metaphor adapted from ACT to distinguish these two constructs (Hayes, Strosahl, & Wilson, 1999):

> "Suppose you really enjoy downhill skiing, and you plan a trip for weeks. Finally, the day of your ski trip arrives; you purchase your lift ticket, wait in line, and arrive at the top of the hill. As you are about to push off, a man steps up and asks you about your goal: 'Where are you trying to get to?' When you reply, 'the bottom of the hill,' he insists he can help you attain that goal and promptly hustles you into a helicopter, flies you to the bottom of the hill, and disappears. Consider how you might feel. Although the goal of skiing is to get to the bottom of the hill, the fun is in the process. Having the goal of getting to the bottom is important because it allows you to engage in the process, but the value in skiing is swooshing down the powdered hill.
>
> "It is similar to falling in love. Imagine that your goal is to commit to a life partner. You attend a party and catch the eye of an attractive and engaging man or woman across the room. Magically, your life fast-forwards through the process and resumes normal speed at the moment you achieve your goal. Next thing you know, you are walking away with this man or woman who is now your life partner. You got to skip the awkward moments, the first fight, and meeting your in-laws, but you also skipped the anticipation of the first kiss, the warm glow that accompanies feelings of true connection, and the experience of professing your love in the company of friends and family during the wedding or commitment ceremony.
>
> "Consider whether this characterization fits with your experience. Goals are useful in that they keep us pointed in valued directions, but we may need to hold them lightly so that the real point of living can remain clear."

A clinical example can be useful in illustrating some of the subtle distinctions between values and goals. Amy, a young female client diagnosed with chronic PTSD related to sexual assault, presented to therapy with the expressed goal of finding a life partner. She was extremely fearful of her thoughts, memories, and emotions related to the assault, and she avoided most interpersonal situations for fear that they would elicit these unwanted experiences. Although her goal of being in an intimate relationship seemed beneficial for treatment, over time it became more apparent that it was not serving a motivational function. Amy was very isolated, and she spent a significant proportion of her time imagining how wonderful life would be if only she had been lucky enough to find the right partner. She would regularly contrast her current self with her idealized future self, and she maintained a mental list of the ways she needed to "be fixed" before she could work on her goal (e.g., she needed to stop ruminating about her sexual abuse, she needed to be happier and less depressed, and she needed to feel whole).

Using many of the methods discussed in this chapter, we took a values approach when working with Amy. We explored the value of "having intimate connections with others" that informed her relationship goal and encouraged her to take some actions consistent with that value (e.g., making eye contact, bringing mindful listening skills to her conversations, disclosing her thoughts and feelings to others) in her current relationships (e.g., with her therapist, her physicians, the other women in her psychotherapy group, and the women she lived with in her residential program) even while she still experienced ruminations, sad feelings, and thoughts of inadequacy. Over time, Amy began to develop more friendships and eventually began dating. Her goal was ultimately met but, more important, the overall quality of her life improved as she began to act in accordance with her value and connect with many people on a daily basis.

Valuing as a Behavior

Most acceptance-based approaches to therapy stress the importance of viewing behavior as independent from internal events such as thoughts or feelings. For instance, emotion regulation skills in DBT describe engaging in "opposite action," in which one intentionally acts in a way counter to the action tendency of a particular emotion. Thus, a client who is experiencing sadness and feeling an urge to isolate him- or herself would intentionally engage with others to separate his or her behavior from this emotional state. Similarly, traditional cognitive-behavioral approaches such as exposure therapy (in which clients are asked to endure urges to escape and avoid while remaining in fear-eliciting situations) and pleasant event scheduling (in which clients are urged to try out activities that once were viewed as pleasurable regardless of what they are currently feeling) encourage clients to act in ways that are inconsistent with their internal experiences.

Valuing itself is defined as an action or behavior that is distinguished from a feeling state or a belief. It is expected that clients will often experience thoughts and feelings that are inconsistent with their stated values. The trouble occurs when a client interprets this inconsistency to mean that he or she is flawed in some way or sees it as a signal that the behavior or the value needs to be changed. Take the example of Sarah, who values engaging in personally challenging activities that promote health and well-being. If Sarah decided to try out for a competitive swim team, we would expect her to have some feelings of fear and uncertainty that she could be encouraged to bring with her as she engaged in a new, values-consistent activity. Sarah would be valuing as a behavior. If, however, Sarah struggled with the inconsistency between her values and her internal state, if she interpreted her feelings to be a sign that swimming was dangerous (and, thus, not values-consistent), if she concluded that she was flawed in some fundamental way for having those thoughts and feelings and ultimately chose to skip tryouts, this response could be considered life-interfering.

When working from an acceptance-based behavioral perspective, it is important to normalize the mismatch between internal experiences and valued actions. In therapy, we offer several examples of ways in which people often behave consistent with their values while having inconsistent thoughts and feelings. For instance, most people who have been involved with exercising can relate to the example of someone who chooses to go to the gym even while experiencing thoughts and feelings that are inconsistent with such an action (e.g., "I would rather be home watching television. I don't feel like doing this"). Similarly, many clients have had the experience of attending a medical or dental appointment even while having thoughts or feelings inconsistent with that behavior ("I don't want to be here. This is really unpleasant"). A more nuanced example that underscores the association between behavior and internal states is that of relationships. One's feelings toward a valued friend likely vacillate on a moment-to-moment or day-by-day basis, yet, in order for a long-term relationship to weather these fluctuations, one needs consistently to behave like a friend.

Building on the mindfulness and defusion skills already acquired in therapy, clients are encouraged to observe disconnections between moment-to-moment internal experiences and longer-held personal values. Whereas a past habit may have been to behave in a way that is consistent with one's mood, clients are urged to consider using values as a compass to direct their behavior.

Values Are Choices

Given the wide repertoire of behaviors available to most individuals, values are useful in directing choices (Hayes, Strosahl, & Wilson, 1999). In ABBT, valuing itself is a highly personal choice that cannot be evaluated or judged. One can freely choose to hold a particular value, and no rational reasoning or justification must be done in order to defend or explain its adoption.

This characteristic of ABBT differs from some approaches to problem solving used in traditional CBT. With some forms of CBT, clients are encouraged to develop a pros and cons list in an attempt to rationally derive the "right" answer to a problem or the "right" decision based on an opportunity. While we agree that there are some benefits to acknowledging and fully processing one's potential choices, this method can paralyze a client who fears making the wrong decisions. Furthermore, if someone holds a particularly strong value, he or she may choose to act in accordance with that value despite a number of logical reasons opposed to doing so. While it can definitely be helpful fully to consider the options, the final choice is exactly that: a choice.

For example, one may be able to enumerate a number of logical reasons not to try to get pregnant while pursuing one's first tenure-track faculty position (e.g., having a baby will interfere with your research productivity; potential interviewers will not take a pregnant applicant seriously or will have concerns about her commitment to the department) and still choose to try to conceive if it is consistent with one's most deeply held values. One could also easily develop a list of reasons to stay in an abusive relationship (e.g., I have nowhere to go; I cannot afford to live on my own; my children will grow up without a father; I am afraid I will never find someone else to love me) and still choose to leave.

In our own practice, we use several exercises from ACT to help clients consider the option of choice. Starting with a relatively trivial preference (e.g., Coca-Cola vs. Pepsi or chocolate vs. vanilla), we ask our clients to defend their choice to value one over another. While the first few queries often elicit quick responses (e.g., because I like the taste), it quickly becomes difficult to generate logical answers to follow-up questions (e.g., Why do you like the taste? Why do you prefer a less creamy taste?), and clients often get to the point of "just because" or "for no reason." Together, we explore the possibility that "just because that is what I choose" is a reasonable explanation supporting all of one's values.

The Relationship between Values and Emotions

We often discuss with clients the complex relationship between our emotions and our values. Emotional pain (such as sadness or anger) can be a signal that we are not living in accordance with our values. For instance, Patricia presented for treatment for help with chronic MDD. She expressed significant self-loathing and viewed herself as psychologically and biologically flawed because of her MDD. Using many of the mindfulness and defusion strategies discussed in Chapters 5 and 6, we encouraged her to dismantle her experience of MDD and to observe passing emotions and thoughts as transient events. Through this method of self-monitoring and -observation she began to notice that her feelings of sadness and boredom were much more prevalent when she was at work. Her typical response had been to judge and avoid those internal experiences by distracting herself or calling in sick; however, as she became more willing to notice and acknowledge them, she came to recognize that she was not engaging in values-consistent activities at work. She was able to see the communicative function of her sad feelings, and she made some behavioral changes (e.g., increased her willingness to engage with others at work, directly addressed conflictual issues with her boss and coworkers, volunteered to challenge herself on a new project) that opened up opportunities for her to experience a fuller range of emotions.

Another way we relate emotions and values is to explore with our clients how efforts to avoid emotional pain often interfere with living a full, engaged, vital life. We validate many of the paradoxes inherent in the human condition. In order to experience love and connection, we need to open ourselves up to potential loss and rejection. Taking risks and reaching for our full potential involves a willingness to experience fear and uncertainty. To determine whether someone is truly trustworthy, we need to expose our vulnerabilities and observe how he or she responds. In other words, there is no way to achieve fullness and vitality without accepting pain and loss.

Often, clients will tell us that they opt to live without love, risk, and trust. They are willing to forgo the ups of life if they can prevent the downs. For instance, one of our clients, who was diagnosed with chronic PTSD related to interpersonal trauma, understandably chose to avoid pursuing relationships in the hope that she could avoid experiencing further emotional pain. From her perspective, past relationships had brought her sadness and anger, and the thought of pursuing new relationships elicited feelings of fear and dread. Therefore, it seemed to make sense that avoiding relationships would prevent her from experiencing more emotional pain. Using mindfulness and acceptance skills, this client came to observe that while avoiding interactions with others decreased the likelihood that she would experience surges in fear, she noticed the presence of a more chronic emotional pain associated with feelings of loneliness and the emptiness that often accompanies a life disconnected from valued action. When she recognized that her attempt to avoid pain was not working, she became more willing to explore alternative actions.

Valuing Is Already in Process

A core assumption underlying acceptance-based approaches is that the client is fundamentally and unconditionally whole (Styron, 2005), motivated to improve (Linehan, 1993a), and in possession of everything that is needed to define and adopt a valued life direction (Hayes, Strosahl, & Wilson, 1999). No client is too impaired, broken, or psychologically wounded to engage in a meaningful life, and no one needs to be "fixed" in order to participate in his or her own life.

However, when the concept of valuing is introduced, some clients feel that they are not yet ready to choose their values or to take value-consistent action. Clients may be unsure about what they value, feel motionless and stuck, or believe that they need to change internally in some way before they can pursue valued action. Yet clients are already valuing as a behavior, even if they are unaware of or numb to it (Hayes, Strosahl, & Wilson, 1999). We constantly make choices about how to behave on a moment-to-moment basis. Early in treatment, those choices are often influenced by the desire to avoid painful thoughts and feelings rather than by valued directions. An initial goal of ABBT is to make clients aware of their own values, to examine the relationship between those values and the choices clients are making about their behavior, to observe the consequences of current behavior, and to explore clients' willingness to consider engaging in other valued behaviors.

INITIAL VALUES ASSESSMENT

As described in Chapter 4, increasing behaviors in valued domains as a central goal of treatment is considered when setting the stage for treatment. In our experience, it can be extremely important to promote a careful discussion of this potential goal as most clients present to treatment with the primary (and often solitary) goal of decreasing the frequency and intensity of negatively evaluated emotions such as sadness, fear, and anger. Many clients are unaware of the subtle shifts they have made in their behavior that have taken them further from their valued directions. Other clients may be painfully aware of the lack of valued direction in their life but believe that radical internal changes are needed before behavioral change can occur. A number of clinical strategies can be used to help clients to gain a clearer perspective on the relationship between their values and their current behavior.

The Valued Living Questionnaire

In our own clinical practice, we begin our exploration of values during the assessment phase by examining the ways in which psychological symptoms such as anxiety, depression, and substance use are interfering in our clients' lives. As discussed in Chapter 2, as part of this initial assessment we administer the Valued Living Questionnaire (VLQ; Wilson & Groom, 2002), a two-part measure that assesses the importance of 10 valued domains of living, including (1) family, (2) marriage/couples/intimate relations, (3) parenting, (4) friendship, (5) work, (6) education, (7) recreation, (8) spirituality, (9) citizenship, and (10) physical self-care. First, clients are asked to rate, on a scale of 1–10, the current importance of each domain, then to rate how consistently they have lived in accord with those values over the past week, also on a scale of 1–10.

Focusing on Key Domains

Therapists and clients have some choices to make in terms of focusing on key valued domains in therapy. One approach could be to use the VLQ to select domains of focus, such as choosing domains that are ranked high in importance and low in consistency. Alternatively, one can ask clients to consider all of the 10 domains and to identify which domains they want to concentrate on in therapy. One potential obstacle with this approach is that clients who are highly avoidant may opt to work on less threatening but potentially less personally meaningful domains. For instance, one client we treated who was struggling with GAD reported significant distress over his career choices. He was interested in pursuing a managerial position, but his significant interpersonal fears were holding him back. He also reluctantly described some serious concerns regarding his relationship with his wife. His inconsistency in engaging in valued behaviors in these two domains was causing him clear distress, but he opted to focus our time-limited therapy on becoming more physically fit. After a few sessions of working on that domain, he realized that things were becoming increasingly worse for him as he was avoiding working on areas of his life that needed significant attention. He acknowledged the role that avoidance was playing in his choice of values and decided to change course.

On the one hand, consistent with an ACT perspective (Hayes, Strosahl, & Wilson, 1999), we absolutely believe in "radically respecting" our clients' choices with regard to their personally held values. On the other, we believe that it is the therapist's job to raise the possibility of avoidance as a factor in choosing a domain for behavioral change. Unfortunately, sometimes it takes time to determine whether avoidance is driving values, which can be a concern particularly when therapy is time-limited.

Another possible approach to values work is to create a hierarchy similar to those used in traditional CBT. For instance, in working with the above-mentioned client, one might choose to work on health-related values early in treatment and move to more challenging domains at a later point in therapy. While this graduated approach can be useful, time constraints on therapy should be considered.

In our own clinical practice, we have grouped the 10 domains described in ACT into three main areas: interpersonal relationships, work/school/community, and self-nuturance and community involvement. Furthermore, rather than asking clients to choose one or two domains as the focus of therapy, all of our early assignments involve a consideration of all three domains. While we certainly attend to initial ratings of importance and consistency in each valued domain, we have found these shift as clients become more aware of their values, patterns of avoidance, and unwillingness. For example, one client we worked with initially indicated that he was living consistently with his relationship values, but as he increased his mindfulness practice, he became aware that, although he spent a significant amount of time hanging out with his friends, he engaged in a number of subtle strategies, such as making jokes and turning the attention to others, that were aimed at keeping people at arm's length. According to his ratings on the VLQ, midway through treatment this client appeared to be living less consistently with his values than he was before treatment began. Therefore, we have found that having clients explicitly consider all three domains of valued living for the first several sessions of therapy, regardless of their initial ratings of importance and consistency, increases their willingness to acknowledge behaviors in need of change more readily.

Values Writing Assignment 1:
Observing How Avoidance Is Restricting One's Life

At the end of the first or second therapy session, we typically ask our clients to complete an outside-of-session assignment aimed at exploring how their presenting issues may be interfering with their personally held values. This writing assignment modeled on the emotional processing task developed by James Pennebaker (1997) and adapted by Kelly Wilson (personal communication, 2000) involves asking clients to set aside 20 minutes a day for 4 days to explore their deepest emotions and thoughts about the ways in which their presenting problems are interfering with their ability to act consistent with their personally held values. On each of the first 3 days, clients are asked to write about the ways in which their presenting issues might be interfering with each of the three domains. We have found that including specific prompting questions helps clients engage more fully in the process. For instance, clients are asked to consider how their issues may be preventing them from asking for what they need in relationships or to explore what sort of self-care activities or hobbies they would consider if they were not struggling with psychological issues. On the fourth day, clients are asked to reflect on anything important that they may have noticed when completing the assignments. These assignments can be personally tailored to the presenting issues of the client. An example of the type of assignment we might suggest to a client struggling with GAD is displayed in Handout 7.2 (pp. 163–164). To introduce this assignment we might say something like:

> "Values refer to the things in life that matter to you, the ways of being that you associate with a meaningful and satisfying life. As we discussed earlier, valued domains can include things such as family or intimate relationships, friendships, career/education, spirituality, community service, and so on. Values reflect what is important, yet our struggle with our emotions, thoughts, and memories can often distract us from those values so that we miss important parts of our experience and/or avoid engaging in activities consistent with our values to avoid more stress.
>
> "We will continue to explore issues related to values over the next few sessions, but this week I would like to suggest that you consider making some time for yourself to think about the ways that your struggles have pulled you away from things you value."

Typical Responses to the Writing Assignment

Not surprisingly, clients have varied reactions to this initial assignment; therefore, it is important to discuss fully potential reactions to the task that may develop over the course of the week and to process the exercise sufficiently during the next therapy session. Some clients feel hopeful and empowered by the process. For others, obvious and subtle patterns of inaction in valued domains are often uncovered. Some clients are surprised by their lack of engagement in what appeared to be a value-consistent lifestyle. Many clients find the exercise elicits strong feelings of sadness as they notice how consumed they have become with internal struggles and how distant they feel from the things that really matter to them. Another common response is to avoid the assignment or to report that it was too difficult or painful to complete. All these responses are validated as we explore with our clients the potential changes they may choose to make in therapy.

Inaction in Valued Domains

Many of the clients we work with have reached a point where their attempts to avoid and control painful thoughts, strong emotions, uncomfortable physical sensations, and difficult memories have significantly narrowed their behavioral repertoires and pulled them away from an array of valued activities. This inaction in valued domains is reflected in their first writing assignment.

For example, Tony, a combat veteran with PTSD whom we saw in therapy, initially reported virtually no current behavior that was consistent with his personally held values. Despite his desire to nurture his relationships with his wife, children, and family of origin, he had moved out of his home and into a small apartment by himself, where he spent the majority of his time "bunkered in." While he valued fostering his creativity, he gave away his treasured guitar and refused to listen to music. He expressed a desire to live a healthy lifestyle yet smoked three packs of cigarettes a day, abused alcohol and Valium, and maintained unhealthy eating habits. In response to this apparent inconsistency between what was important to Tony and how he behaved, he responded that keeping his PTSD symptoms in check was a full-time job that left little time for living.

Kate, a client with social phobia, described the more subtle but insidious ways in which her desire to avoid evaluation had directed her away from engaging in valued activities. She had passed up a number of promotions at work as they would require her to make formal presentations and sales pitches and put her in a position of scrutiny. She often made up excuses (e.g., too much work to do, starting a new diet) to avoid going to lunch with coworkers because she feared that her self-evaluative thoughts would interfere with her ability to make conversation. During the initial assessment, Kate described herself as a quiet person who did not need many challenges in her life and preferred being alone, and she rated several domains of valued living as low in importance; however, during the first writing assignment, she revealed a self-awareness that her fear and anxiety were preventing her from taking risks and being the person she wanted to be.

Mindless Action in Valued Domains

Other clients with whom we have worked appear to be behaving in value-consistent ways, but deeper exploration makes it apparent that they are unable to truly engage in and enjoy these activities. For instance, Marcia, a client we treated for bulimia, was in a long-term loving relationship, pursuing a line of work that was personally meaningful, and raising two children. She seemed to have it all, and her acquaintances saw her as someone who "had it together." Her VLQ profile suggested that she was living consistent with her values, and social desirability did not seem to be a significant factor in her response style. During the first writing assignment, however, she poignantly described feeling like a spectator in her own life, as if she were just going through the motions. Although she chose a career that was consistent with her desire to be challenged at work, she reported that feelings of guilt and thoughts about her children being "neglected" in day care undermined her ability to be psychologically present in the office. In the evenings, when she was home with the children, she would dutifully play with them while ruminating over events from work and worrying about the next project she had to complete.

Loss of Sense of Choice and Purpose

Some of our clients describe having lost the sense of choosing valued directions when they complete the first writing assignment. In other words, life seems full of things that "have to" or that "should" get done. Our client Lei, a graduate student in history, reported a disconnect from the values that had initially pointed her toward graduate school, an interest in challenging herself intellectually and a desire to engage in work aimed at improving the lives of others. She had become increasingly focused on the goal of obtaining her PhD, and she began to view her daily activities (e.g., reading, writing, and conducting research) as representing hoops that she needed to jump through in order to get to where she wanted to be. She felt as if program requirements were controlling her life, and she no longer experienced the inherent value of her work.

Unwillingness/Inability to Complete the Assignment

If a client does not complete this assignment (or any other), our first response is to explore the function and effectiveness of that behavior. We view noncompliance as a behavioral response that can help us better understand our clients and deepen the therapeutic relationship. There are several reasons clients may not complete the values assignments and we explore with them to see which, if any, are relevant. For instance, sometimes clients do not understand the instructions and/or are unclear how this exercise will be useful to them. This is important information that a therapist can use to improve his or her description of the rationale for the assignment. For instance, Maurice was a court-referred client whom we treated after he was arrested for engaging in exhibitionism. Although he agreed to complete the values assignment several times, week after week he claimed to have forgotten it. When the therapist told Maurice that she felt like understanding why he did not bring the assignment in would help her help him meet his therapy goals, he admitted not seeing the link between exploring his values and changing his sexual habits but had been hesitant to bring up his concerns to the therapist because he was ordered by the court to comply with treatment.

A very real concern may be finding time in clients' busy schedules to complete the assignments. We do not underestimate the amount of time and effort it takes to make a radical change and to move from a life driven by avoidance to one motivated by values. Drawing from some acceptance-consistent methods of motivational interviewing (Miller & Rollnick, 2002), we often devote time in session to eliciting change talk in our clients. In other words, we urge them to discuss why they want to change and to connect with the real pain of stagnation and inaction. Fear and avoidance are strong motivators of noncompliance; in response, we encourage clients to apply the methods discussed throughout this volume (e.g., function of emotions, mindfulness, limits of control/avoidance). Clients who struggle with significant self-awareness or who are chronically disconnected from their sense of self may feel unable to articulate their values, but mindfulness practice can assist with values clarification by helping the client to choose valued directions reflexively rather than reactively (Shapiro et al., 2006). Some clients are afraid to commit to one set of values. As we discuss further in Chapter 8, values can change and evolve over time, particularly as clients increase self-awareness and willingness to experience a full range of emotions. Thus, we encourage clients to consider valuing as a process, the content of which might change as a function of growth.

ARTICULATING AND CLARIFYING ONE'S VALUES

Once an initial assessment and the first writing assignment are complete and the client has considered the importance and consistency of valued behavior and become more aware of the ways in which psychological struggles have interfered with valued pursuits, we encourage him or her to work on articulating a set of personally relevant values.

Values Writing Assignment 2

Our second outside-of-session values assignment typically involves asking clients once again to set aside 20 minutes a day for three different days to engage in written emotional processing. The focus of this assignment is for clients to consider their personal values in each of the three domains. Once again, the assignment includes some prompting questions to help clients consider multifaceted aspects of their values and can be modified according to their needs. For instance, clients might be asked to consider what sort of friend or partner they want to be, considering how open or private they would like to be and/or the type of support they would like to give to others. They could also be asked to describe the kind of employee they would like to be with respect to issues such as work habits, relationships with coworkers, and willingness to take on challenges. Finally, clients can be encouraged to write about how they would like to spend their free time, engaging in self-nurturance, recreational activities, or hobbies or becoming more involved with their community (whether or not they perceive themselves as having free time). An example of this values assignment is shown in Handout 7.3 (p. 165).

For most clients, this assignment is only a starting point for the exploration of values. Therefore, a significant amount of time is often spent discussing the assignment in subsequent sessions, and it is not uncommon for some clients to redo the assignment a second time outside of session. A number of issues described below often arise that deserve attention and discussion in session.

Confusing Values and Goals

Even though we spend time in session distinguishing values from goals, it is not uncommon for clients to confuse the two. For instance, one client wrote that her value was to be promoted at work. Another wanted to attend church regularly. While these goals can inform the development of values-consistent actions that can be pursued in therapy (and beyond), our perspective is that it is important clearly to define one's values initially, separate from the goals or valued actions that reflect the values.

Values Involve Changing Emotional States

Often, clients write about valuing particular internal states (e.g., confidence or self-esteem) or emotions (e.g., happiness, calmness). For instance, a client might express the following in the second writing assignment:

> "I would like to be a happy, self-confident person. I think if I were more agreeable
> and optimistic I would have a stronger relationship with my partner. I also would
> like to be more patient with my kids. For instance, when they get into fights with
> each other, I would like to remain cool, calm, and collected instead of flying off the
> handle. If I had higher self-esteem, I think I would have more friends. Basically,

at this point, I don't go out to lunch with my coworkers because I don't feel good enough about myself to spend time with them. Once I work out my esteem issues, I would like to have a stronger circle of friends."

A number of points can be considered when these sorts of values are expressed. Our typical response is to validate the very human desire to feel happy, calm, confident, and so on. We also relate that desire to concepts that have been the focus of previous sessions such as the function of emotion and the limits of attempts at controlling it. We empathically remind clients of their observations about the "human condition"; that with love comes loss and with risk, fear. From a very practical perspective, we believe that if people are engaging in valued activities, they will likely be happier and calmer, but happiness as a constant state is unachievable, and an acceptance of that reality is critical to free up a client to pursue valued activities that are likely to elicit a full range of emotions.

When clients endorse values related to achieving or avoiding emotional states, we often reconceptualize desires to achieve constant happiness, calmness, and high self-esteem (and the related desires to avoid sadness, anxiety, and judgmental negative thoughts) as barriers to valued living. Thus, we ask clients to consider what values they might hold if those obstacles were not present. In other words, we might ask a client to imagine what sort of friend they would want to be if they did not feel held back by sadness and fear.

Drawing from ACT (Hayes, Strosahl, & Wilson, 1999), we often spend some time considering the concept of confidence with our clients, particularly when they acknowledge valuing a state of self-confidence. It is common for people to think about confidence as a trait bestowed on others and as something that is hard to acquire. Self-confidence is often thought of as a state in which the individual has no self-doubt, fear, or negative self-evaluations, but confidence actually involves being true to oneself. In other words, self-confidence involves trusting or having faith in oneself, even in the face of fear. So, we can feel uncertain, doubtful, and/or frightened and still act in ways that demonstrate self-confidence or faith. Confidence is similar to courage, which entails acting while one is scared, not acting without fear. Thus, we encourage our clients to approach this assignment by expressing personally relevant ways of being that will allow them to act with self-confidence.

Values Perfection/Challenges Balancing Multiple Domains

It is not uncommon for this second values assignment to elicit the desire for perfection, as in the following example (which also illustrates a mixing of values and goals and valuing internal states):

> "I would like to be a loving, caring wife who is always there for my husband. I want to be a patient, fun-loving parent who is always attuned to the needs of my children. I want my house to be the place where all the kids hang out—I want to be the cool mom. I want to be a loyal friend. It is really important to me that I am the kind of person that all my friends can depend on—whenever they need me.
>
> "Going back to school is really important to me. If I get accepted to the program, I intend to be a model student and maintain a 4.0 grade point average."

Another example of striving for values perfection arises when a client feels as if action in one domain is pitted against action in another. The client feels unable to live in a way that is consistent with one domain without sacrificing another. For instance:

"On the one hand, I think that on the surface I have it all. I am the vice president of my company, and I earn enough money that my family can live quite comfortably. It is important to me that I am a good provider for the family. I always dreamed of having a large family, and I am thrilled that Debbie and I have five children. We have a pretty good social life—Debbie sets up dinner plans with other couples, I have some golfing partners, and so on—but sometimes I feel like a 'jack of all trades' and a 'master of none.' Even though I have achieved success at work, I am worried that I am viewed as less committed to the company when I take vacation time to spend with my family or if I leave work early to see a school play. I have five great kids, but I wish I could be around more—to coach Mark's baseball team or read to them at night. I know Debbie thinks I am not doing enough with the family. I know it is important to spend time with Debbie and with our friends, but, to tell you the truth, I am often exhausted at night and on the weekend, and I want to sprawl out on the couch and watch television. I value my career, my family, and my friends, but I have no idea how to give it my all in each of these areas. Sometimes I feel like my life is a juggling act—I am just trying to keep all the balls in the air."

Once again, it is important to validate the desire many of us share to be perfect and to discuss how difficult it can be at times to accept the limits associated with being human. We also spend some time exploring the function of "perfection." Often, clients strive to be perfect to be accepted and loved by others and to feel whole and acceptable. We normalize this desire and sometimes encourage clients to practice the accepting yourself on faith exercise described in Chapter 6 to see if they can let go of the need to earn acceptance. We also work with our clients to see if this desire is related to a value, such as developing intimate connections with others. Finally, just as we test the workability of other "rules," we encourage clients to examine whether their attempts to be perfect bring them closer to their values or push those values further away.

It is important to note that, besides the potential association with striving for perfection, the difficulties inherent in balancing valued action across domains are a real, inevitable challenge. We often make choices that are consistent with values in one domain but not another, and there are no clear guidelines for how to choose which domain to attend to in a given moment. At this point in therapy, we simply acknowledge this challenge and note that it is one we experience as well. We note that, in order to achieve a sense of balance across domains, we try to maintain a broad view and ensure that we are attending to each domain at some point across a period of time (a week, a month, or several months, depending on our current life circumstances). We share the metaphor of balancing our sides during yoga practice. We cannot stretch out our right and left leg at the same time. Instead, we stretch out our right leg, bring our awareness and attention only to this action, and then do the same for the other side. In the same way, we try to tend in a focused way to each domain of our lives, often one at a time, but make sure that, over time, none is ignored. Later in treatment, we return to this idea as clients make choices about valued actions, helping them choose in ways that provide overall balance within their lives.

Values That Are Dependent on Others

When people are asked to reflect on the things that matter to them, it is no surprise that the most strongly held values involve others, and while relationships often bring great satisfaction and comfort, they can also involve pain and distress. In the second values assignment, many clients express a strong desire for others to change. For instance:

> "I wish that my partner would really listen to me and be willing to do some of the things I am interested in. We spend so much time going to the movies, which she loves, but she isn't willing to go to concerts or listen to music, which is something I really value."

> "I really value open communication in the workplace, but that is just not possible with my boss. She really is a tyrant. If you disagree with her even the tiniest bit, she flips out. I just have to keep my head in the sand and collect my paycheck."

> "I wish I could have the kind of friendships that were give and take. I feel like all my friends just take, and they are not willing to give. Whenever they have a problem, they call, but no one is there for me when I need a true friend."

Clients can feel stuck and hopeless when they think they cannot pursue their values without depending on others. When these issues come up, we often liken attempts to control others to attempts to control our own internal states. We encourage clients to observe whether attempts to control others are successful and to notice their own emotions and reactions when they engage in attempts to control others. We also gently suggest that they can live consistent with their own values regardless of others' reactions.

For example, Rachel was a client diagnosed with dysthymia who was experiencing feelings of sadness and thoughts about negative self-worth. When she first wrote about her values, she expressed dismay over her current work situation. She often called in sick, and when she was in the office she wasted time surfing the Internet. She described a passive–aggressive pattern of interaction with her boss, whom she felt was an unreasonable and incompetent leader. Once Rachel began to see the connection between her behavior at work and her feelings of sadness, she concluded that she would need to change jobs immediately. She asserted that her current job did not challenge her and that her boss was a bully, but she also began to worry about and doubt her ability to pick the right job in the future, as during her interview for her current job she and her boss got along quite well.

Several sessions were devoted to exploring Rachel's values further. Although she valued being challenged at work, she felt as if the challenges needed to be externally imposed. Together, we explored ways that she might live consistent with her values even when she was in a situation that she did not view as ideal. While she had initially felt her current job was too mundane to involve challenges, using her mindfulness skills (particularly beginner's mind), she became able to define internal challenges that she could try in virtually any context. Consistent with a values-based approach, the emphasis was on the process, not the outcome. For example, she worked on really listening to what her customers, her coworkers, and her boss were trying to communicate. She began to examine processes in her office (such as the system for billing) to see if she could come up with more effective, timely methods of doing business. Rachel began to acknowledge that, whether or not others agreed with her or adopted her suggestions, she could behave in ways that were consistent with her values. Not surprisingly, many things did change for her when she began to engage in these new behavioral patterns.

To clarify, we absolutely supported Rachel's suggestion that she pursue a position that was more consistent with her values. Our philosophy is that if you can make a change that is likely to improve your mood and quality of life and that change is in the service of values and not avoidance-driven, then that change makes perfect sense. Our only concern is when a client expresses the belief that events beyond his or her control (either internal or external) must change in order for him or her to live a meaningful and vital life. From our experience, this perspective is rarely true; throughout history, humans have maintained their dignity and found meaning in the darkest of environments. Of course, there are contexts in which this is more challenging, and it is very important to validate the external realities (particularly those associated with structural inequalities and oppression) that impinge on an individual's well-being, but the therapist can concurrently help the client find ways to live a meaningful life even within real constraints.

Values Driven by Avoidance

When one is entrenched in a chronic pattern of avoidance, it can be difficult to gain enough perspective to see one's values clearly. For instance, a client may state that she would like to be somewhat private in relationships to save herself from getting hurt or to keep her friend or partner from knowing the real person inside. We would work with her to see if she could expand some from that position if anxiety, self-doubt, sadness, and the like could be magically removed. In other words, if the client did not feel compelled to avoid internal experiences (and external experiences guaranteed to raise difficult internal experiences), would her values shift? The goal is to try to get a sense of the client's values separate from her desire to avoid suffering.

One of our clients struggled when considering her career options. On the one hand, Laura valued much about her job as a waitress. She enjoyed interacting with customers, and she appreciated the freedom and flexibility her job gave her to pursue other valued interests, such as music and her relationship with her husband. On the other hand, Laura valued being challenged in her career. She was considering pursuing a management training program at the restaurant where she worked and reported that she was struggling with knowing her own "heart." Laura felt as if her waitressing job was consistent with her values, yet she feared that she might be fooling herself into believing so to avoid the risk associated with pursuing the management training program.

When the client and/or the therapist is concerned as to whether values are driven by avoidance, the most important thing to do is to avoid inaction. It can easily stall therapeutic progress if the therapist and client believe that clarity is needed before action. On the other hand, the pull to just choose a path in order to relieve or avoid the stress and anxiety associated with indecision must also be considered (Wilson & Murrell, 2004). Both of these options—halting action and becoming mired in indecision or impulsively choosing a path just to terminate the distress that often accompanies indecision—can limit the client from experiencing the freedom of choice (Wilson & Murrell, 2004).

Our typical response in this situation is to encourage the client to use all of the skills that he or she has already developed. Practicing acceptance and defusion, observing reality as it unfolds, considering the middle way in the face of what seems to be a black-and-white decision (such as choosing a job as a waitress or a manager), and emotionally processing values through writing assignments and in session can all help the client bring some wisdom to the possibilities of valued action. We also encourage the client to continue taking mindful action while experiencing indecision. For instance, in the case of Laura, we might encourage her to seek ways to challenge herself in her waitressing work, to pursue the other activities that are meaningful to her, and perhaps to seek more information about management/ownership opportunities and challenges. While we generally encourage commitment to a chosen value even in the wake of doubt and uncertainty (as we describe in more detail below), we also believe that exploring multiple opportunities often helps distinguish personally held values from avoidance-driven values.

The Role of Others in Value Development

Hayes, Strosahl, and Wilson (1999) discuss the potentially strong impact of *pliance* on the articulation of values. Pliance occurs when one follows a rule (e.g., "I must volunteer on a regular basis") because of past socially mediated consequences of following the rule (e.g., it pleases others, and I receive positive attention when I volunteer time in my community). Pliance may become an issue when a client endorses values that he or she thinks will elicit approval (or disapproval) of the therapist, the client's parents, other important people in the client's life, or even the larger culture.

While acknowledging that values will always be impacted in part by these forces, Hayes and his colleagues (1999) underscore the importance of an ongoing discussion of the "ownership" of values. For instance, in the case of a client who endorses a value of education and a goal of obtaining a PhD, the therapist may ask the client to consider the imagined consequences of a few different scenarios. How would the value be affected if the client was not able to tell anyone about the PhD? Alternatively, what if the client could tell everyone about the PhD but upon graduation all of his or her acquired knowledge was lost? Values clarification can benefit significantly from this process of observation and introspection. For example, if a client comes to realize that the approval of others related to obtaining a PhD is what is driving the education value, he or she may discover and commit to an even more fundamental value, being loved and loving others.[1]

Unable to Imagine That Change Is Possible

Some clients, particularly those who are in the greatest distress, may find it very difficult to consider that behavioral change is even possible. In these cases, we have found it to be very important to make room for and validate this hopelessness in session; a rush to challenge this assumption can leave clients feeling invalidated, as if the therapist does not understand the extent of the struggle and how stuck they feel. Once again, mindfulness and defusion exercises can be useful in working with these feelings of hopeless-

---

[1]It is important for the therapist to be sensitive to cultural considerations when exploring values. For some clients, particularly those from collectivist cultural backgrounds, acting in a way that is consistent with the wishes of others may be a personally held value and, therefore, an important consideration in choosing valued actions.

ness. Clients are encouraged to consider taking a leap of faith and attempting to engage in behaviors that seem impossible or irrelevant.

Creating Values Statements

In our experience, it can be useful, as the final step in the process of exploring and articulating values, to ask clients specifically to define one or two values in each of the three domains. These stated values will shape and direct much of the remaining work of therapy. We encourage clients fully to engage in this exercise, even if they already feel as if they are behaving consistent with their values. We often use personal examples of how we might be behaving in accordance with a value 95% of the time and yet still have our behavior influenced by experiential avoidance. For instance, one of us (Orsillo) often shares a personal value of being open and available to my children so that I can connect with them and be in tune with their thoughts and feelings. I also share that, while I think I do a reasonably good job of acting consistent with that value, I am aware that when I feel stressed, tired, and overwhelmed I can slip into a state of going through the motions. In other words, I might be there physically, but I am not mindfully present. Sharing an example of how even therapists do not always act in accordance with our values typically encourages clients to open up about their own struggles.

An example of a set of values that might be expressed by a client as part of this exercise might be:

Interpersonal Relationships

"I want to share my thoughts and feelings openly with my partner."
"I want to make time to nurture my relationships with friends."

Work/School/Community

"I want to work cooperatively with my coworkers."
"I want to set challenges for myself so I continue to learn and grow."

Self-Nurturance and Community Involvement

"I want to take good care of my physical health."
"I want to be an active part of my church."

We also ask our clients to consider what obstacles are currently interfering or have interfered with their ability to behave consistent with these values. Clients often acknowledge both internal and external barriers that limit valued behaviors. Internal barriers often include emotional states (e.g., "I am too depressed to connect with my friends"), thoughts (e.g., "I feel too unworthy to ask her out on a date"), urges (e.g., "I want to be there for my children, but the urge to drink is too strong"), and physiological sensations (e.g., "Although I would like to spend more time with my daughter, I need to be careful to not go into situations that might make me feel panicky").

As discussed in Chapter 6, internal obstacles are typically addressed using clinical methods aimed at increasing defusion, mindfulness, and acceptance. External barriers are typically reconceptualized as values-consistent behaviors that deserve consideration. For instance, if a client values taking on challenges at work but is currently unemployed, his unemployment would be seen as an external barrier to his value, but he could take a number of values-consistent actions (e.g., scanning classified ads, working on his résumé, scheduling informational interviews) to work toward eliminating that barrier. Handout 7.4 (p. 166) can be used to help clients to create values statements.

INCREASING AWARENESS OF ACTION AND INACTION IN VALUED DOMAINS

The VLQ asks clients to rate how consistently they act in accordance with their values in different domains. Additionally, we have found that self-monitoring of valued behavior, especially once the client has gained some mindful observing skills, can provide rich information about behavior in valued domains. Using the Valued Activity Log shown in Form 7.1 (p. 167), we ask clients to record several aspects of valued behavior: valued actions taken, extent of mindful engagement in valued activity, missed opportunities to engage in valued behavior, and obstacles that made engagement in valued behavior difficult.

Figure 7.1 provides an example of a client's completed Valued Activity Log. David presented to treatment for concerns related to substance abuse and expressed that intimately connecting with his wife and children and developing and maintaining friendships were valued domains. When he first completed the Valued Activity Log, David noted a day during which he spent some time with his children, consistent with his values, but he rated his mindfulness during that activity as low because he was distracted by ruminations on a conflict he had the night before with his wife Alicia. David also recorded a missed opportunity; his wife arranged for a babysitter so that they could go to dinner and a movie, which was an activity that was consistent with his values, but he cancelled the date, saying that he had a headache, because he feared they might get into another fight over dinner. Later that week, David arranged for some time openly to discuss some issues with his wife that had been simmering between them. He rated this as a valued-consistent activity and noted that he was mindfully present during the conversation. Finally, David marked as a missed opportunity a time at work when all of his coworkers were standing around talking, but he chose to stay in his cubicle because he did not want to feel uncomfortable trying to fit in with them.

Although we use this form to track valued behavior throughout treatment, the first time clients use it we suggest that they not make any changes in their behavior. The goal of the assignment is simply to bring mindful attention to values and behavior to get a clearer sense of the extent to which clients are acting in accordance with their values and the potential obstacles to valued activity. This information is used to set the stage for the rest of therapy, during which clients are asked to consider using defusion and mindfulness skills to increase their willingness to commit to a course of valued action.

VALUED ACTIVITY LOG

Please complete this form at the end of each day.

This week, at the end of each day we would like you to think about an action you took that was consistent with one of your values or an opportunity that you missed to take an action consistent with your value. Briefly describe the action and mark T for taken or M for missed.

On a scale of 0–100, rate how mindful you were during the action or the missed opportunity.

Note any obstacles that you noticed that stopped you from taking action (or could have).

There are no right or wrong answers to this assignment—we all choose not to engage in valued actions for a variety of reasons. This is just a way for us to start to get a better sense of what may be getting in the way for you so that you can make choices as to how you would like to proceed.

Date	Action	Taken (T) or Missed (M)	Mindfulness (0–100)	Obstacles
1/12	Spend time with kids	Taken	10	I was distracted thinking about the fight I had with Alicia.
1/13	Dinner with Alicia	Missed	10	I was afraid if we spent time together we would just continue fighting. I didn't want to feel angry at her or feel bad about myself.
1/17	Spent some time talking with Alicia	Taken	90	
1/18	Hang out with co-workers	Missed	5	I am worried they will think I am a loser. They are all lawyers, and I just barely got my BA at a state school. Being with them makes me feel bad about myself.

FIGURE 7.1. Example of a completed Valued Activity Log.

VALUES

How are values different from goals?

- A goal is an outcome (get your degree, get into a committed relationship).
- A value is a process (learning, being close and loving with others).

Why are values needed?

- Goals are good, but they have some downsides.
- Goals keep us focused on the future; where you are in this moment is never good enough.
- Feeling this way can be motivating, and it also means you cannot be satisfied and content in the moment.

Values are the glue between goals.

VALUES ASSIGNMENT I

Worry and anxiety often interfere with people's relationships, work, and self-nurturance and community involvement. Worrying can distract us so that we are not able to focus on things that matter to us and get less satisfaction from our relationships and activities. Often, in an attempt to avoid more stress and anxiety, we may avoid saying or doing something that is important to us. Sometimes the effects of worry on our life are very obvious. Other times, our responses are so automatic we begin to think we have few choices about change and that "this is just how things have to be."

This assignment is focused on helping you to take some time for yourself to really focus on how your life may be affected by worry and anxiety.

Please set aside 20 minutes on four different days during which you can privately and comfortably do this writing assignment. In your writing, we want you to really let go and explore your very deepest emotions and thoughts about the topics listed below.

As you write, try to allow yourself to experience your thoughts and feelings as completely as you are able. This work is based on the evidence that pushing these disturbing thoughts away can actually make them worse, so try to really let yourself go. If you can't think of what to write next, repeat the same thing over and over until something new comes to you. Be sure to write for the entire 20 minutes. Don't be concerned with spelling, punctuation, or grammar; just write whatever comes to mind.

Day 1

Please write about how you think your anxiety and worry might be interfering with your relationships (family, friends, partner, etc). What are some things that you do when you are anxious that affect your relationships? How does your anxiety and worry hold you back in relationships? What do you need from others in your life? What do you want to give to others? What gets in the way of asking for what you need and giving what you want to give?

Day 2

Please write about how you think your anxiety and worry might be interfering with your work, education, or training or your family/household management if you are a stay-at-home parent. What are some things that you do when you are anxious that affect your job/studies? How does your anxiety and worry hold you back in your work/schooling? Are there changes that you would like to make in this area of your life?

(continued)

Day 3

Please write about how you think your anxiety and worry interfere in your ability to take care of yourself, have fun, and/or get involved with your community. What are some activities in these areas that you would like to spend more time doing? How does your anxiety/worry hold you back?

Day 4

This is your last day of writing, so take some time to reflect on what came up for you over the last few days as you allowed yourself to focus on the issues raised in the first three parts of the writing assignment. Have you noticed any important areas that need more attention? Feel free to write about whatever comes up for you about these three areas of living.

VALUES ASSIGNMENT 2

Often, our attempts to avoid anxiety, worry, and stress cause us to make subtle shifts in our behavior so that we begin doing whatever we are "supposed" to be doing and lose track of what we *want* to be doing, what *personally matters* to us as individuals. In this assignment, we will continue to look at three areas of living to see what changes might be necessary to improve your quality of life.

We would like you to please set aside 20 minutes on three different days during which you can privately and comfortably do this writing assignment. Once again, in your writing, we want you to really let go and explore your very deepest emotions and thoughts about the topics listed below.

As you write, try to allow yourself to experience your thoughts and feelings as completely as you are able. This work is based on the evidence that pushing these disturbing thoughts away can actually make them worse, so try to really let yourself go. If you can't think of what to write next, repeat the same thing over and over until something new comes to you. Be sure to write for the entire 20 minutes. Don't be concerned with spelling, punctuation, or grammar; just write whatever comes to mind.

Day 1: Relationships

Choose two or three relationships that are important to you. You can pick either actual relationships (e.g., my relationship with my brother) or relationships you would like to have (e.g., I would like to be part of a couple, I would like to make more friends). Briefly write about how you would like to be in those relationships. Think about how you would like to *communicate with others* (for example, how open vs. private you would like to be, how direct vs. passive you would like to be in asking for what you need and in giving feedback to others). Think about *what sort of support you would like* from other people and *what sort of support you can give* without sacrificing your own self-care.

Day 2: Work/Education

Briefly write about the sort of work, training, education, or household management you would like to be engaged in and *why it appeals to you*. Next, write about *the kind of worker, student, and/ or household manager* you would like to be with respect to your work habits and your *relationships* with your boss, coworkers, or fellow students. What is important to you about the *product of your work/studies*? How would you like to *communicate to others* about your work? How would you like to *respond to feedback*? What additional *challenges* would you like to take on?

Day 3: Self-Nurturance and Community Involvement

Briefly write about the ways in which you would like to *spend your free time*, whether or not you actually have any free time in your life right now. What would you like to do to have *fun*? What are the ways in which you could *better take care of yourself* (e.g., nutrition, exercise, spirituality)? How might you be more active in your community?

VALUES ASSIGNMENT 3

Over the past few weeks, you have been spending time in and out of session thinking about how your anxiety and worry interfere with the things that personally matter to you, the things that add to your quality of life.

Often, we feel as if we cannot act consistent with our values when we are anxious, sad, stressed, or feeling bad about ourselves. It also often seems as if we have few choices in our life, that we have so many responsibilities that we cannot make the shift to doing what really matters to us. The limits of our ability to control others can make valued action seem like a poor choice or a waste of time, as it may be unlikely that our situation can change. Or we may feel like we are acting consistent with our values, but that worry and anxiety has taken us away from fully enjoying those activities.

In this assignment, we would like you to come up with one or two values in each of the domains of living that we have discussed. Remember that a value is different from a goal in that values are a process—a way of being in the world—whereas goals are an outcome. An example of a value is "I want to open up in my relationships—let others know what I am thinking and how I am feeling" as compared to a goal, such as "I want to find more friends."

Values are ways of being that are important to you. It is often the case that for one reason or another we do not always act consistent with our values. We would like you to think about thoughts, feelings, physical sensations, and life circumstances that can get in the way of your acting consistent with your values. Please think about these obstacles both for values that you are working on pretty consistently and those you may not be ready to work on yet.

Values	Obstacles
Interpersonal Relationships	
Work/School/Community	
Self-Nurturance and Community Involvement	

VALUED ACTIVITY LOG

Please complete this form at the end of each day.

This week, at the end of each day we would like you to think about an action you took that was consistent with one of your values or an opportunity that you missed to take an action consistent with your value. Briefly describe the action and mark T for taken or M for missed.

On a scale of 0–100, rate how mindful you were during the action or the missed opportunity.

Note any obstacles that you noticed that stopped you from taking action (or could have).

There are no right or wrong answers to this assignment—we all choose not to engage in valued actions for a variety of reasons. This is just a way for us to start to get a better sense of what may be getting in the way for you so that you can make choices as to how you would like to proceed.

Date	Action	Taken (T) or Missed (M)	Mindfulness (0–100)	Obstacles

EIGHT

Putting It All Together

Promoting Mindful, Valued Action

In Chapters 5–7, we described several methods for introducing clients to an acceptance-based behavioral model of human functioning, mindfulness and acceptance strategies, and the concept of valuing and behavior change. The ultimate goal of ABBT is to elicit significant and enduring behavioral change, and in this chapter, we describe how we move into a second, action-oriented phase of therapy aimed at integrating all the concepts we have explored and encouraging our clients' motivation and willingness to change.

As we mentioned earlier, we see willingness to change as influenced by reinforcing and punishing properties of behavior. Quite simply, clients will be more likely to engage in behavior change when the rewards associated with new behaviors are more salient than the punishments. When clients present for treatment, they are often sharply focused on the punishing qualities of engaging in their lives. Participating fully in life is guaranteed to elicit a number of painful emotions and thoughts that clients initially consider intolerable and damaging. The rewards associated with connecting with others, taking chances, and trying new activities are often only superficially considered by clients in significant distress, particularly if they feel hopeless about the possibility of change.

ABBT is aimed at decreasing the punishing qualities of uncomfortable internal experiences and increasing the salience of valued activities. Educating clients about the function of emotion, modeling acceptance, validating their experience, and teaching acceptance and defusion strategies can help make internal experiences less threatening. Promoting a reconnection with core values and mindfully evaluating moment-to-moment opportunities to engage in valued activities using the writing assignments and other clinical methods described in Chapter 7 allow clients imaginally to experience the potential rewards associated with valued actions.

Once clients have clearly articulated one or two core values in a few important domains of living (interpersonal relationships, work/school/community, self-nurturance, and community involvement) and mindfully considered how their psychological struggles might be pulling them away from values-consistent action, the next step is to elicit from them a commitment to behavioral change. In this chapter, we discuss the methods we use to encourage clients to live in accordance with their personally held values. We revisit strategies used to address internal and external barriers that interfere with engagement in valued action and share some methods of enhancing willingness to engage mindfully in values-consistent behavior.

PREPARING TO MOVE FROM VALUES ARTICULATION TO VALUES-CONSISTENT BEHAVIOR

In preparation for this discussion, we ask clients to complete a third values writing assignment, specifically aimed at exploring their thoughts, fears, and feelings about making a commitment to behavioral change. Much like in the previous assignments, we ask clients to set aside 20 minutes a day on three different days to write as openly and honestly as they can about a number of important topics that represent a review and consolidation of previously considered material and encourage clients seriously to consider making significant changes. For instance, clients are asked once again to reflect on whether they often feel like they are too busy doing things they *should do* to engage in activities that are consistent with what they *want to do*, if they are just going through the motions or if they are avoiding taking values-consistent actions because of their psychological struggles.

Clients are also encouraged to describe the importance of their values, an exercise similar to one we ask them to complete earlier in the therapy process. At this later point in therapy, once clients have begun to open up and consider their internal experiences and behaviors more honestly and accurately, writing on this topic can serve as a vital catalyst for change. For instance, Marcia, a woman struggling with relationship issues, initially presented for treatment fairly numb to the vacancies in her life. While she was able half-heartedly to describe some potential valued directions, her experiential avoidance prevented her from truly engaging in the initial assignment. Later in therapy, once she had begun to practice mindfulness and to nonjudgmentally observe her inner pain related to the absence of social connectedness in her life, she was more willing to take a risk and articulate her genuine desire to live differently.

Clients are also asked to write about the biggest obstacle they still face with regard to being willing to experience internal events in the service of valued action. Don, a client who sought treatment for his issues with anger, had been using mindfulness quite effectively in a number of challenging contexts, but he wrote that he feared the "800-pound gorilla" lurking in his experiences. In other words, he was concerned that some dangerous and impossible to welcome thought or feeling that he was not currently aware of might arise and prevent him from continuing to move forward. The fear of that possibility held him back from taking some valued actions.

Finally, in this assignment clients are asked to write about their past experiences making commitments, including both successes and failures (see Handout 8.1, p. 179). Most of our clients have made multiple attempts to commit to behavior change in the past, and we have found it very useful to make room for them openly and nondefensively to observe the thoughts and feelings that arise when they consider making a commitment again. Below is a discussion we had about this assignment with Terrell, a client who was struggling with sexual issues.

CLIENT: This assignment was the hardest one yet. I was feeling pretty hopeful about making some changes, but filling this out reminded me of all the times I have failed.

THERAPIST: Tell me a little more about what came up for you.

CLIENT: Well, the writing made me think about how Jazmin and I tried to make a "date night" to improve our sex life. Over the summer, every Saturday night we got a babysitter and went into the city to listen to music or have dinner. We started feeling really close, and I had some hope that our sex life would improve.

THERAPIST: So, what happened?

CLIENT: It's hard to remember how things started to go wrong.

THERAPIST: It can be really painful to remember.

CLIENT: I feel pretty bad about it. I don't know, I think one night I might have had too much to drink, and I wanted us to try to have sex. We had been working with our therapist on taking it slowly—spending time just kissing and touching each other—but I felt good and I wanted to have sex. We started doing it, but I couldn't get hard. I felt like a complete loser, and Jazmin and I got in a pretty nasty fight. I slept downstairs that night.

THERAPIST: What happened after that?

CLIENT: We pretty much stopped going on dates. I never really thought about it too much at the time, but this assignment made me look at it. Work started picking up for me, so we stopped our "date nights." I think money was tight, so I picked up some extra shifts at the restaurant. I get home late, and Jazmin is already asleep. During the day, the kids are around so we can't really get intimate. We just kind of went about our business and let the "sex thing" go.

THERAPIST: So, once you starting thinking about this, writing about it, what did you notice?

CLIENT: I feel afraid. If I say something is really important to me and I don't follow through, it means I am a failure.

THERAPIST: It sounds like, for you, making a commitment means having to get it right all the time. And if you don't act in line with your commitment, you must be a failure.

CLIENT: If I don't keep my word I feel awful. Then, I guess it is just easier to give up.

THERAPIST: This is really important. I am so glad you noticed this. So, if you make a commitment and then miss an opportunity to act in a way that is consistent with your values, you notice some really painful feelings, thoughts that you are a failure, and a behavioral urge to move away from your commitment. Is that right?

CLIENT: Yeah, I guess that is right.

THERAPIST: We will talk more about this, but I want you to know that, although it was really painful for you to notice all this stuff, I think it is going to really help us. The idea of a commitment is scary to most of us, and facing that fear and watching what unfolds can help us respond differently.

MAKING A COMMITMENT TO VALUED ACTIONS AS A PART OF DAILY LIFE

Defining Commitment

Once our clients have had the opportunity to explore their previous experiences with commitment, we spend some time defining this construct. We emphasize that we consider commitment to be a process, or an intention, rather than an outcome. It is critical to underscore that, while one's behavior might not always be consistent with one's commitment or valued intentions, those intentions serve as a road map for directing behavior when slips or lapses occur. Marlatt and Gordon (1985) describe the negative consequences of the abstinence violation effect as it applied to relapse following treatment for substance use problems. They suggest that if a client viewed drinking alcohol as an "all-or-nothing" activity, then having one drink posttreatment would increase the chances that client would continue to drink. Alternatively, if a client viewed a posttreatment drinking episode as a lapse and could learn from the experience and continue to work toward sobriety, then the overall outcome would be more positive.

Drawing from Marlatt and Gordon (1985) and Hayes, Strosahl, and Wilson (1999), we broadly apply this concept to the commitment to a value. To follow up on the example of Terrell described above, he made a commitment to become more intimately connected to his wife, but he had a long-standing and strongly ingrained habit of equating intimacy with sexual intercourse, of judging his own self-worth by his ability to satisfy his partner sexually, and of trying to escape any feelings of failure and inadequacy that were associated with an inability to achieve and maintain an erection. It might take some amount of time (and many lapses) to break such strongly developed habits; however, as Terrell became more able to recommit to his value of intimacy after each lapse and nonjudgmentally allow for the thoughts and feelings associated with values-inconsistent behavior, his behavior became more consistent with his intentions.

We underscore that waxing and waning feelings about committing to a particular direction and ambivalence and doubt about one's valued directions are a normal part of the commitment process. In response to these shifting thoughts and feelings, a client may want to change valued directions. Sometimes this change is an authentic and life-enhancing move, particularly if the client was struggling with avoidance and reduced self-awareness during the early stages of therapy and originally endorsed values that could be considered "safe." For example, one client originally focused on her value of self-care, despite her significant loneliness and lack of friendships and other intimate relationships. As noted above, mindfulness practice can increase clarity, awareness, and willingness such that later in treatment clients may notice their values shifting or evolving.

While the urge to shift values can be a natural outgrowth of therapy, it can also represent a pattern of reacting nonmindfully to one's internal experiences. Barry, a client of ours who was seeking treatment to work on developing intimate relationships, was 45 years old and had never had a relationship with a partner that lasted for more than 6 months. As we discussed his relationship history, it became clear that he had had some abusive and emotionally unavailable partners and had made some healthy and appropriate choices to end those relationships; however, Barry also had a pattern of harshly evaluating his partners after the first 3 months of a relationship and becoming restless and fearful that he had made a poor choice in his dating partner.

The gardening metaphor from ACT can be used to help clients open up to the concept of *considering* sticking with an intention even when doubt arises and change could be justified. In this metaphor, the client is asked to imagine selecting a spot to plant a garden. Once the plot is chosen and you work the soil and plant the seeds, you may begin to notice while you wait for them to sprout that there are other spots just across the yard that look even better for a garden. You might decide to pull up your vegetables and replant your garden elsewhere. As soon as you start working the soil in your new plot, you are bound to notice it is a bit shadier than you thought, or you might encounter a rocky section that will be hard to till. Values are like a spot where you plant a garden. You cannot completely observe and evaluate how a particular spot will perform as a garden if you have to pull up stakes again and again. Of course, if you stick with the same garden for some time, you will notice its imperfections. At times like this, it is perfectly normal to have doubts. The choice is whether you will continue to garden in a particular plot when these difficult thoughts come up. One of the tricky things about gardens is that, while some crops grow very quickly, others require time and dedication. You must choose whether or not you are willing to take a risk on your garden, even with its imperfections, to see if with time, patience, and willingness you can grow some substantial crops.

On the surface, it can be quite difficult to know if a particular shift in values represents growth or avoidance, and no answer applies to all clients or situations. In our experience, considering this metaphor and continuing regular mindfulness practice can often help clients clarify their intentions. An emphasis on values as a process rather than an outcome can also be helpful. For instance, if Barry commits to a relationship, shares intimacies with his partner, and generally behaves like the kind of person he wants to be in relationships, he is living in accordance with his values on a moment-to-moment basis even if the relationship ultimately ends.

OBSTACLES TO COMMITTED ACTION

As noted above, as part of this writing exercise, we ask clients to consider the obstacles that stand in the way of them committing to valued action. In Chapter 7, we introduced the Valued Activity Log (Form 7.1), which clients use to monitor several aspects of valued behavior, including missed opportunities to engage in valued behavior and obstacles that made engagement in valued behavior difficult. Both the writing exercise and the Valued Activity Log highlight the obstacles that need to be addressed in order to motivate clients to engage in behavior change and set the stage for the work to be done in subsequent sessions.

In going over these assignments, we typically classify the obstacles that interfere with valued action as internal or external barriers. External barriers are typically situational circumstances that can be overcome with additional action. For instance, Mark, a male client struggling with depression, noted in his Valued Activity Log that a Saturday evening spent alone was a missed opportunity for engaging in valued social activities. The following discussion ensued:

THERAPIST: So, you noted in your log that you wanted to plan something social for Saturday night, but several obstacles came up. What was one of the obstacles?

CLIENT: Well, you know I have only been living here for about a month. It has always been hard for me to make social plans for the weekend, but at least when I lived in Chicago I knew four or five people I could call.

THERAPIST: And here?

CLIENT: I am getting to know a few people at work. I called two of them Saturday afternoon, but they already had plans.

THERAPIST: You wanted to do something social Saturday night, and the two people you called were busy. That is an example of an external barrier to valued action. When external barriers come up, it can be helpful to make a list of some actions you can take to overcome them. Do you have any ideas about what you might be able to do?

CLIENT: Well, it would be helpful to meet more people.

THERAPIST: That sounds good. And what steps could you take to meet more people?

CLIENT: I know I have to get out of my cubicle more at work and talk to my coworkers.

THERAPIST: That would be a step.

CLIENT: In Chicago, I also belonged to a basketball league. That gave me a place to go a few nights a week and be with other people. I guess I could look into that here.

THERAPIST: Those all sound like good steps toward overcoming some of the external obstacles to your value. Any other ideas?

CLIENT: I probably shouldn't wait until Saturday to make plans for Saturday night.

THERAPIST: I would agree with that! But what if that does happen again? You want to be socially connected with someone, but you can't find anyone to go out with. Can you think of other ways to live consistent with your value in that moment?

CLIENT: OK, I know what you are getting at. Other actions, right?

THERAPIST: Can you think of any?

CLIENT: I guess I could call one of my friends from Chicago to talk. Even if I can't see him, connecting on the phone would be a valued action.

THERAPIST: Great! Any other ideas? What if there is no answer?

CLIENT: I could send him an e-mail. At least I would be taking a step to connect with someone.

THERAPIST: I think you did a really nice job of coming up with a bunch of actions to take that are consistent with your values and that will help with some of these external obstacles.

Internal barriers to taking valued action are also commonly identified by our clients. For instance, in another entry in his log, Mark noted that he missed an opportunity to volunteer to take on a challenging project at work because he felt that doing so would bring up a number of unpleasant thoughts and feelings related to his own perceived incompetence. His experiential avoidance of these particularly painful internal experiences was conceptualized as an important target of therapy.

As has been discussed throughout this volume, by this point in therapy, clients have typically spent a significant amount of time considering the concepts of acceptance and willingness as potential alternatives to experiential avoidance. Most clients have experimented with different forms of mindfulness practice and, thus, have some direct experience with acceptance of a wide range of internal and external events. This second phase of therapy emphasizes explicitly using acceptance, mindfulness, and willingness skills in response to the internal barriers that prevent values-consistent behavior. Specifically, clients are asked to consider making a commitment to their values that involves developing a stance of willingness toward internal barriers.

The "passengers on the bus" metaphor from ACT can be a useful illustration of how internal barriers can interfere with values-consistent behavior and how a client can move in the direction he or she chooses, even with unwanted or uncomfortable thoughts and feelings. In this metaphor, the client is asked to imagine being the driver of a bus filled with passengers that represent the thoughts, worries, emotions, images, and other internal experiences with which the client is struggling. While the initial route of the bus may have been informed by the client's own valued directions and chosen path, the client is asked to consider both the large and subtle detours off-course that have been taken in an attempt to appease the unruly and unwanted passengers. A client may wish to drive her bus toward intimacy, but, in an attempt to avoid the unpleasant passenger of vulnerability, she avoids that route. Another client may have stopped his bus journey toward valued directions to head to the back and deal with his passengers. Both clients have stopped pursuing valued actions in an attempt to control internal experiences. As we discuss in more detail below, taking a willing stance means driving the bus on one's own chosen path even while the passengers threaten, criticize, and complain.

WILLINGNESS TO MAKE A COMMITMENT

As discussed in Chapter 5, acceptance of internal experiences is presented as a possible alternative to control efforts, which have been demonstrated paradoxically to intensify distress and interfere with quality of life. ACT (Hayes, Strosahl, & Wilson, 1999) uses the term *willingness* to describe the acceptance of internal experiences that may arise as a condition of engaging in committed, values-consistent action. Hayes and his colleagues describe several qualities of applied willingness that we find useful to discuss with our clients. The first is that *being willing* to experience the full range of thoughts and emotions that comes along with living is not the same as *wanting* to experience them. Sometimes clients misunderstand the concepts of acceptance and willingness and assume that we are encouraging them fully to embrace or process difficult experiences just for the sake of doing so. We often clarify to clients our stance that there is nothing inherently noble or worthwhile about painful feelings. If there were a way to live a fulfilling, rich, connected life without experiencing pain, vulnerability, loss, and so on, most people (including us) would opt for that route. Taking a stance of willingness simply suggests that one will accept and move forward with the full range of thoughts and feelings that appear when one engages in values-consistent behavior.

In ACT, Hayes, Strosahl, and Wilson (1999) use the metaphor of a swamp to describe the choices regarding willingness that one often makes when pursuing values. They suggest that if you are on a journey to a beautiful mountain and your path is blocked by a disgusting, murky swamp, you might choose to wade through it (even if you do not want to or it does not seem fair that you need to) if you decide that the journey to the mountain is worth it to you. We have found it useful to elaborate and return to the swamp metaphor throughout therapy. For instance, to underscore our perspective that willingness is not wallowing in despair, we might suggest that one does not necessarily have to crawl through the swamp or roll around in it, although there may be times when one does trip and fall, getting dirtier than expected. We also suggest that practice in acceptance, defusion, and mindfulness skills can help one navigate the swamp with somewhat less mess (sort of like wearing boots when wading through). Sometimes swamps surprise you, no matter how much you have practiced dealing with them, so willingness must be flexible and expansive. One can always trip and fall, even after repeated practice; willingness is being able to get back up and keep walking.

It is important to clarify that willingness is an *action*, not a *feeling*. Many clients are uncomfortable acting in ways that are inconsistent with how they feel. For example, a client who is feeling anhedonic may refuse to engage in a previously valued activity, such as painting, because he or she does not feel the joy and passion that previously fueled artistic pursuits. Most of the clients we work with believe that they have to improve their internal flaws and feel strong, competent, and willing before any behavioral changes can be made. As discussed earlier, we strongly emphasize the notion that one can feel completely unwilling to do something and still follow through with a commitment. While thoughts and particularly emotions are strongly associated with action tendencies, they do not dictate action. As noted in Chapter 10, this concept is also discussed in DBT, where it is called *opposite action* (Linehan, 1993b). For instance, if a stay-at-home mother feels guilty leaving her children with a babysitter for one afternoon so she can have lunch with a friend, she would be encouraged to engage in exactly the opposite action of the one the guilt was promoting. It is critical for clients to take the leap of faith that one does not have to feel willing at all to behave in a values-consistent manner.

Hayes, Strosahl, and Wilson (1999) also highlight the all-or-nothing quality of willingness. Frequently, clients assert that they are willing to engage in a values-consistent behavior as long as some personally imposed line is not crossed. An example of this is illustrated in our exchange with Isabella, a client we treated for alcohol dependence.

CLIENT: I am ready to commit to abstinence.

THERAPIST: I know how important this value is to you. What comes up for you when you make that statement out loud?

CLIENT: Well, I feel ready to work on this. I have to. Otherwise, my life will fall apart. I know I can do it, as long as Marcos sticks with me.

THERAPIST: What thoughts are you having about Marcos?

CLIENT: I love him so much. I know I can get through this with his support.

THERAPIST: Things have been pretty bad in your relationship, and you care deeply for Marcos.

CLIENT: I really think I can do this for him, but if he ever left me, I know I would have to drink. There is no way I can be abstinent if we split up. I couldn't handle that alone.

THERAPIST: You are willing to commit to sobriety as long as things with you and Marcos work out.

Another client we worked with, who struggled with social phobia, committed to engage in a conversation with a neighbor at an upcoming party. As we explored his willingness, he committed to staying in the conversation even if he experienced sweaty palms and a shaky voice, but further exploration revealed that if he felt a blush creeping up his neck he would be unwilling to continue with the interaction and would make an excuse to leave.

These terms and conditions of willingness are very common among clients. Unfortunately, our experience shows that placing a limitation on willingness consistently backfires. Although it may be associated with a temporary decrease in distress, it reinforces avoidance and adds to distress. We use a modified metaphor from ACT to illustrate these points.

"Imagine that you are hosting a housewarming party and you choose to invite everyone in the neighborhood. You are thoroughly engaged in the party and enjoying yourself until Joe, your annoying neighbor, shows up. Joe is loud, opinionated, and tacky, and the first reaction you have when you see him is that you have changed your mind and are not actually willing to welcome everyone to your party. Your willingness to engage in this action has some limits. You have a few choices here. You can decide that you are willing to have everyone at your party except Joe, and you can ask him to leave. If you make this choice, you are stuck guarding the door all night to make sure he doesn't return. Another option might be to say that you are willing to have Joe at the party, even though you don't really mean it. In this scenario, you spend the rest of the evening trying to placate and manage Joe and keep him away from all the other guests at the party. Unfortunately, both of these options, which represent the terms and conditions of your willingness, severely limit your ability to participate fully in the party. Instead of enjoying yourself freely, mingling with guests, and truly being part of the party, you are stuck with Joe, monitoring his every move and enduring his negativity. You do have another option. You can be completely willing to have him at the party while you fully participate in the party. You can hold a negative opinion of him and even wish he did not show up and still be willing to have him, continuing to interact with your guests and engage in the event."

In order to benefit from willingness, clients need to embrace its all-or-nothing quality, but they can practice willingness in a graduated manner by choosing the context or situation in which they will practice it. For example, Alik was a woman we treated for PTSD. One of her values was to be more intimately connected with others. At first, she committed to engaging in more honest and open conversations with others as long no thoughts, feelings, memories, or physiological sensations related to her traumatic experience arose. She noted that if that happened she would close down and make an excuse to terminate the conversation. We discussed the potential impact this limit on willingness would have on her therapy goals and offered another possibility. Specifically, we asked her if she could commit to being completely open and available in one relationship, even if painful experiences emerged. She agreed to commit to this behavior with her therapist. Over time, Alik progressed to being willing to allow those experiences in the presence of her partner and, finally, a trusted friend. In this case, Alik did not limit her willingness to be open in relationships; she just practiced this openness in increasingly difficult domains.

Engaging in Regular Valued Action

At this point in the therapy process, if the client is willing, our focus shifts from practicing mindfulness skills and exploring valued directions to applying the skills of acceptance and willingness to encourage active engagement in valued activities. In our approach, each session follows a similar structure. As before, the session starts with a mindfulness exercise, but in these later sessions, the choice of which is dictated by the individual needs of the client. For instance, some clients may benefit from returning to a simple breathing exercise, whereas others may be struggling with mindfulness of thoughts or emotions. Specific skills can also be practiced. One client may benefit from a return to mindfulness exercises that illustrate the utility of beginner's mind, while others may find it helpful to practice self-compassion.

Next, clients are encouraged to describe their out-of-session experiences, specifically their successes and struggles with mindfulness practice, valued actions taken and opportunities missed, and struggles with internal and external barriers. During these discussions, we bring in previously reviewed concepts (e.g., the function of emotions, the problem of control) as relevant. Given the long learning history clients have with experiential avoidance, it is common for them to forget (or misremember) material that was covered in earlier sessions. Reintroducing previously considered handouts, metaphors, and exercises can be a simple but powerful reminder of these concepts.

As discussed above, each week the client is invited to commit to a few valued actions that are monitored using Form 8.1 (p. 181). A significant amount of each session is dedicated to exploring and addressing external and internal barriers to action. For instance, in the case of Mark, who had a limited social circle, time was spent in session developing a number of valued actions that would increase his social contacts, opening up options for his weekend plans. He began asking his coworkers to lunch, joined a basketball league, and enrolled in an adult education course on photography. Another client identified a skills deficit as an external barrier to directly confronting her boss about an issue at work. Time was spent in session developing her social skills and practicing these skills through role playing.

Strategies to Enhance Willingness

As discussed throughout this volume, internal barriers are often the hardest for clients to overcome. The mindfulness and defusion strategies introduced in Chapter 6 can be utilized to enhance willingness to engage in valued actions. For example, if a client is fearful and avoidant of sad feelings, understanding their universal nature and communicative function, realizing that they are not dangerous or pathological, and practicing welcoming them can increase a client's willingness to have them. Additionally, considering the limits of language, differentiating between objective descriptions of experience and judgments, and labeling internal experiences as such are all powerful defusion exercises that can be used to expand willingness to experience uncomfortable thoughts.

Handout 8.2 (p. 180), which summarizes some methods to enhance willingness, is typically given to clients at this point in therapy. To summarize, we suggest that, despite an intent to engage in valued activities, clients will inevitably experience failures to act in ways that are in accordance with their values. An awareness of the factors involved in these failures can increase the probability of future successes. Most commonly, perceived internal barriers and experiential avoidance are the factors that reduce willingness and interfere with valued action. Internal barriers are best responded to with an increased experiential contact with one's values and the futility of previous attempts at *in vivo* and experiential avoidance, as well as with practice in mindfulness and defusion strategies and in participation, which can be positively reinforcing. This form also asks the client to notice how mindful he or she is when engaging in valued activities. As discussed earlier, some clients frequently take actions that are consistent with their values, yet they are not fully aware and engaged when they do so. Participating in valued activities in a mindless and detached way is unlikely to improve well-being and quality of life. If this pattern of behavior persists, it can be useful to return to some of the methods and strategies discussed in Chapter 6 that are aimed at bringing mindfulness to everyday activities.

VALUES ASSIGNMENT 4:
MAKING A COMMITMENT

Please set aside 20 minutes on three different days during which you can privately and comfortably do this writing assignment. As before, in your writing, we want you to really let go and explore your very deepest emotions and thoughts about the topics listed below.

As you write, try to allow yourself to experience your thoughts and feelings as completely as you are able. This work is based on the evidence that pushing these disturbing thoughts away can actually make them worse, so try to really let yourself go.

Write about any or all of the following topics. If you choose to write on only one of the topics, that would be fine. You may write about them in any order you wish. If you cannot think about what to write next, just write the same thing over and over until something new comes to you. Be sure to write for the entire 20 minutes. Please do not spend any time worrying about spelling, punctuation, or grammar—this writing is intended to be a "stream of consciousness"—that is, you may write whatever comes to mind.

- What comes up for you when you think about the idea of making choices in your life and taking action based on what matters to you?
  - Do you often feel like your life is full of what you should do rather than what you want to do?
  - Are you doing what you want to do but feeling disconnected from your actions?
  - Are there things you really want to do but feel unable to do because of your anxiety?
- What is the importance of the values you have chosen? What do they mean to you?
- What comes up for you when you think about the idea of willingness? What is the biggest obstacle that stands between you and the changes that you want to make?
- What negative and positive reactions come up for you when you think about making a commitment? What have been your past experiences in making commitments?

WILLINGNESS

Keep this sheet handy and try some of the suggestions below when you notice you are avoiding certain actions, thoughts, or feelings. These suggestions can help you increase your willingness to take valued action.

- Spend some time thinking about why the value you have chosen matters to you. Find a quiet, comfortable place, close your eyes, and imagine yourself acting in ways that are consistent with this value.
- Think about the time that you have tried to avoid activities or limit your life in order to avoid certain thoughts and feelings. Think about what it has cost you when you have chosen avoidance.
- Think about the times you have tried to control your internal experiences so that you could live a valued life. Consider whether or not that approach has been helpful.
- Read over your mindfulness handouts and think about the concepts that we have discussed, such as nonjudgmental (or compassionate) observation, beginner's mind, acceptance, and letting go.
- Engage in mindfulness practice (one we have done in session or something you have developed outside of therapy) and notice how you can observe your thoughts, feelings, and bodily sensations.
- Fully participate mindfully in some activity (washing dishes, taking a walk, talking with someone) and notice how it feels to participate. Notice the difference between participating and standing back.

VALUES MONITORING ASSIGNMENT

Write down a few commitments that you would like to make for the week. A commitment should include a behavioral action and the willingness to remain present during the action.

_____

_____

_____

_____

Over the week, note some times when you acted consistent with your values and some times that you did not. Include in this monitoring activities related to the commitments that you made. Notice any potential obstacles that got in the way of you engaging in valued activities. Jot down any observations that you notice about your valued action.

Date/Time	Valued Actions	Obstacles	Mindfulness (0–100)

NINE

Evaluating Progress, Relapse Prevention, and Ending Treatment

In this chapter, we discuss some general considerations in monitoring the progress of therapy, decisions about whether to alter a conceptualization and treatment plan based on this assessment, relapse prevention, and ending therapy. The application of each of these will vary a great deal depending on clients' presenting problems and the context in which they are being seen (for instance, when sessions are limited for external reasons), so we focus particularly on the reasons underlying the decisions we make in order to show clinicians that they can adapt suggestions to meet the specific contexts in which they are working.

CONTINUAL ASSESSMENT OF PROGRESS

In our work, we ask clients to complete very brief weekly assessments of symptoms, their relationship to their symptoms, and their functioning. We do this with single-item assessments we develop to specifically assess the targets of treatment (see Form 9.1, Weekly Assessment, p. 200, for an example used with a client with GAD). We also use a more general measure of outcome from the Institute for the Study of Therapeutic Change (*www.talkingcure.com*), which assesses functioning in personal, interpersonal, social, and overall areas with single items (and can be downloaded free). In addition, we administer a more standard symptom measure such as the Depression Anxiety Stress Scales (described in Chapter 2) in order to assess symptom change more reliably.

Although we use these assessments partly for research purposes (due to our interest in studying the trajectory of change in this treatment, as well as predictors of outcome), we also find them clinically important for several reasons. First, these assessments provide an additional form of monitoring, in that clients are asked to reflect on their symptom level and specific aspects of the treatment (e.g., acceptance, mindfulness, engagement in valued action) at least on a weekly basis. Clients who initially have difficulties with daily monitoring will thus engage in this type of reflection once a week and begin to notice fluctuations across these domains. Furthermore, these types of ratings allow clients to see changes as they emerge, such as changes in their relationship to their internal experiences, increases in their valued actions, or reductions in their symptoms. Finally, this assessment allows us to have an overall sense of how these different aspects are changing over time (or not) for clients and to make clinical decisions based on what we observe. For this reason, we ask clients to come in 5–10 minutes before session and complete these forms. We look over them just prior to beginning session, having already reviewed their ratings from previous weeks.

Evaluating the Course of Change

To date, no published studies have empirically examined the process of change in ABBTs, so there is no specific empirical base to rely on in evaluating the progress of treatment from an ABBT perspective; however, data available from CBTs highlights the complexity of the change process. Recent research has highlighted nonlinear, dynamic, variable patterns of change and development in psychotherapy (see Hayes, Laurenceau, et al., 2007, for a review). Hayes and colleagues (2007) suggest that change in psychotherapy may follow a nonlinear, dynamic model because clients are moving from a fixed, stable system, in which problematic behaviors are habitual and predictable, into a new pattern (ideally) in which new behaviors and responses will become habitual and predictable. This kind of change first involves a destabilization of the initial system before individuals can stabilize around the new system, so clients may experience a period in which behavior and responses are more variable and unpredictable, potentially including a worsening of symptoms or behaviors, before the new system can stabilize and become predictable again. Studies are beginning to provide some evidence that temporary increases in symptoms (Hayes, Feldman, et al., 2007) and discontinuous treatment progress (Stultz, Lutz, Leach, Lucock, & Barkham, 2007) may predict positive outcomes for at least some clients.

Clinically, we sometimes explain this kind of process to clients by using the example of trying to change which hand we use to open doors (an example Tom Borkovec often uses with therapists and clients). If we always use our right hand and we decide to try to change to using our left, the process of change is likely to look something like this: First, we keep using our right hand, but after we go through doors we remember we were supposed to try something different and vow to remember next time. This part of the process might go on for a while! Then we may approach doors paying very close attention to which hand we are using and force ourselves to use our left hand. We are likely to have a period of time where we find ourselves fumbling around doors, taking a while to get through them, because we know we do not want to follow our established instincts but we do not yet have new instincts to follow. Things in that moment may look chaotic and ineffective. Eventually, we will use our left hand regularly, probably by paying very close attention. Gradually, if we are consistent, this will become a new habit and we will be able easily to open doors again, although, at times of stress or when we are depleted, we may revert to the previous overlearned habit. Our path to this change would not be linear. The "path up the mountain" metaphor from ACT (presented in Chapter 5), which describes how sometimes trails that lead up a mountain contain a switchback so that it may seem like you are backtracking in your progress, also illustrates nonlinear change.

Evaluating the process of change in ABBTs is further complicated by the emphasis on altering clients' relationships to their internal experiences rather than the experiences themselves. Again, symptoms might increase for a time while clients practice opening themselves up to sadness or fear (similar to the increases in anxiety associated with exposure-based treatments), and this increase might be a sign of improvement rather than decline. For some clients, practicing mindfulness, focusing on the breath or bodily sensations, initially leads to a noticeable decrease in symptoms. Later, practicing mindfulness in more challenging domains or when they begin to engage in values-consistent behaviors that evoke distress may be associated with an increase in symptoms.[1] Therefore, it is important to pick measures that will be sensitive to the kinds of changes you expect to see throughout treatment. It may also be useful to make specific predictions with your client about the patterns of progress that may emerge throughout treatment.

Until more research is available to guide us in determining whether a particular client's current status is likely to predict a positive or negative trajectory, we attend to the following factors in evaluating our clients' progress.

Engagement in the Treatment

Our first concern is whether clients are engaging in the treatment. We pay careful attention to whether clients are using self-monitoring, engaging in mindfulness practice, and attending to valued action as each of these elements is introduced. When clients are not engaging in treatment, we explore with them what might be getting in the way, address these external and internal obstacles (as described in Chapters 5, 6, and 7, following the principles of valued action described in Chapter 8), and evaluate the impact of these alterations. Throughout this work, we maintain a focus on our conceptualization so that we can choose alternative methods that will still serve our intended function.

Sometimes a client's difficulty engaging in treatment can make it impossible to proceed with any other aspects of treatment. In these cases, treatment moves immediately to valued action even though other elements of treatment have yet to be introduced. Jade presented for treatment due to her chronic excessive anxiety and worry, which was interfering with her life so much that she was currently unemployed. She was 30–40 minutes late to her first three sessions. When her therapist asked what was interfering with her ability to get to session, she responded with a stream of apparently external obstacles (she had to return several phone calls, she had job-related letters to send, she ran into a neighbor as she was leaving, she hit unexpected traffic on the way, etc.), but her discomfort at leaving anything unfinished or walking away from a social situation was evident. The therapist therefore focused on this specific context as an example in presenting the model of treatment. He highlighted the way that Jade's anxiety and worry were leading her to take a series of actions (staying later to work on her applications, stopping to talk to a neighbor) that were inconsistent with her stated value of attending to the anxiety that she felt was interrupting her life. While each choice made perfect sense at the time, given the level of anxiety she was experiencing and the relief she felt after attending to these situations, the long-term effect was that she was not able to engage in therapy she really wanted in order to improve her life. The therapist asked

---

[1]Hayes, Feldman, and colleagues (2007) found this type of pattern (an initial decrease associated with skills training and a subsequent spike in symptoms associated with exposure) in their study of the process of change in their treatment for depression.

Jade if, even though it would involve experiencing distress at leaving these situations, Jade might want to commit to leaving early for session and walking away from whatever was in progress in order to act consistent with this stated value. The therapist was careful to very clearly validate Jade's distress and the difficulty of making this kind of radical change so early in treatment. This approach both helped get Jade to attend sessions so she could work on the way her life was unsatisfying when it was guided solely by efforts at relieving anxiety (which were unsuccessful) and gave her an experience of choosing an action despite her internal state, which helped illustrate the concepts of ABBT that her therapist subsequently presented.

Some Evidence of Movement

In terms of monitoring symptom and behavioral change, our experience suggests that what is most important is that clients experience some type of change over time. We do not necessarily expect change until clients have been practicing for a couple of weeks, although often they do experience some type of initial change just from beginning to bring awareness to their internal experiences. At this point, some clients experience a decrease in symptoms, while others experience an increase; both can be indicators of subsequent improvement. Clients who have been restricting their lives significantly may experience more discomfort as they begin to engage more fully, yet this is an indicator of progress. On the other hand, clients who have been continually distressed may find that their distress decreases as they begin to cultivate a mindful presence. Similarly, some clients begin to make behavioral changes right away, while others may become much more aware but continue to feel somewhat stuck behaviorally at first. These clients may not begin to make behavioral changes until they have more fully cultivated mindfulness in their lives.

Based on these observations, we like to give clients several weeks of practicing and applying the principles of therapy and watch the course of their symptoms, their relationship to their symptoms, and their behavioral responses. As long as these are in some type of flux that is consistent with our conceptualization (for instance, increased distress might coincide with increased behavioral engagement if disengagement has been a form of experiential avoidance), then we consider these changes evidence of therapeutic effect. If, after several weeks, there is no evidence of movement in symptoms, relationship to symptoms, or behavioral responses, then we reevaluate our behavioral conceptualization and develop alternative hypotheses for symptom presentations while we try to understand what is maintaining the robust responses.

For instance, Edgar came to treatment reporting chronic dysphoria and social isolation. Despite his strong educational background, he had a history of moving from job to job. When asked about his current relationships, he indicated that he played a passive role in most relationships, often choosing to meet others' needs rather than his own. He described significant anxiety at the thought of sharing his own opinion with friends, his partner, or coworkers. Edgar also had a difficult time completing his values writing assignments, stating that he did not have a clear sense of what was important to him. He and his therapist developed a shared conceptualization tying Edgar's difficulty expressing personal preferences and his habit of choosing to please others rather than himself to his developmental history with affectively intense and demanding parents whom he learned to appease. The therapist developed a treatment plan focused on helping Edgar cultivate a stance of mindfulness toward his experiences, enhancing values exploration assignments to help Edgar gain a better sense of his own desires, and encouraging him to practice stating his needs and preferences in various contexts. Although Edgar engaged in therapy-related activities, he did not experience the predicted change in mood or life satisfaction. The therapist suggested that Edgar specifically apply his mindfulness skills during interpersonal situations to monitor his internal experiences carefully so that the information gathered could be used to potentially modify the conceptualization and treatment plan.

Edgar's mindful monitoring revealed some additional information. Based on the initial conceptualization, the therapist predicted Edgar would feel anxious when expressing his needs for fear that they would not please others, and that a positive response from others would have positive consequences for Edgar. Instead, when Edgar received an accepting or validating response from someone, his anxiety escalated in the moment (which was expected) and continued to linger for several days (which was not expected) and was frequently accompanied by feelings of sadness and even anger. For example, Edgar talked with his temporary employer, Frank, about his dissatisfaction with his current responsibilities. Frank responded positively and offered Edgar a more challenging position that could become permanent. Edgar noticed that he first felt excited and pleased, but more careful monitoring revealed that he also had feelings of anger and dread. A similar mixed response emerged when Edgar's partner responded positively to Edgar's suggestion that they try to spend time together on the weekends. Furthermore, Edgar noticed that he sometimes asserted his needs in a somewhat aggressive way. For instance, when a group of coworkers invited him to lunch, he abruptly told them he had too much work to do. This pattern of responding suggested that the initial conceptualization was incomplete. Edgar became aware that he used his passivity as a means of distancing himself from others. Thus, if his assertions brought praise or closeness, he actually felt more distressed and began to avoid closeness in other ways. Similarly, he sometimes used his new habit of expressing his needs to distance himself from others. Edgar and his therapist concluded that he was fearful and unwilling to be vulnerable in his relationships. When he stated preferences without opening up to his own vulnerabilities, he remained stuck in his pattern of avoidance.

Based on this slightly altered conceptualization, a new treatment plan was derived. Edgar engaged in several values assignments exploring his thoughts and feelings about being deeply connected with others. He considered his unwillingness to deepen his connection to others and practiced acceptance and mindfulness toward his responses both in and out of session (for instance, using the softening toward pain and distress breathing space exercise described on pp. 128–129). As a result of this practice, he chose to strengthen his commitment to pursuing and maintaining intimate relationships, with an emphasis on approaching rather than avoiding interpersonal vulnerability. This choice led to greater fluctuation in his mood (with some temporary increases in sadness, followed by significant decreases), suggesting that he and his therapist had found an important stuck point. Although Edgar's passive way of relating to people had probably served an experientially avoidant function, he had at first moved into a more active way of relating that still avoided his deep feelings of vulnerability so that his symptoms were maintained. Recognizing this helped to move therapy toward an emphasis on his vulnerability so that progress could unfold.

We are careful when evaluating behavioral change not to assume that we know what the optimal behavioral outcome will be for a client. Instead, we attend to the effect the behavioral change has on him or her. Adaptive actions should lead to a greater sense of flexibility and choice and an increased sense of agency, while reactive, avoidant, or detrimental actions will result in an increased sense of being stuck. Sometimes a process needs to unfold before the distinction is apparent.

Matilda came to treatment after a falling-out with a valued friend. She felt the friend had been inconsiderate and hurtful and would not acknowledge his role in her pain. This event was tied to past experiences with her father, leading to very strong feelings of abandonment, anger, and disappointment. The friend was actively engaged in a community in which Matilda was also involved, leading her to feel that she had to leave the community to avoid the pain associated with seeing her friend. Through the course of treatment, Matilda chose several different actions. First, she decided to leave the community. Although she briefly felt relief at this decision, she almost immediately felt pain, sadness, and grief, which were maintained for several weeks. Matilda felt pushed out of the community and had no sense of agency in her choice; it had been reactive. When she observed this response in therapy, she decided to make a different choice and rejoined the community. Throughout this period of time, she worked in and out of session on making room for her feelings of sadness and anger so that, over time, she was able to notice the feelings and the reactions associated with her father and not get as caught up in them. However, Matilda found that her predominant experience at community events was sadness and that she no longer had the sense of connection she had had because it had been so closely tied to her relationship with this friend. She grieved for this loss and the loss of her friend and was able to write him a letter genuinely expressing grief, acknowledging her part in what had happened, expressing (and feeling) compassion for his pain, and telling him what he meant to her. Matilda also decided to leave the community again for a period of time. This time she felt agency and flexibility in her decision. She realized she could tolerate the feelings she had when she was around her former friend and that she could also choose to find other contexts that would be more rewarding for her at the moment. She did not feel that she had to stay away from the community for good, but she wanted to explore other sources of connection. Matilda's discussion of this decision was much more open and flexible than when she had decided to leave the first time, and it was clear that she was opening up to new experiences rather than running away from them.

Need for Skills Building or Other Behavioral Strategies

ABBTs incorporate both acceptance and change strategies, the balance between them varying depending on the conceptualization of the specific client. For example, a client with BPD who presents with intense distress and a long history of having her internal experiences critically judged and invalidated by others will likely need significant skills training. For other clients, mindfulness practice may help them disentangle from their internal experiences and attend to their current environments enough that adaptive, life-enhancing behavioral change evolves naturally without targeted intervention. An initial conceptualization should guide the development of the treatment plan and help the therapist hypothesize the degree to which direct behavioral intervention is needed and the timing of this intervention.

In Chapter 10, we discuss the ways in which ABBTs can be integrated generally with other evidence-based therapeutic approaches. Ongoing assessment of presenting problems can help inform this integration and better address the needs of particular clients.

For instance, in the case of Nicole in Chapter 3, our initial conceptualization suggested that her critical, entangled relationship with her internal experiences was driving her bingeing and purging behavior. This led us initially to develop a treatment plan focused on cultivating acceptance and mindfulness and encouraging further engagement in her life. Although the eating behaviors were not the focus of therapy, we included psycho-education about healthy eating and asked Nicole to monitor these behaviors so that we could track how treatment was affecting them. If these initial strategies did not alter her bingeing and purging behavior, it would be important to integrate other approaches such as the establishment of "regular eating," attention to body checking and avoidance, and exposure to sensations of fullness into her treatment plan.

Similarly, sometimes when clients begin engaging in valued actions, it becomes clear that they have skills deficits in certain areas (e.g., starting a conversation, asserting themselves). This is not surprising, given that they may have very little practice with these highly valued but commonly avoided behaviors. In these cases, therapists can incorporate skills-building exercises in therapy to help clients effectively pursue their desired actions.

RELAPSE PREVENTION

Just as with other treatments, relapse prevention is a critical element of ABBTs and requires careful attention. Clients have made new, often dramatic changes, and new challenges will arise following treatment that will necessitate repeated practice, reminders of the concepts of treatment, and new behavioral plans. Clients need to carry the principles of therapy with them, have multiple ways to remind themselves of these principles if their memories start to diminish, and be prepared to move through the emotional challenges that occur in their lives as well as the apparent setbacks that are an inevitable part of living an engaged life.

Because an acceptance-based stance is often such a radically different way to relate to one's experiences, and experiential escape or avoidance is so often immediately reinforced, we have found that, in the absence of careful attention to potential relapse, some clients lose therapeutic gains and require booster sessions for reminders. Also, because these treatment approaches often include multiple components (exercises, concepts, actions in numerous domains), it can be challenging for clients to develop a coherent model that they remember and follow in the absence of weekly or biweekly sessions. After noticing a slight decline in symptomatic improvement over time in the first open-trial investigation we conducted (Roemer & Orsillo, 2007), we increased our emphasis on relapse prevention throughout treatment, particularly in the last several sessions. Our second study (Roemer et al., 2008) revealed changes that were generally maintained over a 9-month follow-up period, suggesting these alterations were effective. Anecdotally, we have had clients contact us several years posttreatment to comment on how treatment has changed them and the ways these changes have continued over time.

In a sense, ABBTs, like other forms of CBT, incorporate preparation for treatment termination and relapse prevention throughout the course of therapy. Therapists help clients adapt treatment so that it makes sense to them, develop new habits that will support the changes being made in therapy, and take ownership of and responsibility for these changes. We have provided handouts and monitoring sheets throughout this volume, and we find it extraordinarily helpful to give clients a binder to store these documents and to encourage them to review previously discussed concepts and to refer to and retry past exercises. As treatment progresses, therapists intentionally become less directive, allowing clients to guide the focus of sessions, choose mindfulness and behavioral exercises to work on between sessions, and begin to recognize their own active role in therapeutic change and maintenance of this change. We find that it is important for therapists consciously both to step back from a more directive role and to point out clients' agency in their change process. Otherwise, clients may attribute any changes to the therapist rather than seeing their own actions and accomplishments. By increasing clients' awareness of the efficacy of their own actions, therapists can help clients recognize the impact of these actions and motivate them to continue their efforts toward changes that improve their lives.

We also find it helpful to continually review psychoeducational material with clients from early in session as therapy progresses. Often, clients forget concepts presented early on or begin to misremember ideas. Also, sometimes concepts are easier to grasp when clients' lives are more constrained. For instance, some clients really take to the concept of willingness in the abstract, but, when they begin to consider taking new, anxiety-provoking actions in their lives, they automatically become unwilling. Revisiting the concept and ways to enhance willingness (e.g., reviewing Handout 8.2), can help them recommit to being willing while pursuing anxiety-provoking actions. We have also had clients who are very committed to both formal and informal mindfulness practice until they expand their lives, upon which they begin to lose their practice and become very focused on the future and the past again. In these cases, a reintroduction of mindfulness and more focused in-session practice are helpful.

Reintroduction of metaphors or repeated use of metaphors that clients have found particularly helpful can also reduce the risk of relapse. We find that metaphors provide clients with a vivid, easily recalled cue of important aspects of treatment. Clients commonly report reminding themselves to "drop the rope" or asking, "Who's driving the bus?" when they are in an emotionally challenging situation. If clients have not adopted a metaphor, we will reintroduce metaphors that seem appropriate as they address specific areas of their lives so that they can link metaphors with their experience, making them a more potent reminder in the future. The acronyms in DBT skills training serve a similar function by providing concise, easily recalled reminders of important elements of treatment (Linehan, 1993b).

We periodically have clients review handouts from earlier sessions to remind them of particular concepts and provide a model for one way they can bring these elements back into their lives in the future if they find they have begun to lose their connection to them. By engaging clients during the course of therapy in actions that assist with remembering and regenerating learned habits and perspectives, therapists provide clients with experiential learning that will help them recall this method when they are out of therapy and experience similar lapses in their practice or their learning. For instance, Michelle (a client we saw early in the development of our treatment, before we had increased our focus on relapse prevention) had diligently engaged in mindfulness practice throughout therapy and had begun to look for a job and pursue dating opportunities when therapy ended. She found that, in the absence of the structure of therapy, when new challenges arose in her dating life her practice faltered, and she reverted to her old habit of avoiding valued action. As her life became constrained in familiar ways, she felt discouraged and had thoughts that none of her apparent progress had been real. She came in for two booster sessions that focused on mindfulness practice as well as a review of handouts from therapy. As she reviewed the materials, she remembered the way she had incorporated these concepts into her life and developed a new plan for reinvigorating her mindfulness practice and taking more valued action, particularly in pursuing potential intimate relationships. As she described the ways that anxiety had been guiding her actions in recent weeks, she recalled the "passengers on the bus" metaphor and expressed a desire to start driving the bus herself. She also decided to review her therapy materials every few weeks to keep these concepts more present in her life, specifically her commitment to mindfulness and to taking action in the relationship domain, which was important to her. The image of driving her own bus was a helpful reminder of this intention.

Michelle provides an example of the importance of differentiating lapses (i.e., the temporary, inevitable reemergence of a symptom or behavior) from relapse (i.e., returning to baseline levels of functioning for an extended period of time; Marlatt & Gordon, 1985). In DBT, clients often engage in behaviors from which they had previously committed to abstaining. Linehan and colleagues (1999) use the term *dialectical abstinence* to refer to a synthesis of a full commitment to abstaining from a particular behavior with the recognition that it is likely to reoccur and that this reoccurrence will provide a new learning opportunity that will assist with continued commitment to future abstinence. Similarly, when clients avoid valued actions, this can be seen as an opportunity to identify obstacles and determine strategies for engaging in these actions in the future. Thus, all behavioral change strategies used in these approaches emphasize commitment to the stated goal and awareness that these commitments may not be followed behaviorally at all times. As with a refocusing on the breath after the attention inevitably wanders from it, clients can simply notice that they did not act as they would have chosen to, refocus on their commitment to acting a certain way, and proceed accordingly. Continued practice with this pattern throughout treatment helps clients prepare for behavioral lapses that inevitably occur after treatment ends.

As discussed in Chapter 6, clients also often experience lapses into more critical, entangled relationships with their internal experiences and experiential avoidance. Clients who initially open up to their distress often experience relief as their reactivity decreases and their satisfaction increases, but, if they get attached to the calm that can sometimes accompany acceptance and mindfulness, they may struggle when mindfulness brings a different response and return to a pattern of judging and attempting to control feelings of discomfort. We assure clients that this is an understandable, human lapse, reflecting the habitual and automatic nature of a self-critical stance and a tendency toward avoidance. Clients are encouraged to practice awareness and compassion toward this inevitable response and to recommit to regular mindfulness practice.

We specifically attend to relapse prevention during the last several sessions of therapy. In our protocol, in which termination is predetermined at session 16, we address this topic first prior to session 12, when we have clients complete a between-session Treatment Review Writing Assignment (see Handout 9.1, p. 198). This allows clients to begin to turn their attention to the end of therapy, considering what they have learned, how they will maintain the gains they have made, what else they hope to accomplish, and what their fears are about the end of treatment. In the next session, therapists review clients' responses to this exercise, as well as Handout 9.2 (p. 199). Handout 9.2 provides clients with a brief overview of the main elements of treatment, which they can use as a reminder as they review their treatment accomplishments and when they want or need to revisit treatment in order to rejuvenate their practice or their valued actions.

In nonprotocol therapy, we begin this process of review as soon as a decision has been made to terminate therapy. We prefer to have several sessions devoted to treatment review and the termination process, with the last few sessions tapered (i.e., every other week or every third week) so that clients can begin to practice continuing the work of therapy in the absence of a weekly session and address obstacles that arise with their therapist in a subsequent, planned session. Sometimes clients choose to leave therapy more quickly, and the termination process must be completed in the course of one or two sessions. It can also be helpful to include a modified Treatment Review Writing Assignment and version of Handout 9.2 when termination may be indicated but a mutual decision has not yet been made. This provides a context in which therapist and client can collaboratively review accomplishments in treatment and further goals for treatment and can decide whether continued therapy is indicated or the goals can be pursued independently. This type of review of gains and work left to be done should be an informal part of therapy throughout; however, we find that a more formal writing and review process can sometimes be additionally beneficial.

Sessions focused on termination and relapse prevention have several goals: (1) consolidating and reviewing treatment gains, (2) identifying future work to be done independently, (3) predicting lapses (e.g., periods of increased distress and avoidance, decreased practice, apparent setbacks, disconnection from the therapeutic elements of treatment), and (4) developing strategies for addressing lapses. We like to develop a list of strategies (practices, metaphors, examples, handouts, etc.) collaboratively that the client has found particularly helpful. We work with clients to develop a summary sheet of their valued domains to help them remember the areas that they have identified as important so that they can bring their attention back to these domains during difficult times and to develop a plan for consistent mindfulness practice and mindfulness practice reminders. Some of our clients have purchased physical reminders, like stones to put on their desks; others have used books they found particularly inspirational as reminders. (This volume includes an appendix of mindfulness readings that we give clients following treatment, a list that has been supplemented by our clients' suggestions over the years. An excellent, constantly updated source for mindfulness readings is also available on the website of the Institute for Meditation and Psychotherapy, *www.meditationandpsychotherapy.org*.) Some of our clients have pursued formal practice in organized settings, becoming part of meditation groups (sanghas) or enrolling in yoga or tai chi classes. Others commit to regular practice in their homes, sometimes setting aside a corner of a room for this practice to mark its importance.

Clients often express concern that they will not be able to continue the work of therapy without the therapist or the therapy hour to help them remember. In addition to the methods described above, we suggest clients set up a regular time to reflect on their week, with a particular focus on action in valued domains and mindfulness practice. This method can help clients notice when their practice or their functioning begins to fluctuate.

Consistent with Marlatt and Gordon's (1985) model of relapse prevention, we predict fluctuations in functioning and emphasize that these fluctuations are natural, human lapses. We might describe this to a client in the following way:

"As you continue through your life, you will face new challenges and new situations. You will inevitably experience times of increased distress when you find it more difficult to continue your mindfulness practice and act consistently with your values. As we have discussed, mindfulness and valued action are processes—we all need to continue to attend to these areas, notice when things are slipping, when our attention has wandered or we've begun to avoid feelings or situations, and gently bring ourselves back. This can be a very difficult and disheartening process. Often, the first response after noticing this kind of lapse is a feeling of disappointment and a thought like 'I'm right back where I started from' or 'I can't do it on my own.' It can be easy for this to start a cycle of self-critical reactions, increased distress, and experiential avoidance, which feeds back into the sense of disappointment and self-criticism, continuing the cycle. The longer the cycle, the more challenging it becomes to bring self-compassion to the experience, to lessen self-criticism and reactivity, and to reconnect to the practices that have been helpful.

"I find that knowing this kind of lapse is natural and human helps me more quickly notice the pattern of self-criticism and disappointment and add some self-compassion to my reaction. Sometimes it can still take a long time for me to find a way to stop the cycle. At any moment, I can have the thought 'Oh, right, this is the part where I feel like I've lost my ability to be mindful and live a valued life.' I can make room for all the doubts and disappointment, as well as my hope that I can find my way back to the practices that were helpful. I can recommit to doing one thing to begin to bring mindfulness back into my life or find one valued action to take to begin to set myself back on that path. No matter how many times I wander off the path (and I wander often), I am always just one moment of awareness away from stepping back onto it."

We share the ways that a consistent mindfulness practice may help reduce the risk of escalating lapses and review strategies for clients to use when they notice a lapse (review of therapy materials, treatment summaries, and valued action lists; writing assignments to reconnect to or clarify values). We also recommend that clients contact us for booster sessions if their own methods do not seem to reinvoke sufficiently aspects of the treatment that helped them in the past. Often, one or two sessions are sufficient, but sometimes a new issue has emerged that requires additional focus in therapy.

ENDING THE THERAPEUTIC RELATIONSHIP

In the course of therapy within an ABBT framework, clients have often engaged in emotionally vulnerable, sometimes frightening work with the therapist and have expanded their lives in ways that may be novel and unsettling at times. Termination of this strong therapeutic relationship is a significant event that requires attention. Therapists need to be sensitive to individual differences; we are careful neither to overstate the importance of termination for a client who has become less attached to us and is not expressing strong feelings about ending the relationship nor to ignore the significance of termination for a client who has come to rely heavily on us and who will miss us a great deal. Clients often express concerns that, without the support of the therapist, they will lose their newly developed self-compassion or be unable to cope effectively with new challenges. Therapists can validate these fears—it is impossible to know that one can continue this work alone until it has been done, so it is natural to fear this kind of change—but point to the ways clients have already been doing this work alone and help them develop ways to remember the work of the therapy.

Sometimes, clients express a desire to continue the therapeutic relationship as friends. Again, it is important to validate this desire. We ask clients to bring many of the same qualities to the therapeutic relationship that they would to any other intimate relationship, such as openness, honesty, vulnerability, and commitment. Furthermore, acceptance-based behavioral therapists aim to be genuine and unguarded, allowing strong emotions that come up in therapy and self-disclosing in therapeutically useful ways. Given the potential intensity and closeness of the relationship and the ways it can mirror other intimate relationships, it is natural for clients to feel strange about ending the relationship without any conflict or external impetus. It can be useful for therapists to highlight the ways that the therapeutic relationship is different from a friendship, underscoring how these differences are aimed at maximizing the benefits clients may receive from therapy. Clients also may benefit from hearing the therapist's confidence that clients have the skills and abilities necessary to negotiate life's challenges and the rationale that termination will allow clients to experience and recognize their strengths more fully.

In our own practice, we have worked with clients for whom the relationship with the therapist is the most intimate connection they have ever experienced. Many of our particularly isolated clients endorse a value of developing intimate connections and use therapy as a context in which to begin practicing values-consistent behaviors. With clients like these, it is particularly important to expand their social network and support valued actions within those new relationships before therapy is terminated.

When therapy focuses on interpersonal challenges, these themes are likely to arise in the context of the therapeutic relationship and may be particularly salient as the end of therapy nears. Therapists can share these observations and check in with clients to see if they notice a similar connection. For instance, a client who has avoided making a connection to people in his life due to a fear of being abandoned may find termination particularly evocative. Observing this can provide a context for the distress that is emerging, letting the client see how allowing himself to open up to the therapeutic relationship, even though it is ending, has been beneficial for him. This provides experiential evidence for the meaningfulness of pursuing this value even when doing so also brings fear and sadness, which can be a particularly powerful learning experience. As always, these observations about similarities between the therapeutic relationship and outside relationships need to be presented as hypotheses. Some clients may be unable to see these connections, or the therapist may be inaccurate in these observations. Therapists should gently share their observations, allowing the client to refute them and simply encouraging continued awareness.

Clients often choose to give the therapist some kind of token farewell gift, such as a book on mindfulness, a stone to serve as a mindfulness reminder, or a poem reflecting a therapeutic theme. Although some theoretical perspectives discourage the acceptance of any gift and underscore the importance of processing the meaning of such a gesture with clients, we typically accept these gifts (as long as they are not too extravagant) as a token of gratitude for clients' experiences in therapy. These tokens may be particularly common in the context of treatment research because clients are not paying for sessions and, therefore, may particularly want to express their gratitude in some way.

We honor the termination of therapy by expressing our perceptions of the progress clients have made and our appreciation of the effort exerted. We note that we have learned from clients much as they have learned from us. During the final session, we pay particular attention to whether clients seem to be avoiding any negative emotions that arise in the context of saying good-bye and gently bring their attention to these emotions, encouraging an open experience of whatever arises. It is very rare for individuals to have an opportunity to be fully present to a shared termination of an interpersonal relationship; we do our best to take advantage of this opportunity to say an open, emotionally present good-bye.

As noted above, when possible, we invite clients to return for booster sessions as needed. If a client is particularly frightened to leave the security of therapy but appears to have the skills and level of functioning to do so, we will do our best to refrain from any booster sessions for a significant period of time, encouraging the client to rely on his or her own abilities in order to get a clear sense of them. In any subsequent sessions, we continue to emphasize the client's own ability to address challenges that arise, fostering independence and a sense of self-efficacy rather than a renewed reliance on the therapist.

CHALLENGES THAT ARISE DURING TERMINATION

How to Determine When It Is Time to End Therapy

As discussed earlier, assessment of progress is ongoing throughout therapy so that the therapist and client are both attending to the client's progress. Unlike in some traditional approaches to treatment, symptom reduction is not necessarily the central indication that treatment goals have been met. The collaborative treatment plan, which should be continually refined as therapy progresses if new goals emerge or old goals are fine-tuned, will typically contain specific behavioral targets that relate to clients' valued actions in specific domains as well as to clients' ways of responding to their own distress (i.e., with openness, curiosity, and acceptance rather than fear, avoidance, and judgment). These are both process goals; clients will not achieve a steady state of mindful, accepting responses while pursuing valued actions. Therefore, a more pertinent question than whether a client has achieved a certain state is the degree to which a client has acquired the skills to pursue these process goals on his or her own.

Often, the valued directions a client has targeted involve long-term life changes, which require time to unfold after years of living a more constrained life. As discussed in Chapter 8, more proximal actions can be taken on the path in these directions, but long-term outcomes may not be observed in the course of therapy. For instance, a client who values work that makes a difference in people's lives might take steps in exploring different career options, start attending to other people more in his or her current work, and begin some volunteer work over the course of therapy, but not yet have come to a final career decision when treatment ends. Thus, treatment completion is typically indicated more by some consistent pattern of successful valued action in multiple domains rather than by work in these areas feeling complete for the client. As the client begins to exhibit a systematic pattern of approach behavior in intended directions, confronting obstacles relatively independently (with support from the therapist), the therapist should begin to consider termination of therapy so that the client can experience the ability to live his or her life this way independent of therapy. Concurrent with these behavioral changes, therapists should assess the client's ability to consistently return to an accepting, mindful stance, regardless of the frequency of mindless, judgmental responses, which are inevitable. The ability to return to acceptance is the indicator of treatment success.

Clients may also reach a plateau where they have made significant changes, exhibiting increased skills in acceptance and valued action, but still have other areas to explore and that work has stagnated. Therapists and clients may collaboratively choose to take a break from therapy at this point, allowing changes to consolidate and the pattern of valued action to solidify before beginning to address additional issues. It may be that apparently unresolved issues resolve in the course of living a mindful, valued life, or it may be that subsequent sessions are needed. Sometimes a scheduled break from therapy can help determine which of these is the case.

Often, when therapists and clients review progress, they come to an agreement regarding the choice to continue or terminate therapy. As noted above, a writing assignment may help clients reflect on progress and their current state, if the decision is not sufficiently clear. Weekly assessments of experiential avoidance, symptoms, and behavioral actions should be reviewed to assess changes and current status to contribute to this decision.

Ending Therapy When External Factors Require It

Sometimes therapy ends when the therapist and client have not chosen it, such as when a client or therapist is moving and unable to continue with therapy or when other external factors interfere with the client's ability to attend therapy. In these cases, the same process of reviewing progress and the content of therapy, predicting lapses, and putting structures in place to review and maintain the content of therapy remains important. Although clients may not have solidified gains yet, therapists can help them recognize the progress they have made and map out the steps they want to follow to maintain and increase these gains. The suggestion to set aside time for weekly reflection and commitment to practice is particularly important in these cases, as it will help clients maintain focus on their progress and implement aspects of therapy on their own.

Ending Therapy When the Client Does Not Feel Ready

Sometimes clients do not feel ready to end therapy even though they have made significant gains. They may not recognize the gains that have been made, or they may be afraid that they cannot maintain these gains in the absence of the therapist. Reviewing progress and changes in assessment over time can help illustrate the gains that have occurred. Sometimes a longer series of tapered sessions can be helpful; clients can begin coming to therapy every other week or every third week, so that they have the opportunity to see what it is like not to have therapy weekly and to experience their own ability to cope with what emerges without the stress of leaving therapy altogether. However, it is important not to continue this process for too long. Clients may never feel completely ready to leave therapy, and this unwillingness may be another example of experiential avoidance, with clients not wanting to experience the anxiety of losing the safety net of weekly therapy. Framing it this way to clients can be helpful, and they often see that terminating therapy is another valued action that may not feel comfortable but that they can nonetheless choose.

Sometimes clients continue to hold on to unrealistic goals for therapy, such as being symptom-free. In these cases, reviewing the model of treatment and data that show symptoms often persist intermittently after efficacious treatment (although disorders do not continue) can help clients see that they will not experience a symptom-free life.

Ending Therapy When the Client Has Not Responded to Treatment

Sometimes clients are simply not responding to the treatment approach, and an alternative form of therapy should be sought. In these cases, it is still important to review whatever gains have been made as well as the obstacles that seem to have occurred. Clients may be seeking a different approach to therapy, in which case a referral should be made to someone who practices from that perspective (unless the therapist feels skilled in this approach as well and wants to shift focus). Sometimes clients do not feel they are a good fit with therapists who have a particular interpersonal style or cultural identity and may ask for a referral to a different provider. Although these therapy challenges can elicit uncomfortable thoughts and feelings in therapists (such as "I am not good enough" or "Why doesn't she like me?"), mindfulness and acceptance skills can help facilitate responses consistent with one's values as a therapist. When these situations arise, clients should be praised for recognizing that the therapy was not a good fit and for being willing to discuss their concerns openly and encouraged to pursue an approach or therapist who may be a better fit. The therapist can review different approaches to treatment at this point and help the client select an appropriate new therapist.

Sometimes clients are not willing to make the kinds of changes that are part of therapy. For example, a client may not be experiencing sufficient distress to motivate him or her to do the challenging work of therapy, or a client may have serious life stressors such as poverty, unemployment, or a medical condition that require significant time and attention. It is sometimes the case that clients are aware of their own avoidance and the changes they want to make to live a more fulfilling life but are simply unwilling to do so. (In our own work, it is helpful for us to think about changes in our lives that we as therapists are aware of but not currently working on.) When a client is not willing to fully engage in therapy for any of these reasons, it is important that the therapist help the client realize and articulate this rather than allowing him or her to continue to attend sessions without actively working. Keeping clients in therapy when progress is at a standstill can lead them to believe that therapy is not helpful and may inhibit them from seeking services in the future. Clients can be encouraged to return to therapy when they are willing and able to commit to the work. In all of these cases, therapists should first work with clients to identify the obstacles to their engagement in therapy, altering treatment so as to optimize their engagement and making sure that clients share therapists' conceptualization and approach. Often, what appears to be disengagement is really the absence of a collaborative treatment plan. Other times, a client is truly not interested in therapy and is pursuing it due to someone else's wishes or a sense that it "should" be done. This is not a good use of the client's time, and it is best to help him or her realize this and make a valued choice regarding engagement in therapy. Sometimes termination is the most therapeutic choice.

Clients Experiencing So Little Distress That It Is Difficult to Prepare for Lapses

For many clients, engagement in a valued life offers several opportunities to open up to difficult thoughts and emotions that can be used to help them prepare for posttherapy challenges. Occasionally, at the end of treatment clients are experiencing so few symptoms that it is difficult for them to imagine a lapse and to prepare for it. In these cases, we ask clients to brainstorm about upcoming events or activities to elicit some thoughts and emotions that can be approached with acceptance and compassion. Imaginal exercises that involve remembering difficult situations from the past or imagining future challenges can also help clients get in touch with difficult thoughts and feelings and practice responding to them so that they are more prepared for the inevitable emotional challenges they will experience.

Need for Therapy in the Future

Regardless of the course of treatment, clients may seek therapy again in the future. If possible, we prefer to have clients who have responded to treatment with us come back into therapy with us so that we can continue with an approach that has been helpful for them. Sometimes booster sessions only are warranted, but sometimes clients require a more extended dose of treatment due to new issues that have emerged or old issues that have reemerged. When clients call to schedule a booster session, we refer them to their binder and ask them to bring it to session. Often, by the time they come in for the appointment, they are already back on track.

Sometimes it is not possible for clients to return to their previous therapist (due to job changes, moves, or lack of openings). In these cases, it can be challenging to find an appropriate referral, particularly when the client is seeking more ABBT. Websites provide directories of clinicians who practice DBT (*www.behavioraltech.com/resources/crd.cfm*) and ACT (*www.contextualpsychology.org/therapist_referrals*), and the MBCT website (*mbct. com*) provides suggestions for locating classes. There is also a mindfulness listserv for the Association for Behavioral and Cognitive Therapies (go to *listserv.kent.edu/archives/ mindfulness.html to join*); posts to this listserv can result in identification of therapists who use mindfulness within a CBT tradition. Clients may find themselves seeing therapists who do not specialize in an acceptance-based behavioral approach. In this case, they can share materials from their previous therapy as well as what worked for them. Although it is not often made explicit, acceptance, enhanced awareness, and intentional, valued action are aspects of many approaches to treatment. Skillful therapists trained in a number of theoretical traditions will respond well to clients' descriptions of the work they have done and will be able to continue to foster that work. Clients can be coached on how to assess whether a specific therapist is responding well to the approach they are hoping to take in treatment so that they do not end up with someone who emphasizes experiential control in a way that would not fit well with their previous work.

TREATMENT REVIEW WRITING ASSIGNMENT

Please set aside 20 minutes during which you can privately and comfortably do this writing assignment. In your writing, we want you to really let go and explore your very deepest emotions and thoughts about the topics listed below.

Write about any or all of the following topics. If you choose to write on only one of the topics, that would be fine. You may write about them in any order you wish. If you cannot think about what to write next, just write the same thing over and over until something new comes to you. Be sure to write for the entire 20 minutes. Please do not spend any time worrying about spelling, punctuation, or grammar—this writing is intended to be a "stream of consciousness"—that is, you may write whatever comes to mind.

- What have you learned about yourself over the course of treatment?
- What methods have you learned that have been helpful to you?
- What methods do you need to continue to practice most once treatment ends?
- What new commitments do you need to make with regard to valued action?
- What concerns do you have (if any) about treatment ending?

TREATMENT REVIEW

In this treatment you learned:

- **Techniques to increase your present-moment focus, such as:**
  - Self-awareness (monitoring thoughts and emotions).
  - Mindfulness (focus on present-moment nonjudgmental observation of your actual experience).
- **The problem of control and willingness as a solution.**
  - Emotions and thoughts (positively and negatively evaluated) are part of the human experience and have adaptive value.
  - Attempts to control thoughts and feelings can backfire.
  - Increasing your willingness to experience all thoughts, feelings, and bodily sensations can open you up to more choices in your life.
- **Making valued choices about your behavior adds "color" to life.**
  - You completed an assessment of the areas in life you value.
  - You chose to make a commitment to live your life in a certain way.
  - You learned the difference between values and goals, process and outcome.

Awareness, mindfulness, willingness, and valued action are all concepts that one can continue to work toward. They are processes, not goals that one meets and/or completes.

WEEKLY ASSESSMENT

The following questions are designed to give us a sense of how your week has been in terms of the kinds of things we are focusing on in therapy. There are no right or wrong answers. We just want to get *your* impression of your week.

What percentage of the time did you find yourself worrying over the past week?

0 —— 10 —— 20 —— 30 —— 40 —— 50 —— 60 —— 70 —— 80 —— 90 ——100

What percentage of the time were you mindful over the past week? By "mindful," we mean aware of your current experience, focused on where you were at that moment and what you were doing, as opposed to what you did earlier or would do later?

0 —— 10 —— 20 —— 30 —— 40 —— 50 —— 60 —— 70 —— 80 —— 90 ——100

What percentage of the time did you feel accepting of your internal experience (thoughts and feelings) as opposed to trying to push it away?

0 —— 10 —— 20 —— 30 —— 40 —— 50 —— 60 —— 70 —— 80 —— 90 ——100

What percentage of the time did you feel you were spending time on the things that are important to you?

0 —— 10 —— 20 —— 30 —— 40 —— 50 —— 60 —— 70 —— 80 —— 90 ——100

What percentage of the time did you feel like your thoughts and feelings were getting in the way of what you wanted/needed to be doing?

0 —— 10 —— 20 —— 30 —— 40 —— 50 —— 60 —— 70 —— 80 —— 90 ——100

TEN

Incorporating Other Evidence-Based Interventions with Acceptance-Based Behavioral Therapies

In the introduction to this volume we provided an overview of studies that support the integration of acceptance and mindfulness with previously established cognitive and behavioral clinical methods in treating anxiety disorders, depression, substance abuse, eating disorders, BPD, and psychosis. While ABBTs show significant promise, data on the efficacy and effectiveness of these approaches and studies aimed at determining the mechanisms of change are still accruing.

Research on traditional forms of CBT has demonstrated its usefulness for a variety of clinical issues, including mood, anxiety, personality, eating, and substance use disorders. For many disorders, CBT has been shown to be more effective than other approaches. Despite these promising findings, the gains achieved in research have not fully translated into widespread clinical use. Research studies on CBT methods are often criticized by seasoned therapists on numerous counts. Most notably, while they have provided information about significant average reductions in symptoms from pre- to posttreatment enjoyed by research participants, they do not always account for individual clients who refuse randomization, who are excluded on the basis of the severity or complexity of their presentation, or who fail to complete treatment. Furthermore, outcome is often defined more narrowly in research than it is in clinical practice. Many studies focus on symptom reduction and ignore the more clinically salient but difficult to measure potential impact of treatment on quality of life. Although these criticisms have begun to impact the way in which treatment research is designed, the shortcomings of earlier studies have led some clinicians away from the use of CBT methods in practice, despite significant support for the use of certain CBT methods. We view the integration of acceptance and mindfulness approaches with cognitive-behavioral methods as one of many innovations in CBT that have the potential to address some of its limitations. This perspective's emphasis on helping clients live in accordance with their personal values and increasing their quality of life is likely to increase willingness to enter into and remain in treatment. Acceptance and mindfulness practice directly aimed at providing clients with skills to manage their thoughts and emotions may be particularly useful in addressing the fear and avoidance that surround many CBT techniques. Finally, like more traditional forms of CBT, ABBTs are not disorder-specific. Given that many topographically distinct behaviors (e.g., avoidance of fear-eliciting situations, use of alcohol, engagement in self-injurious behaviors) are conceptualized as forms of experiential avoidance, ABBTs may be particularly useful for clients with comorbid conditions and complex presentations.

In this chapter, we describe how acceptance and mindfulness approaches can be integrated with traditional CBT to produce clinically meaningful improvements in psychological functioning. Scientist-practitioners who work primarily in clinical settings are frequently charged with balancing the need to provide immediate evidence-based mental health services with the reality that findings from treatment-outcome research accrue slowly and do not always provide definitive guidelines on how to treat a particular client. ABBTs and the CBT tradition they draw from help practitioners in this bind in that they offer empirically based principles that can be flexibly modified to meet the individual needs of a particular client. Therapists can also increase their confidence in their choice of clinical methods by empirically evaluating their client's progress using the methods described in Chapter 9.

In this chapter, we explore the ways in which traditional CBT and ABBTs are similar and different and make recommendations for enhancing CBT with methods aimed at promoting acceptance. In addition to discussing cognitive therapy generally, we provide a description of how acceptance-based approaches can be used in conjunction with exposure therapy, behavioral activation, relaxation training, and skills development.

COGNITIVE THERAPY[1]

Although both acceptance-based and cognitive approaches acknowledge the role of life experiences in producing thoughts that many clients find troubling and distressing, they differ in the presumed role of cognitions in the development and treatment of psychological disorders. The conceptual model underlying traditional cognitive therapy (CT) is that maladaptive thoughts cause emotional distress and behavioral inaction. Therefore, CT is aimed at identifying distorted cognitions and examining their veracity through logical analysis and empirical hypothesis testing (e.g., Beck, 1976; Clark, 1986). In contrast, from an acceptance standpoint, thoughts are seen as transient reactions to different experiences, and the attempt to change their form or frequency is assumed to be a form of experiential avoidance. Thus, at the theoretical level, CT and ABBT may seem diametrically opposed, but it is important to note that CT and CBT are often used as general labels for a variety of techniques, some of which are inconsistent with acceptance-based approaches and some of which are not. Furthermore, a recent review of the literature suggests that those aspects of CBT that seem most inconsistent with an acceptance-based approach (e.g., cognitive restructuring) may not be necessary ele-

[1]Some confusion in the literature stems from the use of the term *cognitive-behavioral therapy* to refer to a wide range of approaches, some of which emphasize a causal role of cognitions in symptoms and some of which do not. We choose to use the term *cognitive therapy* to describe those approaches that emphasize the primacy of cognition in intervention, although these treatments also include behavioral elements, and some CBTs also address cognition.

ments of psychotherapy (Longmore & Worrell, 2007). There is some evidence that both CT and acceptance-based approaches work via the same mechanism of action. At least one study found that increases in metacognitive awareness (the ability to view thoughts and feelings from a decentered perspective) were associated with decreasing depressive relapse in both mindfulness-based and traditional CT (Teasdale et al., 2002). Thus, from our perspective, CT and acceptance-based approaches share a number of clinical similarities and can be successfully integrated.

CT typically consists of three types of clinical methods: (1) self-monitoring, or the identification and labeling of thoughts; (2) logical analysis, which involves restructuring or changing the content of a dysfunctional cognition through Socratic questioning; and (3) hypothesis testing, or the evaluation of the validity of dysfunctional cognition through the design and implementation of behavioral experiments (Jarrett & Nelson, 1987).

Self-Monitoring

The first component of CT, self-monitoring, is highly consistent with an acceptance-based approach. Both CBT and acceptance-based models underscore the role of narrowed, restricted attention in psychopathology. Clients with anxiety disorders often focus primarily on perceived threats, whereas those struggling with depression are more attuned to negative events and experiences. Treatment from both perspectives involves broadening a client's attention and facilitating awareness and differentiation of particular internal events. For example, where a client might initially only perceive herself as experiencing intense negative affect, self-monitoring can help her become aware of nuances in her emotional responding. Clients are also often unaware of the habitual behaviors they engage in that may contribute to their distress. Self-monitoring brings awareness to behavior and allows clients to make choices about the actions they take.

While traditional CT often uses self-monitoring as a first step in the cognitive-restructuring process, this clinical method has many other benefits. A broadening of awareness can presumably increase clients' contact with present-moment contingencies, reinforcing and supporting more flexible, effective, and values-driven behavior. Additionally, continued observation of internal experiences as transient events separate from one's sense of self promotes cognitive defusion, which should reduce a client's urgency to engage in experiential avoidance.

ABBT involves a number of clinical methods that can be used to help develop and support the self-monitoring skills that originated with traditional CBT. Given that many clients present to treatment with a decreased awareness of their internal experiences, a lack of practice in this skill, and a natural inclination toward experiential avoidance, simply assigning the task of self-monitoring may not be sufficient. ABBTs include a wide range of mindfulness practices (described in Chapter 6) that can be used to develop and sharpen observational skills. Mindfulness practice can impact qualitative aspects of self-monitoring that may help maintain the behavior and facilitate overall improvements. Recent research suggests that simple awareness of internal experiences may not be clinically beneficial (Lischetzke & Eid, 2003; Salters-Pedneault, Roemer, & Tull, 2006; Tull, Barrett, McMillan, & Roemer, 2007; Tull & Roemer, 2007), and the cultivation of a compassionate, curious, nonjudgmental, and accepting response to one's observation of internal experiences may be most clinically useful (Teasdale, 2004).

Logical Analysis/Cognitive Restructuring

Logical analysis, the second component of CT, involves a process of systematic questioning aimed at changing the content of a thought and seems the most inconsistent with an acceptance-based approach; however, cognitive restructuring itself consists of a number of disparate methods, some which are easily compatible with ABBT. For instance, one method of working with a maladaptive thought as part of cognitive restructuring is to challenge the content directly. When working with a client with panic disorder, the therapist might challenge the thought "If I have a panic attack I will die" by asking the client to consider the probability of such an event occurring based on past experience and available medical data. The client is encouraged to replace the seemingly irrational thought with another, more rational thought such as "There is no evidence that a panic attack could be fatal" to decrease anxiety and associated avoidance.

Other clinical methods of cognitive restructuring encourage a change in the *relationship* a client has to his or her thoughts, a key feature of ABBTs. For instance, in both cognitive restructuring and ABBTs, clients can be encouraged to consider thoughts as internal events that may or may not be based in fact. Also, flexibility in viewing thoughts may be emphasized rather than the importance of content change (e.g., "How many ways are there to see this?"; Borkovec & Sharpless, 2004, p. 223). Another method common to both cognitive restructuring and ABBTs is to have clients recognize that thoughts and feelings can be separate from behavior. Often, clients feel compelled to act in ways that are consistent with how they feel. For instance, when a client feels sad and low in energy she may believe she should stay in bed. A client who feels anxious in a new situation may respond by leaving, and one who feels angry may lash out. Both cognitive restructuring and ABBTs ask clients to consider acting in ways that are inconsistent with the action tendencies elicited by different emotional states. In DBT, this is referred to as *opposite action*. For example, a "workaholic" client who feels guilty about leaving work early for an important doctor's appointment might be encouraged to do so, even while experiencing those feelings. Another client might experiment with approaching and remaining in a social situation even while feeling anxious.

Many of the mindfulness and defusion methods described throughout this book can be used to enhance traditional cognitive-restructuring methods. For example, as discussed in Chapter 6, Hayes, Strosahl, and Wilson (1999) suggest that therapists adopt a number of verbal conventions in session that are aimed at helping clients change their relationships with internal experiences and ask their clients to use them as well. One is to overtly label thoughts and emotions as such. For example, if a client were to say, "I could never get through a family event without drinking," he would be encouraged to describe his experience more accurately as, "I am having the thought that I could never get through a family event without drinking" or "When I have urges to drink, it feels like I have no control over my behavior." Also, we recommend that clients consider replacing broad, pathological descriptors of their experience such as "depression" with more specific terms. Another simple, but potentially powerful convention from ACT encourages therapists and clients to consider substituting the word "but" for "and" to see if it provides a more accurate description of events and experiences. For instance, rather than saying "I want to go out to lunch with people at work, but I am anxious," the client would be encouraged to say, "I want to go to lunch with my coworkers and the thought of doing so is associated with feelings of anxiety."

Consider the following example of how we might help a client change his or her relationship with internal experience by the way we talk about events.

CLIENT: I couldn't go to work on Thursday because my depression came back.

THERAPIST: It sounds like Thursday was a hard day. I was wondering if we could take a few minutes to explore your experience on Thursday more fully. Remember we talked about becoming an expert observer of your thoughts, emotions, physical sensations, and behaviors? Let's see if we can break down "depression" into all the experiences you had and the choices you made.

CLIENT: OK.

THERAPIST: I want you and me both to develop a good understanding of all the experiences that you had on Thursday and how they unfolded. I think this might be helpful in making you feel less confused and out of control, which I know you have been struggling with.

CLIENT: OK, how should I start?

THERAPIST: Well, see if you can imagine yourself in bed Thursday morning. What did you first notice?

CLIENT: I felt depressed.

THERAPIST: What emotion do you experience when you are "depressed"?

CLIENT: Sadness.

THERAPIST: OK, so you noticed feelings of sadness. Any other emotions?

CLIENT: I guess a little anger. I really can't stand going into work anymore and dealing with my boss.

THERAPIST: Got it. So you noticed feelings of sadness and anger. Were there any physical sensations that you experienced?

CLIENT: I was exhausted.

THERAPIST: How could you tell?

CLIENT: My whole body felt heavy.

THERAPIST: This is really helping me get a feel for your experience. OK, so you mentioned that you had the thought "I can't stand going into work and dealing with my boss." Did you notice any other thoughts that emerged?

CLIENT: Just that I couldn't go to work. Is that a thought?

THERAPIST: Did you have a thought that was something like "I know it is time to go to work, but I feel too depressed"?

CLIENT: Well, I guess. I don't really think of it as a thought. More of a conclusion.

THERAPIST: It is definitely the case that it often seems like when we feel a certain way, we absolutely have to act a certain way. Those feelings can be really, really strong for two reasons. Remember, when we talked about the function of emotion, we talked about action tendencies? That we are hardwired or prepared to act in a certain way when we feel an emotion? Like how our body prepares us to flee a dangerous situation?

CLIENT: Right. We get a really strong urge to act in certain ways when we feel certain emotions, but we don't always have to follow through. Like the fact that I am frequently pissed off by my boss, but I don't hit him.

THERAPIST: Exactly. The other thing is that when we get in the habit of acting a certain way every time we feel a certain way, it almost becomes automatic. You have developed a strong habit that you should avoid activity when you feel sad and tired. So, when you woke up on Thursday and noticed feelings of sadness and anger, sensations of being heavy, and thoughts and very strong urges to stay home, what choice did you make about your behavior?

CLIENT: To call in sick and stay home. But it didn't feel like a choice at the time.

THERAPIST: The urge to stay in bed was really, really strong. Do you think it is possible that you could wake up with all those thoughts, feelings, and sensations and still go to work?

CLIENT: I guess it is possible. Of course it is.

THERAPIST: OK, are you willing to keep that possibility open?

CLIENT: To tell you the truth, I don't feel like it is possible, but I know it is. I have done it before.

THERAPIST: Great. One more thing I want to point out about a very common habit many of us have.

CLIENT: OK.

THERAPIST: A lot of times, when we say we want or need to do something that we didn't follow through with, we use the word "but" to describe how some emotion or thought stood in our way. Like if someone asks me to give a talk in front of a large audience, my first reaction might be "I want to, but I am too nervous." "But" makes it sound like my nervousness is preventing me from giving the talk. In that example, it is actually my unwillingness to feel nervous that is getting in the way of the talk. I could feel nervous and give a talk in front of an audience. I have before, and lots of other people do too. So, the "but" is not exactly right. In our attempt to observe things exactly as they are, sometimes it is more accurate to replace the word "but" with "and." "I want to give the talk, and I am nervous." That is a little more accurate. I am going to ask us both to watch for when we use the word "but." When that happens let's consider whether "and" is more accurate, OK?

CLIENT: I never really thought about that before. It seems so automatic.

THERAPIST: I know. So much of what we will do together involves noticing automatic patterns and considering new options. So, we started session with you saying you couldn't go to work on Thursday because your depression came back, and you have done a great job breaking that down into all the experiences that unfolded. So, what I am going to ask you to do right now is to see if you can describe what happened on Thursday to me including the emotions, thoughts, and sensations you noticed and the behavioral choice you made. Tell me what you noticed in each area.

CLIENT: On Thursday morning, I woke up and noticed feelings of sadness and anger.

I noticed I had the thought that I couldn't stand dealing with my boss and that I couldn't go to work when I was feeling so sad, angry, and tired. I made the choice to call in sick and stay in bed.

THERAPIST: That was great. I have such a better understanding of what you went through.

CLIENT: I guess it is helpful to talk about it that way, but I feel worse now about calling in sick.

THERAPIST: You're noticing . . .

CLIENT: I am noticing feelings of guilt and thoughts that I am a faker and should have gone to work.

THERAPIST: I can understand how thinking about behavior as choices can be painful, but the goal here is to help you open up to possibilities, to feel like you have some choices that you can make, not to encourage you to judge or berate yourself for the choices you make. We all make choices sometimes that seem driven by our feelings. Noticing the pull that thoughts, sensations, and feelings have on our behavior is the first step in opening up the possibility that we can do something differently.

CLIENT: OK, I can see that.

THERAPIST: Let's try together to see if we can both talk about your experiences in the way we just did. So instead of using shorthand labels like "depression," let's both try to label all the thoughts and feelings that you have and the behavioral choices you make. Let's also try to look out for the word "and."

CLIENT: OK, I can try.

THERAPIST: It might feel really awkward at first. Once you develop a habit, doing anything differently can feel strange or difficult.

Behavioral Experiments

The final component of CT involves testing the validity of maladaptive cognitions through behavioral experiments or hypothesis testing. For example, a client who believes "I will pass out or go crazy if I get dizzy" might be encouraged to engage in an exercise that elicits feelings of dizziness (like spinning in a chair) and to notice that the uncomfortable sensations eventually subside. Behavioral interventions are also a key characteristic of ABBTs, but these interventions are not solely conducted to produce cognitive change. The central aim of behavioral strategies in ABBTs is to encourage clients to engage in valued activities, even while experiencing uncomfortable thoughts and feelings. As with CT, clients are encouraged to practice engaging in activities with an expanded attention. For example, a client with panic disorder who fears the sensation of dizziness may be encouraged to go on an amusement park ride with her daughter if sharing that experience is part of her values. While in that situation, the client is encouraged to notice her full range of internal and external experiences rather than just focusing on threat cues. For instance, she might notice that her daughter is smiling and giggling and that it is a beautiful spring day. This broadened attention encourages the client to be a more present participant in her own life.

Behavioral interventions are among the most powerful components of CBT. Fortunately, there has been significant theory and research aimed at integrating acceptance and mindfulness with this efficacious approach. Given the relative importance of this work, two particular forms of behavioral engagement, exposure therapy for anxiety and behavioral activation for depression, are discussed in additional detail below.

EXPOSURE THERAPY

Exposure therapy, which involves progressively exposing clients to feared situations, is one of the most effective components of CBT for anxiety disorders. Yet, despite growing research support for this approach, relatively few clients receive this treatment in clinical practice (e.g., Cook, Schnurr, & Foa, 2004; Goisman et al., 1993). Although one obstacle to dissemination is the misconceptions therapists and clients share about exposure therapy (Cook et al., 2004), there is some evidence that exposure therapy is less effective with clients with more severe problems (e.g., Barlow, 2002) or greater emotional avoidance (Foa et al., 1995; Jaycox et al., 1998).

ABBTs offer a number of specific clinical methods that can be used to reduce the experiential avoidance that prevents clients from pursuing or fully engaging in exposure therapy. As discussed in Chapter 6, clients first practice acceptance and mindfulness in neutral and nonthreatening contexts such as mindfulness of breath, mindfulness of sounds, or the raisin exercise. (Of course, these domains might be frightening for clients with panic disorder who fear their internal sensations. While we offer a general progression to be used here, the order of exercises should always be adapted to the specific needs of the client depending on his or her presenting concerns.) Once clients develop experience directing their attention toward different internal experiences, noticing the tendency to judge and avoid certain sensations and cultivating a curious and compassionate stance toward internal events, they may be more willing to apply these skills in progressively more difficult domains. A second step might be to practice acceptance and mindfulness with the full range of thoughts and emotions elicited by everyday events before applying these skills to specifically threatening experiences (such as traumatic thoughts or socially threatening situations).

Explicitly connecting approach or exposure with values may increase the willingness of a previously reluctant client to experience private events, as the purpose and benefit of doing so may be more obvious and salient than in traditional behavioral approaches. Traditional exposure therapy is based on the principle of extinction and this rationale is provided to clients at the beginning of therapy.[2] Clients are encouraged to expose themselves repeatedly to every stimulus they have grown to fear and to resist the urge to escape or avoid the stimuli until anxiety is reduced. Anxiety-eliciting stimuli can include internal experiences (e.g., images, thoughts, memories, physiological sensations), external objects (e.g., dogs, snakes), and specific activities (e.g., being involved

---

[2]It was initially believed that fearful associations were actually removed or extinguished in the course of repeated exposure, but research has demonstrated that new, nonfearful associations are learned, but existing threatening associations are never completely removed. This is why fearful responses can be easily relearned or can recur spontaneously (LeDoux, 1996).

in a conversation, driving over a bridge). Depending on the nature of the feared object, exposure can be imaginal (e.g., a client with PTSD is asked to recall a traumatic event), interoceptive (e.g., a client with panic disorder purposively brings on panic-reminiscent feelings of dizziness by spinning in a chair), or *in vivo* (e.g., a client with social phobia gives a speech in front of a small audience). Although exposure therapy, like all methods of CBT, is a collaborative process between the therapist and the client, it is also highly directive. In most cases, the therapist will choose the target for exposure based on a hierarchy of feared situations and events generated specifically for the client. The therapist also typically sets up the details of the exposure situation and encourages the client to stay in the exposure until anxiety dissipates.

Although acceptance-enhanced exposure therapy is not inconsistent with traditional CBT, it has a number of subtle differences that may increase the efficacy and acceptability of this powerful component of CBT. Acceptance-enhanced exposure therapy explicitly connects exposure exercises and increased quality of life. When clients fully participate in valued activities, these actions will inevitably elicit painful thoughts, feelings, images, sensations, and urges to avoid. Clients are encouraged to accept and allow the presence of these experiences in the service of living a fulfilling life. While it is likely that repeated exposure to feared situations might result in an extinction of fear as the client learns that the situation is not as dangerous as previously feared, the primary rationale for exposure in ABBTs is engagement in inherently valuable activities.

To illustrate the differences in the two approaches, we will use Marcela as an example. If Marcela were seeking exposure therapy for panic disorder, she would be systematically questioned to develop a hierarchy of feared stimuli. At the top of the hierarchy might be going to a store in the middle of a busy shopping mall. Marcela would be encouraged to visit the mall, noting her fear level and urge to avoid every few minutes and staying for 30 minutes or until her subjective units of discomfort declined. Marcela would be told that the goal of the mall visit is for her to gain mastery and control over her emotions and for her anxiety to be reduced.

From an acceptance-based perspective, Marcela would be asked to explore which activities were personally meaningful to her. If she expressed a desire to become more intimately connected with others, we would examine barriers that prevented her from engaging in activities consistent with this value. She might describe an invitation to go shopping at the mall with friends as a potential opportunity to act on her values. We would validate and normalize the anxiety and anxiety-related thoughts elicited by taking such a risky action, use mindfulness and defusion methods to encourage her to view those internal experiences as tolerable transient events, and encourage her to consider going on the shopping trip. During the shopping trip, Marcela would be encouraged to use mindfulness skills to stay in the moment and to engage and participate actively in the interaction, while having self-compassion for any anxiety that arises.

This type of acceptance-enhanced exposure therapy is inherent in the values work that is central to ABBT, but other clinicians have conducted acceptance-enhanced exposure therapy in a slightly more traditional manner. Batten, Orsillo, and Walser (2005) discuss the possibility of conducting systematic prolonged exposure with clients struggling with PTSD in the traditional manner with a slight variation. Specifically, they modify the rationale for exposure by suggesting that approaching instead of avoiding traumatic memories and associated thoughts and emotions changes the nature of the relationship that the client has with these experiences. This change in context allows for more behavioral flexibility and increased ability to move in valued directions. Similarly, Levitt and Karekla (2005) introduce traditional interoceptive exposure to clients with panic disorder after first teaching them mindfulness and defusion skills and exploring valued directions.

BEHAVIORAL ACTIVATION

Behavioral activation (BA) was first proposed as a clinical method by Peter Lewinsohn (1974), based on his theory that a decrease in the frequency of pleasant events and/or an increase in the frequency of aversive events contributed to the development and maintenance of depression. Thus, BA involved teaching clients to monitor the frequency of different activities and, most important, using activity scheduling to directly increase clients' engagement in pleasant events.

More recently, Jacobson and his colleagues (Jacobson, Martell, & Dimidjian, 2001; Martell, Addis, & Jacobson, 2001), conceptualizing MDD from a behavior analytic framework, developed a more idiographic and acceptance-based approach to BA that differs from traditional BA in a number of important but subtle ways. At the most basic level, to ensure that pleasant activity scheduling is an effective and enriching clinical method, a functional analysis of contingencies of reinforcement for each client is conducted to guide the process of developing a personalized list of potential activities. While reading a good book is often generically considered a pleasant event, it may be counterproductive if it is assigned to a client who uses reading as an avoidance strategy and who often feels more disconnected and lethargic after reading. A careful assessment ensures that scheduled activities are more likely to be reinforcing. The process of uncovering which activities are personally meaningful to the client in BA is very similar to the values assessment described throughout this volume.

Additionally, when using this new approach to BA, clients are encouraged to consider the *function* rather than the *content* of certain patterns of thinking. For example, Jonah went out to lunch with his coworkers, an activity that he had identified as potentially reinforcing, but in the next session, he reported feeling miserably depressed during and after the meal and questioned whether BA would be useful for him. A careful analysis revealed that, while Jonah physically attended the lunch, he did not mindfully participate. As his coworkers interacted, Jonah experienced a number of thoughts about his loneliness and perceived inadequacies. When those thoughts arose, Jonah shifted his attention internally, became consumed and entangled with his thoughts, and completely withdrew from the conversation. Thus, his depressogenic thoughts actually served an avoidant function. Whereas a more traditional cognitive therapist might focus on challenging and changing the content of the depressogenic thoughts, Jonah's therapist focused on increasing his awareness of the function they served. Specifically, his therapist pointed out that, even if Jonah followed through with different behavioral assignments designed to improve his mood, engaging in rumination during events was a form of avoidance that would interfere with his enjoyment. Thus, Jonah was encouraged to bring his full attention to the next event he engaged in and to participate fully in the activity, even if he noticed the emergence of painful thoughts.

RELAXATION TRAINING

Many cognitive-behavioral treatment programs include elements such as diaphragmatic breathing, progressive muscle relaxation (PMR), and applied relaxation that are promoted as coping strategies clients can use to gain control over their anxious feelings. The research suggests that these approaches may be useful, particularly for clients struggling with GAD (Siev & Chambless, 2007). On the surface, it may seem that strategies aimed at gaining control of anxious symptoms are inconsistent with ABBT, but in our experience they can be integrated in a way that is clinically quite useful. When these methods are used as part of an ABBT approach, their focus is not to control or change the experience of anxiety (in fact, some research suggests that the use of breathing retraining with exposure therapy may actually decrease the efficacy of exposure (Schmidt et al., 2000), likely because it could be conceptualized as teaching avoidance (Barlow, 2002). Instead, the goal is to observe and allow the presence of certain internal experiences and to practice letting go of the struggle with physical sensations.

In PMR, originally developed by Jacobson (1934), clients are taught first deliberately to apply tension to isolated muscle groups and then to let the muscles relax, while noticing the difference between tension and relaxation. In our own practice, as discussed in Chapter 6, we use PMR with a few modifications as a mindfulness exercise. Once again, the rationale for the use of this clinical technique is important. We stress the use of PMR as an exercise to practice attention to and awareness of one's physical sensations and to anchor oneself to the present moment rather than as a method of anxiety control. We encourage clients to focus on their experience of breathing (and tension), to notice fully the sensations involved, and to make a subtle change and observe what happens (e.g., to let go of the tension in their shoulders).

We also find it useful to acknowledge the complexities of practicing a method such as PMR. Sometimes it elicits feelings of calmness and relaxation, but other times it is paradoxically associated with an increase in anxiety or even sadness. We encourage clients to be open to whatever experiences arise and note that PMR can reduce stress and anxiety at times, particularly when that stress and anxiety is related to one's reactions to and attempts to struggle with and change one's inner experience. Accepting and allowing one's internal experience can be associated with a sense of peace and calmness. Other times, feelings of anxiety and thoughts about painful experiences represent a realistic response to a difficult life circumstance or challenge. While some anxiety management techniques, such as PMR, might temporarily reduce those internal experiences, the situation eliciting them has not changed. Some feelings of anxiety or sadness cannot be changed without taking action. Other feelings and thoughts are an inevitable response to life (e.g., falling in love, taking a risk at work) and cannot be avoided by using anxiety management. Thus, it is important that clients and therapists not cling to an outcome of anxiety reduction when engaging in these practices and that a focus on living a meaningful, engaged life underlies choices made regarding these strategies. Again, the ultimate goal is for clients to change the relationship they have with their internal experiences such that thoughts, feelings, and sensations are seen as transient natural events rather than threatening reflections of their psychopathology that must be suppressed or eliminated.

SKILLS TRAINING

One of the most beneficial aspects of CBT is that it can be used to teach clients to develop and refine life skills that can be applied to a wide variety of domains. *Skills training* is a broad term used to describe methods taught to clients to help them solve problems, manage social/interpersonal interactions, become more assertive, and cope with emotions.

Acceptance and mindfulness techniques can be easily integrated with skills training. As discussed in Chapter 8, once a client has identified valued directions, he or she may note internal and external obstacles to engaging in valued activities. Internal obstacles are typically thoughts, feelings, images, and physical sensations that the client wishes to avoid that can be addressed with the application of clinical methods aimed at increasing acceptance, mindfulness, and willingness. External barriers to pursuing activities consistent with one's valued directions often include deficits in resources and skills. For instance, a client who wants to be challenged in the workplace may lack the interpersonal skills needed to interview for and secure a new job. A client who values interpersonal connections may lack some of the social skills necessary to cultivate friendships. Thus, once a client has identified valued life directions and developed a willingness to be open to internal experiences, traditional skills training can be quite useful in promoting valued action.

The most notable example of the integration of traditional CBT and ABBT is dialectical behavior therapy (DBT), an approach that balances acceptance and change by teaching and reinforcing effective skills in the context of acceptance and validation (Linehan, 1993a). Skills training in DBT involves learning core mindfulness skills such as observing and describing one's experience, fully participating in activities, taking a nonjudgmental stance toward internal and external events, focusing on one thing in the moment, and choosing to engage in effective behaviors. Additionally, clients are taught interpersonal skills (aimed at increasing social effectiveness), distress tolerance skills (i.e., learning to bear pain skillfully), and skills aimed at increasing emotion regulation (e.g., identifying and labeling affect, increasing mindfulness of current emotion, increasing positive emotion events, reducing vulnerability to "emotion mind").

Some therapists struggle with what can seem like opposing concepts: the acceptance of internal experiences and emotion regulation. Clinically, the term *emotion regulation* is often used to describe attempts to manage or change one's emotional experience. These strategies can seem at odds with that of ABBT, which suggest that internal efforts to change thoughts, emotions, and sensations paradoxically increase distress, amplifying negative responses and interfering with behavioral action, but emotion regulation is actually a much broader concept, including the strategic and automatic processes individuals use to influence which emotions they have, when they have them, and how they are experienced and expressed (Gross, 1998). Whereas emotion regulation strategies aimed at manipulating one's internal response may seem inconsistent with ABBT, a number of other emotion regulation strategies may not be. For instance, in the case of

BA discussed above, clients may choose to engage in activities that are more likely to evoke pleasant emotions. Expanding one's attention beyond threat cues may modulate the level of anxiety one has in an anxiety-eliciting situation. Maintaining healthy habits such as eating nutritious meals, getting adequate rest, and engaging in regular exercise may modulate the intensity of emotion.

In our experience, it is important that clients be willing to experience the full range of emotions that are part of the human experience. While there are a number of actions one can take that may increase the probability of experiencing positive emotions and minimizing negative ones, clients will be most satisfied if they can remain open and unattached to the outcomes of different choices. Remember the swamp metaphor from ACT discussed in Chapter 8: It is perfectly acceptable to wear boots and water-repellent clothes during the journey as long as you accept that you still might get dirty and wet along the way.

It is also important to acknowledge the potentially reciprocal relationship between emotion regulation and mindfulness. When one is aware and accepting of one's internal experiences, it may be easier to engage in strategies that may improve mood. Similarly, engagement in certain emotion regulation strategies may promote mindfulness. When we first introduce the concept of acceptance to our clients, they are often very reluctant to consider welcoming the intense and overwhelming distress they are experiencing. As they engage in better self-care and learn some emotion modulation strategies, their emotional reactions tend to be less powerful and extreme, making the prospect of acceptance more palatable. Of course, as we have discussed throughout this volume, it is often the case that emotion regulation strategies are ineffective in reducing painful and difficult emotions, thoughts, and sensations when we most need them. Thus, it is critical that, even while clients learn different methods to respond to their responses, they cultivate an attitude of nonattachment to outcome and remain willing to experience the full range of human responses.

MEDICATION

Often, clients present for psychological services while they are concurrently being treated with psychotropic medications, particularly antidepressants and/or antianxiety medications. At first glance, it may seem that taking medication in order to attenuate one's emotional experience is inconsistent with an acceptance or mindfulness stance, but these two forms of treatment can be successfully integrated. A client who is experiencing a significant vegetative depression or one whose anxiety is debilitating may find it extremely difficult to commit to a regular mindfulness practice. Similarly, a client who is experiencing intense and extreme shifts in affect may be too frightened by her experience to consider allowing emotions to be present. It may also be difficult to clarify one's values when one's symptoms are particularly strong and debilitating. Psychotropic medication may either sufficiently energize a client or modulate negative affect enough to increase willingness to participate in treatment. Often, the clients we have seen in ABBT who are receiving concurrent pharmacotherapy decided to reduce or discontinue their medication over time, as their stance toward their internal experience shifted and their mindfulness skills increased. We encourage clients to consult with all their treatment providers about any potential change in medication.

SUMMARY

From our perspective, acceptance-based behavioral approaches represent some of the many advancements and refinements within the larger field of CBT. Although there is preliminary support for these approaches, research is still needed to demonstrate the ways in which acceptance and mindfulness may increase the efficacy of CBT. In our experience, integrating acceptance and mindfulness with other empirically supported approaches to treatment has increased our clients' willingness more fully to engage in and to benefit from these strategies. As discussed throughout this volume, we encourage practitioners to openly discuss alternative treatment options with all clients before beginning treatment, to track progress throughout therapy, and to stay abreast of new developments in the research literature that may inform practice.

ELEVEN

Cultural Considerations in Acceptance-Based Behavioral Therapies

WITH JONATHAN K. LEE AND CARA FUCHS

Throughout this volume, we have provided an overview of the clinical methods that we use when working from an ABBT perspective. As we have noted, a careful and comprehensive assessment and case conceptualization is necessary to inform the development of a flexible and individualized treatment plan for each client. Cultural identification is a critical element to consider in this process. While we have made careful effort to highlight examples of the ways in which maintaining a culturally responsive stance can enhance treatment, we have chosen to dedicate a chapter to specifically addressing issues related to cultural competence. The goal of the current chapter is to highlight some of the ways in which acceptance-based behavioral approaches may be particularly applicable to people from diverse backgrounds and to offer some practical suggestions as to how ABBTs might be adapted and used successfully with these clients. Considerably more research is needed in this area, so this discussion of these important issues should be considered preliminary.

Throughout the chapter, we use the word "culture" to refer to the lens through which people view and interact with the world. Pederson and Ivey (1993) define culture as follows:

> Like personal constructs, culture is within the person, develops as a result of accumulated learning from a complexity of sources, depends on interaction with others to define itself, changes to accommodate the experiences in a changing world, provides a basis for predicting future behavior of self and others, and becomes the central control point for any and all decisions. (p. 2)

Jonathan K. Lee, MA, is a doctoral student in clinical psychology and a member of the Acceptance, Mindfulness and Emotion Lab at Suffolk University in Boston.

Cara Fuchs, MPH, MA, is a doctoral student in clinical psychology and member of the Emotions Research Lab at the University of Massachusetts Boston.

The definition highlights three important elements of culture: (1) it is shaped by our past experience, (2) it is dynamic and constantly in flux, and (3) it influences the way in which we view and relate to the world around us. A number of different frameworks for understanding culture in the context of psychotherapy have been proposed in the literature (e.g., Leong, 1996; Pederson & Ivey, 1993; Sue, 1998; Sue & Sue, 2003), as have guidelines for culturally competent practice (American Psychological Association, 2003). For the purpose of this chapter, we have selected a general framework for identifying the salient dimensions that influence a client's cultural identity. Pamela Hays (2008) offers a multidimensional approach for achieving this goal that can be remembered using the acronym ADDRESSING. The elements of the framework are having an understanding of the client's (1) **A**ge and generational influences, (2) **D**evelopmental and acquired **D**isabilities, (3) **R**eligion and spiritual orientation, (4) **E**thnicity, (5) **S**ocioeconomic status, (6) **S**exual orientation, (7) **I**ndigenous heritage, (8) **N**ational origin, and (9) **G**ender. We also supplement this framework with specific attention to race as a socially constructed identity in addition to ethnicity and awareness of the ways that structural and individual racism may play a role in the client's experiences and challenges. The extent to which a client assigns values and meanings to any given dimension will vary, and the clinician should explore these dimensions with the client to understand fully how each dimension fits into the client's daily life. It is important to note that the dimensions of the ADDRESSING framework should not be considered mutually exclusive, as the average person will identify with multiple dimensions. The dimension(s) that is (are) most salient in a given moment will vary depending on the context. Individuals carry multiple identities and that the ways these identities intersect are important to consider when engaging in culturally competent therapy.

THE RELEVANCE OF ABBTs TO CLIENTS FROM DIVERSE BACKGROUNDS

Racial and ethnic minorities represent the fastest growing sector of the American population (President's New Freedom Commission on Mental Health, 2003). Despite the fact that ethnic and racial minorities are less likely to meet criteria for a psychological diagnosis than White Americans (Breslau et al., 2006), among those who are in need of psychological treatment, ethnic and racial minorities are significantly more likely either to receive poorer quality mental health services or to remain untreated (Wang et al., 2005). Furthermore, ethnic minorities who do receive mental health services are at an increased risk of premature termination (Sue, 1998). To explain these trends, some psychologists have argued that White therapists are insensitive to the cultural backgrounds of these clients (Sue & Zane, 1987). In the extreme, there are those that propose that Western psychotherapy may not be a suitable intervention for minorities. For example, feminist psychologists argue that CBTs serve as a vehicle for promoting "valued functions, processes, and structures of white, male European-Americans" and that they "may neither fit nor be responsive to diverse ways of knowing and to the preferred processes and alternative world views of non-whites, non-males, or non-Europeans" (Kantrowitz & Ballou, 1992, p. 80). Based on this premise, it has been proposed that psychological interventions are needed to make room for clients' worldviews, which may be different from those of therapists.

The Therapeutic Model

The basic stance from which clients and their presenting concerns are viewed within ABBT seems to address these concerns directly. ABBTs acknowledge that clients' experience is shaped in part by sociohistorical and sociopolitical forces that contribute to their psychological distress. ABBTs such as ACT "view psychological events as ongoing actions of the whole organism interacting in and with historically and situationally defined contexts" (Hayes et al., 2006, p. 4). ABBTs focus on the ubiquity of human suffering, the normalization of psychological distress, and the importance of viewing the client and his or her struggles in a broad context, which may be particularly appealing to a client who already feels labeled and disempowered because of race, sexual orientation, economic disadvantage, physical disability, language, or other characteristics.

Destigmatizing Therapy

In many cultures, being labeled with a psychological diagnosis is highly stigmatizing and assumed to reflect personal failure or weakness of character, which can be a major deterrent for individuals who are considering psychotherapy. Often, this stigma and shame is extended to the entire family of a member struggling with psychological issues. The therapeutic stance described above is one way in which psychological difficulties may be destigmatized. Additionally, for these clients, the educational/skills-based nature of ABBTs might be particularly appealing. For instance, Roth and Robbins (2004) found that describing MBSR as an educational intervention increased the willingness of some inner-city Spanish-speaking clients with medical problems who were initially apprehensive about entering the program to engage in treatment.

The use of metaphor, which is a central component of ABBTs, may also be particularly useful when working with clients who are from a culture where emotional distress and related life difficulties are rarely discussed with people outside of the extended family. In our work with Pacific Island men, we have found that the use of metaphor in therapy provides clients an opening to begin to discuss their struggles in a culturally acceptable way.

The Client–Therapist Relationship

It has been suggested that ascribed credibility (cultural beliefs in the value of Western psychotherapy) and achieved credibility (individual perception that therapy is beneficial) are important elements to address early in treatment. The former is related to the low rates of mental health service utilization by people who do not subscribe to the values of Western cultures and the latter to the high rates of premature termination by ethnic minorities (Sue, 2006). While ascribed credibility is dictated by a client's cultural norms, achieved credibility is influenced by the therapist–client interaction. Depending on the ascribed credibility of Western psychotherapy in a client's culture, it is reasonable to believe that a client may have arrived at the decision to seek treatment through careful contemplation and may be uncertain about the benefits of treatment. Addressing achieved credibility in a timely fashion may, therefore, prevent premature termination, particularly with ethnic minority clients who have doubts about the effectiveness of Western psychotherapy. Sue and Zane (1987) term this *gift giving* (referring to the gift-giving ritual that is common in interpersonal relationships in Asia) and suggest it can be accomplished by giving the client a meaningful gain early in therapy to increase rapport and the therapeutic alliance.

Several of the initial practices and information provided in ABBTs are directly aimed at increasing the client's understanding of his or her experience, at providing a strong rationale for why the approach may be beneficial, and at giving immediate experiences of the potential for therapeutic benefit. For example, in our own work, in the initial therapy sessions, we provide clients with a rationale for the treatment that is specifically drawn from the shared conceptualization of the client's presenting concerns. We engage in a breathing exercise with clients and encourage them to use the practice throughout the week. In session two, clients struggling with anxiety are offered an adapted form of PMR, a powerful practice that most of them find quite useful. In that early session, we also have clients specifically consider the ways in which presenting concerns are interfering with their own values. Although no data exist yet, these efforts may help promote achieved credibility. We are careful to attend to clients' specific values and beliefs in this process in order to ensure that the gifts being presented are appropriate and well received. In fact, we begin treatment by assessing clients' understanding of their presenting problems, as well as their families', and their hopes for treatment. This helps us construct early sessions that are most likely to be perceived as beneficial.

Like CBT, ABBTs involve taking a collaborative approach to treatment, which can be particularly helpful when the power/privilege difference between therapist and client is significant. The "two-mountain metaphor" described in Chapter 4 provides an opportunity for the therapist to demonstrate humility and genuineness and to communicate that he or she is not judging or pathologizing the client. Therapeutically useful self-disclosures, which are encouraged in ABBTs, may also help minimize the power imbalance inherent in the therapeutic context, particularly when the therapist is from a dominant cultural background and the client identifies with one or more oppressed groups.

Acceptance of and Defusion from Internal Biases

As discussed throughout this volume, therapists who deliver ABBTs are encouraged to incorporate acceptance, mindfulness, and values into their own lives and particularly into their roles as therapists. A preliminary study suggests that ACT may be useful in helping individuals become aware of and defuse from prejudiced thoughts (Lillis & Hayes, 2007). Furthermore, in this study, increased acceptance and decreased believability of prejudicial thoughts were associated with increases in self-reported behavioral intentions to increase exposure to culturally diverse situations. Thus, ABBTs may offer therapists an effective way to work with the biases and prejudiced thoughts that often emerge when working with a client from a different cultural background.

ABBTs also provide a means by which clients may acknowledge their own internalized racism, heterosexism, ageism, or gender-role stereotyping and notice the extent to which these beliefs may be affecting their current values and actions. For example an African American female client may hold the belief that she needs to appear strong and suppress the display or experience of emotions such as fear or sadness to achieve or maintain power or privilege. If she values serving as a role model and mentor to her children, she might view teaching her children that showing or feeling distress is a sign of weakness as a valued action. ABBT allows the client to express this value within a framework that allows for curiosity and exploration. Through a dialectical stance, the therapist can validate the experiences that led to these conclusions and encourage the client to notice and observe potential costs that emerge when she behaves in ways consistent with this value. The therapist might also provide the client with psychoeducation about the ways that the suppression of negative emotions is often encouraged in the United States and that people who identify as racial minorities may be particularly encouraged not to show their emotions as an aspect of oppression. Through this work, the client may come to see ways that rigid adherence to this guideline can be harmful for her and her children and can, in fact, be disempowering. This could lead her to redefine her idea of what it means to be a good mother. This process would incorporate the realities of her experience so that she might instead conclude that there are contexts in which showing distress can have negative consequences and that she wants to teach her children to recognize these and respond accordingly. After noticing negative consequences of rigid expressive suppression, however, she may come to value expressive flexibility for both herself and her children. She also may notice that, even when she chooses not to express her emotions, recognizing them and accepting them is beneficial and something she would like to teach her children.

Acknowledging and Encouraging Personally Held Values

One of the most central ways in which ABBTs might be particularly relevant for clients from a range of backgrounds is the emphasis in therapy on client-defined values. The values component of treatment promotes the need for understanding the client's worldview, as values are proposed to be a salient indicator of cultural identity (Hofstede, 1980; Schwartz, 2006). In ABBTs, therapists do not define or judge which actions or choices might be viewed as adaptive or maladaptive. Instead, every suggestion proposed by the therapist or the client is evaluated as to the extent to which it brings the client closer to or further from his or her own values.

ABBTs also allow for an examination of systemic, cultural, and familial obstacles to engaging in valued actions (which should be a part of any culturally competent therapy). For example, values writing assignments can help a client explore the ways in which family members or the client's broader social network may be impacted before any commitment is made. They can also empower clients to form an understanding of the ways that systemic oppression has restricted them and discover steps they can take to create changes despite those obstacles. The dialectical stance of ABBTs provides a context in which the therapist can validate the systemic barriers that have prevented the client from being able to take valued actions and the distress associated with that while helping the client discover the ways that he or she can take valued actions within these constraints. For example, while working with a client with a physical disability and symptoms of anxiety, we would help the client begin to differentiate between the systemic obstacles to making valued changes and the obstacles caused by anxiety. This helps the client identify areas in which valued action can be pursued despite external constraints. Furthermore, actions aimed at changing the systemic obstacles can be conceptualized as consistent with the client's values and become an active part of therapy as well.

While these are all ways that ABBTs can lend themselves to culturally responsive therapy, it requires careful attention to and knowledge of contextual factors to use the treatment in this way. Therapists need to familiarize themselves with characteristics of specific cultural identities, particularly when they differ from the therapists'. Consultation with other professionals is often an important aspect of culturally competent care. Below, we discuss some examples of considerations that may arise when using this approach to treatment.

ADAPTING ABBTs FOR CLIENTS
FROM DIVERSE BACKGROUND

Cultural sensitivity involves fully assessing potentially important components of a client's background and identity, integrating culturally relevant information into the case conceptualization, and offering clinical methods that respect and complement a client's culture. In this section, we discuss some of the ways in which cultural factors influence our conceptualization and treatment approach from an acceptance-based behavioral perspective. We also note unique challenges that may arise when adapting ABBT to meet the needs of particular clients. Readers should see Hays and Iwamasa (2006) for a book-length review of culturally responsive CBT, which provides guidelines for specific racial and ethnic groups. Of course, it is critical that therapists avoid drawing broad, stereotypical conclusions about a client based on factors such as age, gender, race, socioeconomic background, and ethnicity. As noted above, individuals often view themselves from many intersecting perspectives, reflecting different cultural influences, so it is important to be extremely sensitive to the ways in which these identities should inform a client's treatment plan. A deeper appreciation of the client can be gained by understanding when to generalize versus when to individualize a client's sense of cultural identity, often referred to as *dynamic sizing* (Sue, 1998, 2006).

For example, Aisha, a young adult immigrant we worked with, presented with social anxiety, substance use issues, and feelings of depression. Knowing that immigration experiences can be influential, we asked more about her experience moving to the United States for graduate school. We learned that Aisha's trip was delayed due to flight restrictions in the wake of September 11, leading her to miss orientation and the vital social-networking opportunities it provided. Subsequently, she became isolated and withdrawn. The only friendships she developed were with a group of students of the same ethnicity who happened to drink alcohol regularly. Although she realized that regularly drinking was interfering with her ability to live consistent with her values, she felt limited by her restricted social options. As Aisha's white, American-born therapist, it was important to think and inquire about the possible ways that her identity as an immigrant to the United States during a time when the nation was mourning a tragedy and sharing in a period of strong national unity were relevant to her presenting concerns, likely contributing to her sense of isolation. Also, given her immigrant status, it was important to be sensitive to the ways her cultural identity was likely to be in a state of confusion through her process of acculturation. Values work would be particularly important and challenging as she was discovering for herself which American values she wanted to adopt and/or which values from her country of origin remained salient and important to her. Acknowledging and exploring this state of flux is an important form of validation that can help clients navigate complex cultural contexts during transitional times.

Encouraging Nonjudgmental, Compassionate Awareness

Earlier, we discussed the ways in which acceptance-based behavioral approaches to treatment may destigmatize some aspects of seeking and accepting treatment for emotional difficulties, but clients whose families or cultures strongly discourage the experience and expression of emotion may still struggle with the concept of changing their relationship to their internal experience. While some therapists may view such rules about emotional experience and display as restrictive and judgmental, clients may face enormous difficulty if asked to consider changing them. For example, Emilio is a Puerto Rican married male with four children who experiences frequent and disruptive periods of depression. He presented to treatment extremely angry and frustrated with himself for not being able to control his internal emotional and physiological responses, and he was deeply embarrassed as he believed his wife and children viewed him as "weak." As Emilio's depression intensified, he grew increasingly concerned that he would not be able to continue to work and that he would be unable to fulfill his value of financially supporting his family.

A client with this presenting perspective may be extremely reluctant to consider developing a compassionate and nonjudgmental stance toward his inner experiences. It is critical for the therapist to both validate the client's concerns and encourage the client to explore whether changing this stance would actually make him "weaker" or allow him to engage in actions more consistent with his values. Through monitoring, he may come to see that his efforts to control his feelings of sadness are associated with increased rather than decreased dysphoria. He might be able then to consider the possibility that compassion for his emotions would actually make him more rather than less able to fulfill his role as the economic provider for his family, even though it *feels* like acceptance and self-compassion will make the problem worse. When working with a client from a culture that places a strong emphasis on familial cohesion and gender-role responsibilities, particularly if there are strong cultural and family obstacles that may prevent a client from considering this self-accepting stance, it may also be useful to involve the family in treatment. For example, we might provide Emilio's wife with some psychoeducation about emotional responding, the paradoxical effects of control, and the rationale for Emilio's treatment plan. This may help Emilio feel less judged by his wife and better able to develop a different relationship to his distress.

Mindfulness as Culturally or Religiously Incongruent

As noted in Chapter 6, it is important to present the concept of mindfulness as separate from the Buddhist tradition from which it developed. This is particularly relevant for clients who feel less comfortable with spirituality or who have a firmly established spiritual identity and may be threatened by feeling forced to change it. For instance, Muñoz and Mendelson (2005) describe a Latina client who refused to practice deep muscle relaxation techniques out of a concern that it too closely resembled yoga. Of course, a client's willingness to accept any clinical method should always take precedence in therapy; at the same time, therapists are encouraged to consider developing individual, culturally relevant practices that serve the same function as traditional mindfulness exercises. Several religions, including Christianity, Judaism, and Islam, contain some opportunities for contemplative practice. For example, for a client who is a devout Catholic and may not be willing to engage in "meditation" exercises because it may be a violation of his or her faith, alternative exercises can be suggested to practice present-moment awareness. Hinton (personal communication) suggests encouraging such a client to bring gentle awareness to the physical sensations in the fingertips as each rosary bead is touched in sequence. Passage meditation is a form of meditation in which practitioners focus on and slowly repeat a memorized passage from a scripture or by a major spiritual figure that has been shown to be quite similar to MBSR in function and form (Oman et al., 2007). Encouraging a client to practice mindfulness in the context of his or her own spiritual tradition may strengthen the therapeutic alliance by demonstrating the therapist's respect for the client's culture, enhance the impact of the practice, and increase the possibility that the client will continue the practice after treatment is terminated.

The content of mindfulness exercises can also be modified to capture culturally relevant images. For example, in his work with Cambodian and Vietnamese refugees with orthostatic panic, Hinton and colleagues (Hinton et al., 2001; Hinton, Pham, Chan, Tran, & Hinton, 2003) asked clients to visualize a lotus bloom that spins in the wind at the end of a stem during mindfulness exercises, a culturally relevant metaphor emphasizing flexibility.

Therapists should also be sensitive to the possibility that clients might react negatively to the use of mindfulness in therapy due to its congruence with an aspect of their background. That is, clients from a Buddhist background or an Asian background with cultural ties to Buddhism (such as family members who practice) or with their own history of any form of meditation may have a reaction to the use of mindfulness in treatment. In this case, clients may object to something personal becoming a part of a standard intervention or to the ways that its application in treatment may seem to be uprooted from the rich spiritual, religious, or cultural associations it has in their own lives. We are careful to assess and discuss these issues with clients early to develop a shared view of our use of mindfulness in therapy. In these discussions, we share our view that particular aspects of this tradition may be useful in the specific context of therapy, while many other aspects are vitally important in other contexts. In this way, we are careful to validate the personal meanings of these practices for clients while explaining their particular utility in the context of therapy.

Client-Relevant Behavioral Change

One of the stated limitations of using CBT with clients from diverse backgrounds is the traditional emphasis on individual-level behavioral change (Hays & Iwamasa, 2006). This limited emphasis fails to acknowledge the social and systemic factors that may make behavior change more challenging. As noted above, there are often structural barriers such as oppression and poverty that may inhibit a client's success in making changes that both therapist and client feel would be adaptive. The expectations and desires of the client's family members and larger support group may also serve as obstacles to change. Although the framework of ABBTs allows for acknowledgement and consideration of these barriers, it may be challenging for therapists to fully understand and appreciate these complex societal forces.

For example, Maria was a Mexican American client who was struggling with completing her schoolwork. She described her problem as reflecting procrastination. Her inability to get her assignments done outside of class was so chronic that Maria was on academic probation and at risk of losing her financial aid. Despite the fact that she identified education as a value, Maria was struggling with the idea of being able to commit to a consistent effort on her schoolwork. Our initial assumption was that Maria had developed a habit of procrastination, but when we explored with Maria what might be preventing her from completing her schoolwork, she admitted that it was concerns about spending time with her mother. By Maria's report, her mother expected Maria to spend a significant amount of time with her each week, and she was concerned that it would be difficult for her mother to adjust to her being less available. When we asked Maria whether she had directly discussed her concerns with her mother, it became clear that this conversation was more complicated than we initially imagined. Maria explained that her mother was unfamiliar with the U.S. school system and unaware of the time commitment associated with obtaining a college degree. It was evident that Maria had not told her mother about the amount of time her schoolwork required outside of being at school, precluding any opportunity for her mother to understand the time commitment involved in a college education. Therefore, we discussed ways she might talk to her mother about her school-related time commitments, as well as the possibility of Maria trying to get more of her schoolwork done at school so that her time at home could be more easily spent with her mother, given her commitment to being connected to and available to her mother. Had we not explored these potential external challenges, Maria might have failed in her attempts at behavioral change and incorrectly labeled herself as lazy.

Although ABBTs allow for individually derived values, therapists still need to be extremely sensitive to the ways in which cultural factors may affect a client's ability to articulate a set of values. One dimension on which cultures vary is the degree to which members give priority to individuals versus groups—that is, collectivist versus individualistic orientations (e.g., Markus & Kitayama, 1991). A client with a strong group orientation may have difficulty articulating "personal" needs as part of a values exercise. Moreover, if a client's values differ in orientation from the therapist's, a lack of understanding of the historical and social context in which values are assigned meaning can detrimentally affect treatment, particularly if the therapist attempts to influence the client to adapt to the therapist's culturally based values.

For example, Kim, a young Chinese American woman, shared her struggle with an aspect of the instructions associated with a values exercise. Specifically, in our attempt to help clients identify what is personally relevant, we suggested that they should consider their own values, not those imposed by others. On the one hand, Kim explained that she did not distinguish between individual and group values within her family, seeing her family's values as shared among all members. At the same time, she partially identified with American culture and had a desire to explore her own values as separate from those of her family. This issue came up most frequently around her choice of career. Her family's shared value was to financially support and provide for extended family members. Kim was pursuing an advanced degree in business that she believed would help her earn enough money to act consistent with that value, but she was struggling with a sense that a career in business would not be personally fulfilling or allow her to have a positive impact on society. Kim's therapist became aware of her own biases, coming from a culture that values personal fulfillment and meaningful work and is less concerned with financially providing for family members. This awareness allowed the therapist to recognize and defuse from thoughts that she should try and influence Kim to act in a way that was consistent with the therapist's values. Instead, the therapist provided a safe context in which Kim could consider the ways in which her personal and familial values were both valid. After several weeks of exploration, Kim decided to continue pursuing a career in business while making a concerted effort to engage in nonwork activities that were personally meaningful to her. Kim also moved toward accepting that, as a Chinese American, she would face the struggle of holding personal values that were sometimes in competition with and sometimes merely in addition to the values of her family and her Chinese cultural background.

The case of Kim also illustrates a common values struggle that can be seen among American children of first-generation immigrants. Often, children of immigrants (depending on the age of the child at the time of immigration) acculturate at a more rapid pace than their parents and, thus, are quicker to adopt American values. During this process of acculturation, friction may emerge between parents and children as the parents adhere to values from their country of origin, while the children adopt or integrate new values. At the same time, these children may struggle to find a way to maintain values from their country of origin as an important aspect of their identity while finding ways to function in new contexts that often demand acculturation and abandonment of these values. Therapists need to be sensitive to the complexities of this process for all members of the family as they work with clients to examine what is most meaningful to them and how they want to be living their lives. In these contexts, acknowledging the dynamic nature of valuing and the ways that one's values may fluctuate and evolve is particularly important.

Another example of the role of culture in values is illustrated by my (Lee) work with David, a 25-year-old white American I was treating for substance use issues. A major barrier to David's recovery was his homelessness. I encouraged David to invite his mother to a session and to ask her if he could temporarily live in her house while he was working on his recovery. As the therapist, I was trying to elicit familial support for David from his mother, but during the session, it became clear that both David and his mother valued the idea of David being able to live independently and support himself financially, seeing it as a sign of personal growth and maturity. David disclosed that he thought that being employed and working toward gaining some financial stability would make it easier for him to view substance use as a strategy that might interfere with his ability to live consistent with his values. This interaction made me realize that, as a Korean American, I had extended my culturally influenced value of interdependence to David and his mother.

We acknowledge that our approach to values clarification might seem to contain an individualistic bias in that we specify a domain of self-nurturance and community involvement. While the latter part of that category can be seen as emphasizing interdependence, the first part has a more individualistic orientation. We are careful to examine our use of language with clients when we describe this domain and to articulate our reasoning for including it. Even among those for whom group needs are valued above individual needs, nurturance of the individual can be an important component of maintaining the well-being of the collective. We try to be sensitive to the cultural lens of clients in our exploration of this domain to ensure that we are not imposing individualistic values on them by focusing on the self. We also intentionally incorporate community involvement to provide an avenue for more group-focused values within this domain.

Culture can also influence the choice of specific actions that might reflect a client's values. For example, Hinton, Pich, Chhean, Safren, and Pollack (2006) describe working with a Buddhist client who was struggling with survival guilt related to PTSD. The client was searching for current actions that might reflect his value of honoring others who had died. The therapist encouraged the client to participate in religious activities considered to be "merit making," as it is believed that the earned merit promotes a good rebirth for the deceased.

Flexibility in Outside-of-Therapy Assignments

Flexibility is also needed when considering the amount and type of outside-of-session practice that is required of a client. In general, we assume that the more time a client can devote to self-monitoring, mindfulness practice, and values exercises, the greater the therapeutic benefit, but economic conditions, family obligations, school and work demands, and cultural expectations may all limit the amount of personal time available to a client. Clients may also live in conditions that can make it difficult to find a space in which they can concentrate on reading material, reflect on their experiences, or set aside time for mindfulness practice. It is critical that we both validate the real constraints on our clients' time and generate creative suggestions as to how clients might overcome these obstacles (or manage them the best they can) and offer any support we can to facilitate the process. For instance, one of us advocated for the inclusion of babysitting services at a mental health clinic that served primarily low-income women. Offering child care is one concrete way that clinics can increase the probability of clients attending therapy sessions or coming in between sessions to complete out-of-therapy assignments.

Several strategies can be used to help clients who are having difficulty completing out-of-session assignments. Assignments can be streamlined to make them more manageable. Clients can be asked to complete monitoring forms at one set time during the day rather than throughout the day. Practice can be abbreviated to make it more possible to fit in; we would rather a client practice mindfulness for 2 minutes each day with regularity than plan for 15 minutes but never be able to fit it in or do it only once a week. As discussed in Chapter 6, remembering the function of the assignment is important when these adjustments are made. If we are interested in increasing the habit of mindfulness, any length of practice is preferable to no practice.

When formal practice is not possible at home, it can be a regular part of session, and informal practice can be emphasized at home, as it can be done in conjunction with any daily task. Similarly, if formal monitoring cannot be managed, clients can be encouraged to increase awareness during the week, and sessions can be used to recall imaginally specific situations and notice thoughts, feelings, efforts to control internal experiences, or whatever is the focus of treatment that week.

Even as we acknowledge the real constraints on clients that may underlie their difficulties in completing assignments, we are also careful to continue to attend to the possibility that experiential avoidance may contribute to these difficulties. We share our own experiences of avoiding practice at times and finding monitoring challenging to ensure that this suggestion does not appear blaming in any way, and we do not persist in this suggestion if it does not resonate with clients, given that external obstacles may be the cause of their inability to complete assignments. Either way, practicing mindfulness and monitoring in session may provide experience with these methods that facilitates using them between sessions as well.

It is also important to consider the ways in which clients' experiences and abilities may render certain aspects of treatment more personally challenging. In conducting DBT groups with individuals with intellectual disabilities, Lew, Matta, and Tripp-Tebo (2006) found that, because of this population's adverse experiences with schoolwork, the use of the term *homework* for outside-of-session practice carried a negative connotation. Instead, these therapists referred to homework as "practice," and skills were practiced with films, pictures, or any medium that clients preferred. In our own clinical work, we encourage clients who struggle with written assignments because of language, educational, or physical disability–related barriers to use recording devices to capture their out-of-session thoughts and experiences.

Developmental Considerations

While this volume focuses on the provision of ABBT to adults, there is some evidence that these approaches may be adapted and successfully used with children and adolescents. For instance, developmentally appropriate metaphors and concrete examples may be especially helpful in trying to convey some of the main concepts in ABBT. A case study of an adolescent female suffering from anorexia found that using a map to illustrate the commitment to valued directions was especially helpful in concretizing metaphors like the "passengers on the bus" metaphor (Heffner et al., 2002). Similarly, another study found that asking children to write down their daily worries on a piece of paper and place them in an actual "worry warts basket" helped the children understand the more complex concept of distancing from their anxious thoughts (Semple, Reid, & Miller, 2005). Semple and her colleagues (2005) describe making a number of adaptations to mindfulness-based treatment aimed at keeping children interested and engaged. Groups are limited to six to eight children and two co-leaders, whereas the typical adult MBCT program runs with a 12-to-1 participant-to-leader ratio. Children are given notebooks to decorate and fill with cartoon stickers that are provided as rewards for session attendance and between-session mindfulness practice. Frequent meditations of 3–5 minutes replace the typical 20- to 40-minute sitting meditations that are characteristic of groups run with adults. Furthermore, a variety of mindfulness exercises are introduced in each session, with an emphasis on active practices such as drawing pictures, making music, and tasting different foods. Finally, parents are introduced to mindfulness exercises in a pretreatment session and they are asked to support their children's between-session practice.

Family involvement is presumed to be a critical factor when providing ABBTs to children. As discussed earlier, attitudes about emotions and their appropriate expression are typically learned within a family context. If a therapist is working with a child to increase his or her acceptance of painful thoughts and feelings, these efforts might be thwarted by parents who regard emotional control as a marker of good mental health. Similarly, if a therapist is trying to encourage a young client to allow anxiety, well-meaning parents may block the opportunity for practice if they habitually respond to their child's anxiety with distraction and reassurance.

In the mindfulness treatment described above (Semple et al., 2005), parents are invited to an orientation session where they are encouraged to practice mindfulness exercises with their children at home. Also, at the end of treatment, a "review and dialogue" session is held for the parents where they can discuss their experiences and ways in which they can continue to cultivate and support their child's mindfulness practice at home.

ABBTs may also be useful in working with older adults, particularly those who are contemplating existential issues such as the meaning of life or the inevitability of death and dying. With such clients, a focus on present-moment awareness and self-compassion may provide a space in which to approach such emotionally laden issues. Smith (2006) discusses the cultivation of mindfulness among older adults who are struggling with depression with concerns about attaining their goals and little hope for the future. He describes mindfulness as the "path to alive mind" that offers these clients an opportunity to live in the present moment and discover that they have more to live for. Lynch and colleagues (2007) describe their adaptation of DBT for older adults with depression and personality disorders, which specifically targets skills deficits and behavioral inflexibility in these clients. One adaptation is presentation of a dialectic between "fixed mind" and "fresh mind" to help clients synthesize information gathered over their lives with new information available in the current context—in other words, to promote flexibility. They have also added skills modules on "looking forward" (values, goal setting, and goal planning) and "looking back" (forgiveness and creating a life story). In these ways, therapy focused on developing a present-moment openness to experience and behavior in values-consistent ways can be adapted to address developmentally relevant themes and challenges.

Although we have primarily described ABBT as an individual treatment, many have argued that groups may be beneficial, particularly for clients within distinct age groups. For example, Smith (2006) argues that a group format may provide a social network for older adults who are at greater risk for more severe depression and social isolation. Seeing other older adults engage in mindfulness exercises may destigmatize the practice and increase a client's willingness to try new methods of coping with difficult emotions. Also, reunion or program graduate groups can support the continued practice of mindfulness (Smith, 2006; Wagner, Rathus, & Miller, 2006).

Developmental adaptations to the structure of ABBTs may also be necessary. For example, Semple and colleagues (2005) found that it was necessary initially to shorten the length of the breathing exercises to 3-minute sessions when working with children as it was difficult for them to maintain attention on their breath for a longer period. To accommodate older adults who may have less endurance, Smith (2006) suggests that it might be beneficial to reduce session length. Smith recommends sharing an awareness of this potential issue with clients at the beginning of therapy and checking in frequently to prevent overexertion. If the length of sessions will have to be shortened, it may be necessary to increase the number and/or frequency of sessions to present the material successfully.

SUMMARY AND CONCLUSIONS

Research is needed to examine the clinical effectiveness of acceptance-based approaches when working with people of different cultures, specifically examining adaptations that are made to ensure that the treatment is delivered in a culturally competent manner. It seems, however, that the focus on the clients' values and the context may make ABBTs helpful in treating a diverse range of clients. The literature base on the use of acceptance- and mindfulness-based treatments with diverse populations is steadily growing, and a current review suggests promising findings. We recently conducted a metanalytic review of 15 acceptance- and mindfulness-based treatment studies that included predominantly individuals who were nonwhite, non-European American, non-English-speaking children/adolescents, older adults, nonheterosexual, low-income, and/or incarcerated. This resulted in 15 studies from 13 peer-reviewed articles and included 700 participants who were treated with some ABBT approach. Studies that included no comparison group, on average, demonstrated the largest effect sizes ($d = 1.35$, $n = 5$). Studies that compared a mindfulness- or acceptance-based treatment to treatment as usual or a no-contact group showed moderate effects on average ($d = 0.64$, $n = 6$, and $d = 0.45$, $n = 2$, respectively). Only two studies compared the treatment of interest to an empirically established approach, yielding the smallest effect on average ($d = 0.20$, $n = 2$) (Fuchs, Lee, Orsillo, & Roemer, 2007). While these initial findings provide some support for the utility of ABBTs with people from diverse backgrounds, more rigorous clinical research is needed. In our current research, we are collecting qualitative data from clients of different ethnic backgrounds in order to obtain some preliminary information on the perceived appropriateness and cultural relevance of the clinical methods we are using.

APPENDIX: MINDFULNESS BOOKS

Bayda, E. (2009). *Zen heart: Simple advice for living with mindfulness and compassion.* Boston: Shambhala.

Bayda, E., & Bartok, J. (2005). *Saying yes to life (even the hard parts).* Somerville, MA: Wisdom.

Beck, C. J. (1989). *Everyday Zen: Love and work.* New York: HarperOne.

Boccio, F. J. (2004). *Mindfulness yoga: The awakened union of breath, body, and mind.* Somerville, MA: Wisdom.

Brach, T. (2004). *Radical acceptance: Embracing your life with the heart of a Buddha.* New York: Bantam Dell.

Chödrön, P. (2000). *When things fall apart: Heart advice for difficult times.* Boston: Shambhala.

Chödrön, P. (2002). *The places that scare you: A guide to fearlessness in difficult times.* Boston: Shambhala.

Germer, C. K. (2009). *The mindful path to self-compassion: Freeing yourself from destructive thoughts and emotions.* New York: Guilford Press.

Gunaratana, B. H. (2002). *Mindfulness in plain English.* Somerville, MA: Wisdom.

Kabat-Zinn, J. (1994). *Wherever you go there you are: Mindfulness meditation in everyday life.* New York: Hyperion.

Kabat-Zinn, M., & Kabat-Zinn, J. (1998). *Everyday blessings: The inner work of mindful parenting.* New York: Hyperion.

Nhat Hanh, T. (1976). *The miracle of mindfulness.* Boston: Beacon Press.

Nhat Hanh, T. (1992). *Peace is every step: The path of mindfulness in everyday life.* New York: Bantam Books.

Orsillo, S. M., & Roemer, L. (2011). *The mindful way through anxiety: Break free from chronic worry and reclaim your life.* New York: Guilford Press.

Salzberg, S. (2002). *Faith: Trusting your own deepest experience.* New York: Riverhead Books.

Salzberg, S. (2005). *Lovingkindness: The revolutionary art of happiness.* Boston: Shambhala.

Sharples, B. (2006). *Meditation and relaxation in plain English.* Somerville, MA: Wisdom.

Siegel, R. D. (2010). *The mindfulness solution: Everyday practices for everyday problems.* New York: Guilford Press.

Williams, J. M. G., Teasdale, J. D., Segal, Z. V., & Kabat-Zinn, J. (2007). *The mindful way through depression: Freeing yourself from chronic unhappiness.* New York: Guilford Press.

SPECIFICALLY FOR THERAPISTS

Bien, T. (2006). *Mindful therapy: A guide for therapists and helping professionals.* Somerville, MA: Wisdom.

Christensen, A., & Jacobson, N. (1998). *Acceptance and change in couple therapy: A therapist's guide to transforming relationships.* New York: W. W. Norton and Company.

Dimeff, L., & Koerner, K. (Eds.). (2007). *Dialectical behavior therapy in clinical practice: Applications across disorders and settings.* New York: Guilford Press.

Germer, C. K., & Siegel, R. D. (forthcoming). *Compassion and wisdom in psychotherapy.* New York: Guilford Press.

Germer, C. K., Siegel, R. D., & Fulton, P. R. (Eds.). (2005). *Mindfulness and psychotherapy.* New York: Guilford Press.

Hayes, S. C., Follette, V. M., & Linehan, M. M. (Eds.). (2004). *Mindfulness and acceptance: Expanding the cognitive-behavioral tradition.* New York: Guilford Press.

Hayes, S. C., Strosahl, K. D., & Wilson, K. G. (1999). *Acceptance and commitment therapy: An experiential approach to behavior change.* New York: Guilford Press.

Kozak, A. (2009). *Wild chickens and petty tyrants: 108 metaphors for mindfulness.* Boston: Wisdom.

Linehan, M. M. (1993). *Cognitive-behavioral treatment of borderline personality disorder.* New York: Guilford Press.

Linehan, M. M. (1993). *Skills training manual for treating borderline personality disorder.* New York: Guilford Press.

Olendski, A. (2010). *Unlimiting mind: The radically experiential psychology of Buddhism.* Boston: Wisdom.

Segal, Z. V., Williams, J. M. G., & Teasdale, J. D. (2002). *Mindfulness-based cognitive therapy for depression: A new approach to preventing relapse.* New York: Guilford Press.

References

American Psychological Association. (2003). Guidelines on multicultural education, training, research, practice and organizational change for psychologists. *American Psychologist, 58*, 377–402.

Antony, M. M., Orsillo, S. M., & Roemer, L. (Eds.). (2001). *Practitioner's guide to empirically based measures of anxiety*. New York: Kluwer Academic/Plenum Press.

Bach, P., & Hayes, S. C. (2002). The use of acceptance and commitment therapy to prevent the rehospitalization of psychotic patients: A randomized controlled trial. *Journal of Consulting and Clinical Psychology, 70*, 1129–1139.

Baer, R. A., Smith, G. T., & Allen, K. B. (2004). Assessment of mindfulness by self-report: The Kentucky Inventory of Mindfulness Skills. *Assessment, 11*, 191–206.

Baer, R. A., Smith, G. T., Hopkins, J., Krietemeyer, J., & Toney, L. (2006). Using self-report assessment methods to explore facets of mindfulness. *Assessment, 13*, 27–45.

Bagby, R. M., Parker, J. D. A., & Taylor, G. J. (1994). The twenty-item Toronto Alexithymia Scale: I Item selection and cross-validation of the factor structure. *Journal of Psychosomatic Research, 38*, 23–32.

Barks, C., with Moyne, J., Arberry, A. A., & Nicholson, R. (Trans.). (1995). *The essential Rumi*. San Francisco: Harper.

Barlow, D. H. (1991). Disorders of emotion. *Psychological Inquiry, 2*, 58–71.

Barlow, D. H. (2002). *Anxiety and its disorders: The nature and treatment of anxiety and panic* (2nd ed.). New York: Guilford Press.

Barlow, D. H. (Ed.). (2008). *Clinical handbook of psychological disorders: A step-by-step treatment manual* (4th ed.). New York: Guilford Press.

Barlow, D. H., Allen, L. B., & Choate, M. L. (2004). Toward a unified treatment for emotional disorders. *Behavior Therapy, 35*, 205–230.

Batten, S. V., Orsillo, S. M., & Walser, R. D. (2005). Acceptance and mindfulness-based approaches to the treatment of posttraumatic stress disorder. In S. M. Orsillo & L. Roemer (Eds.), *Acceptance- and mindfulness-based approaches to anxiety: Conceptualization and treatment* (pp. 241–269). New York: Springer.

Beck, A. T. (1976). *Cognitive therapy and the emotional disorders*. New York: International Universities Press.

Bernstein, D. A., Borkovec, T. D., & Hazlett-Stevens, H. (2000). *New directions in progressive relaxation training: A guidebook for helping professionals*. Westport, CT: Praeger.

Bishop, S. R., Lau, M., Shapiro, S., Carlson, L., Anderson, N. D., Carmody, J., et al. (2004). Mindfulness: A proposed operational definition. *Clinical Psychology: Science and Practice, 11*, 230–241.

Blackledge, J. T., Ciarrochi, J., & Bailey, A. (2007). *Personal Values Questionnaire*. Unpublished measure.

Borkovec, T. D., Alcaine, O. M., & Behar, E. (2004). Avoidance theory of worry and generalized anxiety disorder. In R. G. Heimberg, C. L. Turk, & D. S. Mennin (Eds.), *Generalized anxiety disorder: Advances in research and practice* (pp. 77–108). New York: Guilford Press.

Borkovec, T. D., & Hu, S. (1990). The effect of worry

on cardiovascular response to phobic imagery. *Behaviour Research and Therapy, 28,* 69–73.

Borkovec, T. D., & Sharpless, B. (2004). Generalized anxiety disorder: Bringing cognitive-behavioral therapy into the valued present. In S. C. Hayes, V. M. Follette, & M. M. Linehan (Eds.), *Mindfulness and acceptance: Expanding the cognitive-behavioral tradition* (pp. 209–242). New York: Guilford Press.

Bowen, S., Witkiewitz, K., Dillworth, T. M., Chawla, N., Simpson, T. L., Ostafin, B. D., et al. (2006). Mindfulness meditation and substance use in an incarcerated population. *Psychology of Addictive Behaviors, 20,* 343–347.

Brach, T. (2003). *Radical acceptance: Embracing your life with the heart of a Buddha.* New York: Bantam Dell.

Breslau, J., Aguilar-Gaxiola, S., Kendler, K. S., Su, M., Williams, D., & Kessler, R. C. (2006). Specifying race–ethnic differences in risk for psychiatric disorder in a U.S. national sample. *Psychological Medicine, 36,* 57–68.

Brown, K. W., & Ryan, R. M. (2003). The benefits of being present: Mindfulness and its role in psychological well-being. *Journal of Personality and Social Psychology, 84,* 822–848.

Buchheld, N., Grossman, P., & Walach, H. (2001). Measuring mindfulness in insight meditation (vipassana) and meditation-based psychotherapy: The development of the Freiburg Mindfulness Inventory (FMI). *Journal for Meditation and Meditation Research, 1,* 11–34.

Buysse, D. J., Reynolds, C. F., Monk, T. H., Berman, S. R., & Kupfer, D. J. (1989). The Pittsburgh Sleep Quality Index: A new instrument for psychiatric practice and research. *Psychiatry Research, 28,* 193–213.

Carson, J. W., Carson, K. M., Gil, K. M., & Baucom, D. H. (2004). Mindfulness-based relationship enhancement. *Behavior Therapy, 35,* 471–494.

Chapman, A. L., Gratz, K. L., & Brown, M. Z. (2006). Solving the puzzle of deliberate self-harm: The experiential avoidance model. *Behaviour Research and Therapy, 44,* 371–394.

Chiles, J. A., & Strosahl, K. D. (2005). *Clinical manual for assessment and treatment of suicidal patients.* Washington, DC: American Psychiatric Publishing.

Chodron, P. (2001). *The places that scare you: A guide to fearlessness in difficult times.* Boston: Shambhala.

Chodron, P. (2007). *Practicing peace in times of war.* Boston: Shambhala.

Christensen, A., Atkins, D. C., Berns, S., Wheeler, J., Baucom, D. H., & Simpson, L. E. (2004). Traditional versus integrative behavioral couple therapy for significantly and chronically distressed married couples. *Journal of Consulting and Clinical Psychology, 72,* 176–191.

Christensen, A., Atkins, D. C., Yi, J., Baucom, D. H., & George, W. H. (2006). Couple and individual adjustment for two years following a randomized clinical trial comparing traditional versus integrative behavioral couple therapy. *Journal of Consulting and Clinical Psychology, 74,* 1180–1191.

Christensen, A., & Jacobson, N. S. (2000). *Reconcilable differences.* New York: Guilford Press.

Clark, D. M. (1986). A cognitive approach to panic. *Behaviour Research and Therapy, 24,* 461–470.

Cocoran, J., & Fischer, K. (2000). *Measures for clinical practice: A sourcebook* (3rd ed.). New York: Free Press.

Cook, J. M., Schnurr, P. P., & Foa, E. B. (2004). Bridging the gap between posttraumatic stress disorder research and clinical practice: The example of exposure therapy. *Psychotherapy: Theory, Research, Practice, Training, 41,* 374–387.

Derogatis, L. R., & Melisaratos, N. (1979). The DSFI: A multidimensional measure of sexual functioning. *Journal of Sex and Marital Therapy, 5,* 244–281.

Derogatis, L. R., & Spencer, P. M. (1982). *The Brief Symptom Inventory: Administration, scoring, and procedures manual.* Minneapolis, MN: National Computer Systems.

DiNardo, P. A., Brown, T. A., & Barlow, D. H. (1994). *Anxiety Disorders Interview Schedule for DSM-IV.* Albany, NY: Graywind.

Eifert, G. H., & Forsyth, J. P. (2005). *Acceptance and commitment therapy for anxiety disorders: A practitioner's treatment guide to using mindfulness, acceptance, and values-based behavior change strategies.* Oakland, CA: New Harbinger.

Eifert, G. H., & Heffner, M. (2003). The effects of acceptance versus control contexts on avoidance of panic-related symptoms. *Journal of Behavior Therapy and Experimental Psychiatry, 34,* 293–312.

Emmons, R. A. (1986). Personal strivings: An approach to personality and subjective well-being. *Journal of Personality and Social Psychology, 51,* 1058–1068.

First, M. B., Gibbons, M., Spitzer, R. L., & Williams, J. B. W. (1996). *Structured Clinical Interview for DSM-IV Axis I Disorders, Clinician Version (SCID-CV).* Washington, DC: American Psychiatric Press.

Foa, E. B., & Kozak, M. J. (1986). Emotional processing of fear: Exposure to corrective information. *Psychological Bulletin, 99,* 20–35.

Foa, E. B., Riggs, D. S., Massie, E. D., & Yarczower, M. (1995). The impact of fear activation and anger on the efficacy of exposure treatment for posttraumatic stress disorder. *Behavior Therapy, 26,* 487–499.

Forman, E. M., Herbert, J. D., Moitra, E., Yeomans, P. D., & Geller, P. A. (2007). A randomized controlled effectiveness trial of acceptance and commitment therapy and cognitive therapy for anxiety and depression. *Behavior Modification, 31,* 772–799.

Frijda, N. H. (1986). *The emotions.* New York: Cambridge University Press.

Frisch, M. B., Cornell, J., Villanueva, M., & Retzlaff, P. J. (1992). Clinical validation of the Quality of Life Inventory: A measure of life satisfaction for use in treatment planning and outcome assessment. *Psychological Assessment, 4,* 92–101.

Fuchs, C., Lee, J. K., Orsillo, S. M., & Roemer, L. (2007, November). *A meta-analytic review of mindfulness- and acceptance-based treatments used with diverse, underserved populations.* Poster session presented at the annual meeting of the Association for Behavioral and Cognitive Therapies, Philadelphia.

Fulton, P. R. (2005). Mindfulness as clinical training. In C. K. Germer, R. D. Siegel, & P. R. Fulton (Eds.), *Mindfulness and psychotherapy* (pp. 55–72). New York: Guilford Press.

Gaudiano, B. A., & Herbert, J. D. (2006). Acute treatment of inpatients with psychotic symptoms using acceptance and commitment therapy: Pilot results. *Behaviour Research and Therapy, 44,* 415–437.

Germer, C. K. (2005). Anxiety disorders: Befriending fear. In C. K. Germer, R. D. Siegel, & P. R. Fulton (Eds.), *Mindfulness and psychotherapy* (pp. 152–172). New York: Guilford Press.

Germer, C. K., Siegel, R. D., & Fulton, P. R. (Eds.). (2005). *Mindfulness and psychotherapy.* New York: Guilford Press.

Gifford, E. V., Kohlenberg, B. S., Hayes, S. C., Antonuccio, D. O., Piasecki, M. M., Rasmussen-Hall, M. L., et al. (2004). Acceptance-based treatment for smoking cessation. *Behavior Therapy, 35,* 689–705.

Gilbert, P. (Ed.). (2005). *Compassion: Conceptualisations, research, and use in psychotherapy.* New York: Routledge.

Goisman, R. M., Rogers, M. P., Steketee, G. S., Warshaw, M. G., Cuneo, P., & Keller, M. B. (1993). Utilization of behavioral methods in a multicenter anxiety disorders study. *Journal of Clinical Psychiatry, 54,* 213–218.

Goldstein, A. J., & Chambless, D. L. (1978). A reanalysis of agoraphobia. *Behavior Therapy, 9,* 47–59.

Gratz, K. L., & Gunderson, J. G. (2006). Preliminary data on an acceptance-based emotion regulation group intervention for deliberate self-harm among women with borderline personality disorder. *Behavior Therapy, 37,* 25–35.

Gratz, K. L., & Roemer, L. (2004). Multidimensional assessment of emotion regulation and dysregulation: Development, factor structure, and initial validation of the Difficulties in Emotion Regulation Scale. *Journal of Psychopathology and Behavioral Assessment, 26,* 41–54.

Greenberg, L. S. (2002). *Emotion-focused therapy: Coaching clients to work through their feelings.* Washington, DC: American Psychological Association.

Greenberg, L. S., & Safran, J. D. (1987). *Emotion in psychotherapy.* New York: Guilford Press.

Gregg, J. A., Callaghan, G. M., Hayes, S. C., & Glenn-Lawson, J. L. (2007). Improving diabetes self-management through acceptance, mindfulness, and values: A randomized controlled trial. *Journal of Consulting and Clinical Psychology, 75,* 336–343.

Gross, J. J. (1998). The emerging field of emotion regulation: An integrative review. *Review of General Psychology, 2,* 271–299.

Gross, J. J., & John, O. P. (2003). Individual differences in two emotion regulation processes: Implications for affect, relationships, and well-being. *Journal of Personality and Social Psychology, 85,* 348–362.

Gross, J. J., & Levenson, R. W. (1993). Emotional suppression: Physiology, self-report, and expressive behavior. *Journal of Personality and Social Psychology, 64,* 970–986.

Gross, J. J., & Levenson, R. W. (1997). Hiding feelings: The acute effects of inhibiting negative and positive emotion. *Journal of Abnormal Psychology, 106,* 95–103.

Grossman, P., Niemann, L., Schmidt, S., & Walach, H. (2004). Mindfulness-based stress reduction and health benefits: A meta-analysis. *Journal of Psychosomatic Research, 57,* 35–43.

Hayes, A. M., Feldman, G. C., Beevers, C. G., Laurenceau, J.-P., Cardaciotto, L., & Lewis-Smith, J. (2007). Discontinuities and cognitive changes in an exposure-based cognitive therapy for depression. *Journal of Consulting and Clinical Psychology, 75,* 409–421.

Hayes, A. M., Laurenceau, J.-P., Feldman, G., Strauss, J. L., & Cardaciotto, L. (2007). Change is not always linear: The study of nonlinear and discontinuous patterns of change in psychotherapy. *Clinical Psychology Review, 27,* 715–723.

Hayes, S. C. (2004). Acceptance and commitment therapy and the new behavior therapies: Mindfulness, acceptance, and relationship. In S. C. Hayes, V. M. Follette, & M. M. Linehan (Eds.), *Mindfulness and acceptance: Expanding the cognitive-behavioral tradition* (pp. 1–29). New York: Guilford Press.

Hayes, S. C., Barnes-Holmes, D., & Rosche, B. (2001). *Relational frame theory: A post-Skinnerian account of human language and cognition*. New York: Springer.

Hayes, S. C., Batten, S. V., Gifford, E. V., Wilson, K. G., Afari, N., & McCurry, S. M. (1999). *Acceptance and commitment therapy: An individual psychotherapy manual for the treatment of experiential avoidance*. Reno, NV: Context Press.

Hayes, S. C., Bissett, R., Roget, N., Padilla, M., Kohlenberg, B. S., Fisher, G., et al. (2004). The impact of acceptance and commitment training and multicultural training on the stigmatizing attitudes and professional burnout of substance abuse counselors. *Behavior Therapy, 35*, 821–835.

Hayes, S. C., Follette, V. M., & Linehan, M. M. (Eds.). (2004). *Mindfulness and acceptance: Expanding the cognitive-behavioral tradition*. New York: Guilford Press.

Hayes, S. C., Luoma, J., Bond, F., Masuda, A., & Lillis, J. (2006). Acceptance and commitment therapy: Model, processes, and outcomes. *Behavioral Research and Therapy, 44*, 1–25.

Hayes, S. C., & Shenk, C. (2004). Operationalizing mindfulness without unnecessary attachments. *Clinical Psychology: Science and Practice, 11*, 249–254.

Hayes, S. C., & Smith, S. (2005). *Get out of your mind and into your life: The new acceptance and commitment therapy*. Oakland, CA: New Harbinger.

Hayes, S. C., & Strosahl, K. D. (Eds.). (2004). *A practical guide to acceptance and commitment therapy*. New York: Kluwer/Plenum Press.

Hayes, S. C., Strosahl, K. D., & Wilson, K. G. (1999). *Acceptance and commitment therapy: An experiential approach to behavior change*. New York: Guilford Press.

Hayes, S. C., Strosahl, K. D., Wilson, K. G., Bissett, R. T., Pistorello, J., Toarmino, D., et al. (2004). Measuring experiential avoidance: A preliminary test of a working model. *Psychological Record, 54*, 553–578.

Hayes, S. C., Wilson, K. G., Gifford, E. V., Bissett, R., Piasecki, M., Batten, S. V., et al. (2004). A preliminary trial of twelve-step facilitation and acceptance and commitment therapy with polysubstance-abusing methadone-maintained opiate addicts. *Behavior Therapy, 35*, 667–688.

Hayes, S. C., Wilson, K. G., Gifford, E. V., Follette, V. M., & Strosahl, K. (1996). Experiential avoidance and behavioral disorders: A functional dimensional approach to diagnosis and treatment. *Journal of Consulting and Clinical Psychology, 64*, 1152–1168.

Hays, P. A. (2008). *Addressing cultural complexities in practice: Assessment, diagnosis and therapy* (2nd ed.). Washington, DC: American Psychological Association.

Hays, P. A., & Iwamasa, G. Y. (Eds.). (2006). *Culturally responsive cognitive-behavioral therapy: Assessment, practice, and supervision*. Washington, DC: American Psychological Association.

Hays, R. D., & Stewart, A. L. (1992). Sleep measures. In A. L. Stewart & J. E. Ware (Eds.), *Measuring functioning and well-being: The Medical Outcomes Study approach* (pp. 235–259). Durham, NC: Duke University Press.

Heffner, M., Sperry, J., Eifert, G. H., & Detweiler, M. (2002). Acceptance and commitment therapy in the treatment of an adolescent female with anorexia nervosa: A case example. *Cognitive and Behavioral Practice, 9*, 232–236.

Hinton, D. E., Chau, H., Nguyen, L., Nguyen, M., Pham, T., Quinn, S., et al. (2001). Panic disorder among Vietnamese refugees attending a psychiatric clinic: Prevalence and subtypes. *General Hospital Psychiatry, 23*, 337–344.

Hinton, D. E., Pham, T., Chau, H., Tran, M., & Hinton, S. D. (2003). "Hit by the wind" and temperature-shift panic among Vietnamese refugees. *Transcultural Psychiatry, 40*, 342–376.

Hinton, D. E., Pich, V., Chhean, D., Safren, S. A., & Pollack, M. H. (2006). Somatic-focused therapy for traumatized refugees: Treating posttraumatic stress disorder and comorbid neck-focused panic attacks among Cambodian refugees. *Psychotherapy: Theory, Research, Practice, Training, 43*(4), 491–505.

Hofstede, G. (1980). *Culture's consequences: International differences in work-related values*. Beverly Hills, CA: Sage.

Holowka, D., & Roemer, L. (2007, November). *Psychometric evaluation of the Experiential Awareness Measure*. Poster session presented at the annual meeting of the Association for Behavioral and Cognitive Therapies, Philadelphia.

Holowka, D. W. (2008). *Experiential awareness and psychological well-being: Preliminary investigation of a proposed common factor*. Doctoral dissertation, University of Massachusetts, Boston.

Jacobson, E. (1934). *You must relax*. New York: McGraw-Hill.

Jacobson, N. S., & Christensen, A. (1996). *Acceptance and change in couple therapy: A therapist's guide to transforming relationships.* New York: Norton.

Jacobson, N. S., Christensen, A., Prince, S. E., Cordova, J., & Eldridge, K. (2000). Integrative behavioral couple therapy: An acceptance-based, promising new treatment for couple discord. *Journal of Consulting and Clinical Psychology, 68,* 351–355.

Jacobson, N. S., Martell, C. R., & Dimidjian, S. (2001). Behavioral activation treatment for depression: Returning to contextual roots. *Clinical Psychology: Science and Practice, 8,* 255–270.

Jain, S., Shapiro, S. L., Swanick, S., Roesch, S. C., Mills, P. J., Bell, I., et al. (2007). A randomized controlled trial of mindfulness meditation versus relaxation training: Effects on distress, positive states of mind, rumination, and distraction. *Annals of Behavioral Medicine, 33,* 11–21.

Jarrett, R. B., & Nelson, R. O. (1987). Mechanisms of change in cognitive therapy of depression. *Behavior Therapy, 18,* 227–241.

Jaycox, L. H., Foa, E. B., & Morral, A. R. (1998). Influence of emotional engagement and habituation on exposure therapy for PTSD. *Journal of Consulting and Clinical Psychology, 66,* 185–192.

Kabat-Zinn, J. (1990). *Full catastrophe living: Using the wisdom of your body and mind to face stress, pain, and illness.* New York: Delta.

Kabat-Zinn, J. (1994). *Wherever you go there you are: Mindfulness meditation in everyday life.* New York: Hyperion.

Kabat-Zinn, J. (2005). *Coming to our senses: Healing ourselves and the world through mindfulness.* New York: Hyperion.

Kantrowitz, R. E., & Ballou, M. (1992). A feminist critique of cognitive-behavioral therapy. In L. S. Brown & M. Ballou (Eds.), *Personality and psychopathology: Feminist reappraisals* (pp. 70–87). New York: Guilford Press.

Kashdan, T. B., & Steger, M. F. (2006). Expanding the topography of social anxiety: An experience-sampling assessment of positive emotions, positive events, and emotion suppression. *Psychological Science, 17,* 120–128.

Kenny, M. A., & Williams, J. M. G. (2007). Treatment-resistant depressed patients show a good response to mindfulness-based cognitive therapy. *Behaviour Research and Therapy, 45,* 617–625.

Kingston, T., Dooley, B., Bates, A., Lawlor, E., & Malone, K. (2007). Mindfulness-based cognitive therapy for residual depressive symptoms. *Psychology and Psychotherapy: Theory, Research and Practice, 80,* 193–203.

Koons, C. R., Robins, C. J., Tweed, J. L., Lynch, T.

R., Gonzalez, A. M., Morse, J. Q., et al. (2001). Efficacy of dialectical behavior therapy in women veterans with borderline personality disorder. *Behavior Therapy, 32,* 371–390.

Koszycki, D., Benger, M., Shlik, J., & Bradwejn, J. (2007). Randomized trial of a meditation-based stress reduction program and cognitive behavior therapy in generalized social anxiety disorder. *Behaviour Research and Therapy, 45,* 2518–2526.

Laumann, E. O., Paik, A., & Rosen, R. C. (1999). Sexual dysfunction in the United States: Prevalence and predictors. *Journal of the American Medical Association, 281,* 537–544.

LeDoux, J. (1996). *The emotional brain: The mysterious underpinnings of emotional life.* New York: Simon & Schuster.

Leong, F. T. L. (1996). Toward an integrative model for cross-cultural counseling and psychotherapy. *Applied and Preventive Psychology, 5,* 189–209.

Levitt, J. T., Brown, T. A., Orsillo, S. M., & Barlow, D. H. (2004). The effects of acceptance versus suppression of emotion on subjective and psychophysiological response to carbon dioxide challenge in patients with panic disorder. *Behavior Therapy, 35,* 747–766.

Levitt, J. T., & Karekla, M. (2005). Integrating acceptance and mindfulness with cognitive behavioral treatment for panic disorder. In S. M. Orsillo & L. Roemer (Eds.), *Acceptance and mindfulness-based approaches to anxiety: Conceptualization and treatment* (pp. 165–188). New York: Springer.

Lew, M., Matta, C., Tripp-Tebo, C., & Watts, D. (2006). Dialectical behavior therapy (DBT) for individuals with intellectual disabilities: A program description. *Mental Health Aspects of Developmental Disabilities, 9,* 1–12.

Lewinsohn, P. M. (1974). A behavioral approach to depression. In R. M. Friedman & M. M. Katz (Eds.), *The psychology of depression: Contemporary theory and research* (pp. 157–185). New York: Wiley.

Lillis, J., & Hayes, S. C. (2007). Applying acceptance, mindfulness, and values to the reduction of prejudice: A pilot study. *Behavior Modification, 31,* 389–411.

Linehan, M. M. (1993a). *Cognitive-behavioral treatment of borderline personality disorder.* New York: Guilford Press.

Linehan, M. M. (1993b). *Skills training manual for treating borderline personality disorder.* New York: Guilford Press.

Linehan, M. M., Armstrong, H. E., Suarez, A.,

Allmon, D., & Heard, H. L. (1991). Cognitive-behavioral treatment of chronically parasuicidal borderline patients. *Archives of General Psychiatry, 48*, 1060–1064.

Linehan, M. M., Comtois, K. A., Murray, A. M., Brown, M. Z., Gallop, R. J., Heard, H. L., et al. (2007). Two-year randomized controlled trial and follow-up of dialectical behavior therapy vs. therapy by experts for suicidal behaviors and borderline personality disorder. *Archives of General Psychiatry, 63*, 757–766.

Linehan, M. M., Dimeff, L. A., Reynolds, S. K., Comtois, K. A., Welch, S. S., Heagerty, P., et al. (2002). Dialectical behavior therapy versus comprehensive validation therapy plus 12-step for the treatment of opioid dependent women meeting criteria for borderline personality disorder. *Drug and Alcohol Dependence, 67*, 13–26.

Linehan, M. M., Goodstein, J. L., Nielsen, S. L., & Chiles, J. A. (1983). Reasons for staying alive when you are thinking of killing yourself: The Reasons for Living Inventory. *Journal of Consulting and Clinical Psychology, 51*, 276–286.

Linehan, M. M., Heard, H. L., & Armstrong, H. E. (1993). Naturalistic follow-up of a behavioral treatment for chronically parasuicidal borderline patients. *Archives of General Psychiatry, 50*, 971–974.

Linehan, M. M., Schmidt, H., Dimeff, L. A., Craft, J. C., Kanter, J., & Comtois, K. A. (1999). Dialectical behavior therapy for patients with borderline personality disorder and drug-dependence. *merican Journal on Addictions, 8*, 279–292.

Lischetzke, T., & Eid, M. (2003). Is attention to feelings beneficial or detrimental to affective well-being?: Mood regulation as a moderator variable. *Emotion, 3*, 361–377.

Longmore, R. J., & Worrell, M. (2007). Do we need to challenge thoughts in cognitive behavior therapy? *Clinical Psychology Review, 27*, 173–187.

Lovibond, S. H., & Lovibond, P. F. (1995). *Manual for the Depression Anxiety Stress Scales*. Sydney: Psychology Foundation of Australia.

Lundgren, T., Dahl, J., & Hayes, S. C. (2008). Evaluation of mediators of change in the treatment of epilepsy with acceptance and commitment therapy. *Journal of Behavior Medicine, 31*, 225–235.

Lundgren, A. T., Dahl, J., Melin, L., & Kies, B. (2006). Evaluation of acceptance and commitment therapy for drug refractory epilepsy: A randomized controlled trial in South Africa—A pilot study. *Epilepsia, 47*, 2173–2179.

Lynch, T. R., Cheavens, J. S., Cukrowicz, K., Thorp, S. R., Bronner, L., & Beyer, J. (2007). Treatment of older adults with co-morbid personality disorder and depression: A dialectical behavior therapy approach. *International Journal of Geriatric Psychiatry, 22*, 131–143.

Lynch, T. R., Morse, J. Q., Mendelson, T., & Robins, C. J. (2003). Dialectical behavior therapy for depressed older adults: A randomized pilot study. *American Journal of Geriatric Psychiatry, 11*, 33–45.

Ma, S. H., & Teasdale, J. D. (2004). Mindfulness-based cognitive therapy for depression: Replication and exploration of differential relapse prevention effects. *Journal of Consulting and Clinical Psychology, 72*, 31–40.

Markus, H. R., & Kitayama, S. (1991). Culture and the self: Implications for cognition, emotion, and motivation. *Psychological Review, 98*, 224–253.

Marlatt, G. A., & Gordon, J. R. (Eds.). (1985). *Relapse prevention: Maintenance strategies in the treatment of addictive behaviors*. New York: Guilford Press.

Marlatt, G. A., & Witkiewitz, K. (2005). Relapse prevention for alcohol and drug problems. In G. A. Marlatt & D. M. Donovan (Eds.), *Relapse prevention: Maintenance strategies in the treatment of addictive behaviors* (2nd ed., pp. 1–44). New York: Guilford Press.

Martell, C. R., Addis, M. E., & Jacobson, N. S. (2001). *Depression in context: Strategies for guided action*. New York: Norton.

Martin, J. R. (1997). Mindfulness: A proposed common factor. *Journal of Psychotherapy Integration, 7*, 291–312.

May, R. (1996). *The meaning of anxiety*. New York: Norton.

Mayfield, D., McLeod, G., & Hall, P. (1974). The CAGE questionnaire: Validation of a new alcoholism screening instrument. *American Journal of Psychiatry, 131*, 1121–1123.

Mennin, D. S. (2006). Emotion regulation therapy: An integrative approach to treatment-resistant anxiety disorders. *Journal of Contemporary Psychotherapy, 36*, 95–105.

Miller, W. R., & Rollnick, S. (2002). *Motivational interviewing: Preparing people for change* (2nd ed.). New York: Guilford Press.

Morgan, W. D., & Morgan, S. T. (2005). Cultivating attention and empathy. In C. K. Germer, R. D. Siegel, & P. R. Fulton (Eds.), *Mindfulness and psychotherapy* (pp. 73–90). New York: Guilford Press.

Mowrer, O. H. (1960). *Learning theory and behavior*. New York: Wiley.

Muñoz, R. F., & Mendelson, T. (2005). Toward evidence-based interventions for diverse populations: The San Francisco General Hospital prevention and treatment manuals. *Journal of Consulting and Clinical Psychology, 73*, 790–799.

National Sleep Foundation. (2007). *Sleep in America Poll.* Retrieved January 25, 2007, from www.sleepfoundation.org/atf/cf/%7BF6BF2668-A1B4-4FE8-8D1A-A5D39340D9CB%7D/Summary_Of_Findings%20-%20FINAL.pdf.

Neff, K. D., Rude, S. S., & Kirkpatrick, K. L. (2007). An examination of self-compassion in relation to positive psychological functioning and personality traits. *Journal of Research in Personality, 41*, 908–916.

Nezu, A. M. Ronan, G. F., Meadows, E. A., & McClure, K. S. (2000). *Practitioner's guide to empirically based measures of depression.* New York: Kluwer.

Nowlis, V. (1965). Research with the Mood Adjective Check List. In S. S. Tompkins & C. E. Izard (Eds.), *Affect, cognition, and personality* (pp. 352–389). New York: Springer.

Oman, D., Shapiro, S. L., Thoresen, C. E., Flinders, T., Driskell, J. D., & Plante, T. G. (2007). Learning from spiritual models and meditation: A randomized evaluation of a college course. *Pastoral Psychology, 55*, 473–493.

Orsillo, S. M., & Roemer, L. (Eds.). (2005). *Acceptance and mindfulness-based approaches to anxiety: Conceptualization and treatment.* New York: Springer.

Orsillo, S. M., Roemer, L., & Barlow, D. H. (2003). Integrating acceptance and mindfulness into existing cognitive-behavioral treatment for GAD: A case study. *Cognitive and Behavioral Practice, 10*, 223–230.

Orsillo, S. M., Roemer, L., & Holowka, D. W. (2005). Acceptance-based behavioral therapies for anxiety: Using acceptance and mindfulness to enhance traditional cognitive-behavioral approaches. In S. M. Orsillo & L. Roemer (Eds.), *Acceptance and mindfulness-based approaches to anxiety: Conceptualization and treatment* (pp. 3–35). New York: Springer.

Orsillo, S. M., Roemer, L., Lerner, J. B., & Tull, M. T. (2004). Acceptance, mindfulness, and cognitive-behavioral therapy: Comparisons, contrasts, and application to anxiety. In S. C. Hayes, V. M. Follette, & M. M. Linehan (Eds.), *Mindfulness and acceptance: Expanding the cognitive-behavioral tradition* (pp. 66–95). New York: Guilford Press.

Patel, S. R. (2006, March). *Mindfulness-based treatment for OCD: A case report.* Paper presented at the 5th annual Mindfulness-Based Stress Reduction International Conference, Worcester, MA.

Pederson, P. B., & Ivey, A. (1993). *Culture-centered counseling and interviewing skills: A practical guide.* Westport, CT: Praeger.

Pennebaker, J. W. (1997). Writing about emotional experiences as a therapeutic process. *Psychological Science, 8*, 162–166.

Persons, J. B. (1989). *Cognitive therapy in practice: A case formulation approach.* New York: Norton.

President's New Freedom Commission on Mental Health. (2003). *Achieving the promise: Transforming mental health care in America. Report of the President's New Freedom Commission on Mental Health.* Rockville, MD: Author.

Purdon, C. (1999). Thought suppression and psychopathology. *Behaviour Research and Therapy, 37*, 1029–1054.

Reiss, S., Peterson, R. A., Gursky, D. M., & McNally, R. J. (1986). Anxiety sensitivity, anxiety frequency and the predictions of fearfulness. *Behaviour Research and Therapy, 24*, 1–8.

Robins, C. J., Schmidt, H., III, & Linehan, M. M. (2004). Dialectical behavior therapy: Synthesizing radical acceptance with skillful means. In S. C. Hayes, V. M. Follette, & M. M. Linehan (Eds.), *Mindfulness and acceptance: Expanding the cognitive-behavioral tradition* (pp. 30–44). New York: Guilford Press.

Roemer, L., & Borkovec, T. D. (1994). Effects of suppressing thoughts about emotional material. *Journal of Abnormal Psychology, 103*, 467–474.

Roemer, L., & Orsillo, S. M. (2005). An acceptance-based behavior therapy for generalized anxiety disorder. In S. M. Orsillo & L. Roemer (Eds.), *Acceptance and mindfulness-based approaches to anxiety: Conceptualization and treatment* (pp. 213–240). New York: Springer.

Roemer, L., & Orsillo, S. M. (2007). An open trial of an acceptance-based behavior therapy for generalized anxiety disorder. *Behavior Therapy, 38*, 72–85.

Roemer, L., Orsillo, S. M., & Salters-Pedneault, K. (2008). Efficacy of an acceptance-based behavior therapy for generalized anxiety disorder: Evaluation in a randomized controlled trial. *Journal of Consulting and Clinical Psychology, 76*, 1083–1089.

Rogers, A. E., Caruso, C. C., & Aldrich, M. S. (1993). Reliability of sleep diaries for assessment of sleep/wake patterns. *Nursing Research, 42*, 368–372.

Rogers, C. R. (1961). *On becoming a person: A therapist's view of psychotherapy.* Boston: Houghton Mifflin.

Roth, B., & Robbins, D. (2004). Mindfulness-based stress reduction and health-related quality of life: Findings from a bilingual inner-city patient population. *Psychosomatic Medicine, 66,* 113–123.

Safer, D. L., Telch, C. F., & Agras, W. S. (2001). Dialectical behavior therapy for bulimia nervosa. *American Journal of Psychiatry, 158,* 632–634.

Salters-Pedneault, K., Roemer, L., Tull, M. T., Rucker, L., & Mennin, D. S. (2006). Evidence of broad deficits in emotion regulation associated with chronic worry and generalized anxiety disorder. *Cognitive Therapy and Research, 30,* 469–480.

Salters-Pedneault, K., Tull, M. T., & Roemer, L. (2004). The role of avoidance of emotional material in the anxiety disorders. *Applied and Preventive Psychology: Current Scientific Perspectives, 11,* 95–114.

Schmidt, N. B., Woolaway-Bickel, K., Trakowski, J., Santiago, H., Storey, J., Koselka, M., et al. (2000). Dismantling cognitive-behavioral treatment for panic disorder: Questioning the utility of breathing retraining. *Journal of Consulting and Clinical Psychology, 68,* 417–424.

Schwartz, S. H. (2006). Basic human values: Theory, measurement, and applications. *Revue française de sociologie, 47,* 929–968.

Segal, Z. V., Williams, J. M. G., & Teasdale, J. D. (2002). *Mindfulness-based cognitive therapy for depression: A new approach to preventing relapse.* New York: Guilford Press.

Semple, R. J., Reid, E. F. G., & Miller, L. (2005). Treating anxiety with mindfulness: An open trial of mindfulness training for anxious children. *Journal of Cognitive Psychotherapy, 19,* 379–392.

Shafran, R., Thordarson, D. S., & Rachman, S. (1996). Thought-action fusion in obsessive compulsive disorder. *Journal of Anxiety Disorders, 10,* 379–391.

Shapiro, S. L., Astin, J. A., Bishop, S. R., & Cordova, M. (2005). Mindfulness-based stress reduction for health care professionals: Results from a randomized trial. *International Journal of Stress Management, 12,* 164–176.

Shapiro, S. L., Carlson, L. E., Astin, J. A., & Freedman, B. (2006). Mechanisms of mindfulness. *Journal of Clinical Psychology, 62,* 373–386.

Siev, J., & Chambless, D. L. (2007). Specificity of treatment effects: Cognitive therapy and relaxation for generalized anxiety and panic disorders. *Journal of Consulting and Clinical Psychology, 75,* 513–522.

Smith, A. (2006). "Like waking up from a dream": Mindfulness training for older people with anxiety and depression. In R. A. Baer (Ed.), *Mindfulness-based treatment approaches: Clinician's guide to evidence base and applications* (pp. 191–216). Burlington, MA: Elsevier.

Stulz, N., Lutz, W., Leach, C., Lucock, M., & Barkham, M. (2007). Shapes of early change in psychotherapy under routine outpatient conditions. *Journal of Consulting and Clinical Psychology, 75,* 864–874.

Styron, C. W. (2005). Positive psychology: Awakening to the fullness of life. In C. K. Germer, R. D. Siegel, & P. R. Fulton (Eds.), *Mindfulness and psychotherapy* (pp. 262–282). New York: Guilford Press.

Sue, D. W., & Sue, D. (2003). *Counseling the culturally diverse: Theory and practice.* New York: Wiley.

Sue, S. (1998). In search of cultural competence in psychotherapy and counseling. *American Psychologist, 53,* 440–448.

Sue, S. (2006). Cultural competency: From philosophy to research and practice. *Journal of Community Psychology, 34,* 237–245.

Sue, S., & Zane, N. (1987). The role of culture and cultural techniques in psychotherapy: A critique and reformulation. *American Psychologist, 42,* 37–45.

Tanaka-Matsumi, J., Seiden, D. Y., & Lam, K. N. (1996). The culturally informed functional assessment (CIFA) interview: A strategy for cross-cultural behavioral practice. *Cognitive and Behavioral Practice, 3,* 215–233.

Teasdale, J., Segal, Z. V., & Williams, J. M. G. (2003). Mindfulness and problem formulation. *Clinical Psychology: Science and Practice, 10,* 157–160.

Teasdale, J. D. (2004). Mindfulness-based cognitive therapy. In J. Yiend (Ed.), *Cognition, emotion and psychopathology: Theoretical, empirical and clinical directions* (pp. 270–289). New York: Cambridge University Press.

Teasdale, J. D., Moore, R. G., Hayhurst, H., Pope, M., Williams, S., & Segal, Z. V. (2002). Megacognitive awareness and prevention of relapse in depression: Empirical evidence. *Journal of Consulting and Clinical Psychology, 70,* 275–287.

Teasdale, J. D., Segal, Z. V., Williams, J. M. G., Ridgeway, V. A., Soulsby, J. M., & Lau, M. A. (2000). Prevention of relapse/recurrence in major depression by mindfulness-based cognitive therapy. *Journal of Consulting and Clinical Psychology, 68,* 615–623.

Telch, C. F., Agras, W. S., & Linehan, M. M. (2001). Dialectical behavior therapy for binge eating disorder. *Journal of Consulting and Clinical Psychology, 69,* 1061–1065.

Thompson, R. A. (1994). Emotion regulation: A theme in search of definition. *Monographs of the Society for Research in Child Development, 59,* 25–52.

Tull, M. T., Barrett, H. M., McMillan, E. S., & Roemer, L. (2007). A preliminary investigation of the relationship between emotion regulation difficulties and posttraumatic stress symptoms. *Behavior Therapy, 38*, 303–313.

Tull, M. T., & Roemer, L. (2007). Emotion regulation difficulties associated with the experience of uncued panic attacks: Evidence of experiential avoidance, emotional nonacceptance, and decreased emotional clarity. *Behavior Therapy, 38*, 378–391.

Turner, R. M. (2000). Naturalistic evaluation of dialectical behavior therapy—oriented treatment for borderline personality disorder. *Cognitive and Behavioral Practice, 7*, 413–419.

Van den Bosch, L. M., Koeter, M. W., Stijnen, T., Verheul, R., & Van den Brink, W. (2005). Sustained efficacy of dialectical behaviour therapy for borderline personality disorder. *Behaviour Research and Therapy, 43*, 1231–1241.

Verheul, R., Van den Bosch, L. M., Koeter, M. W., de Ridder, M. A., Stijnen, T., & van den Brink, W. (2003). Dialectical behaviour therapy for women with borderline personality: 12-month, randomised clinical trial in the Netherlands. *British Journal of Psychiatry, 182*, 135–140.

Wagner, E. E., Rathus, J. H., & Miller, A. L. (2006). Mindfulness in dialectical behavior therapy (DBT) for adolescents. In R. A. Baer (Ed.), *Mindfulness-based treatment approaches: Clinician's guide to evidence base and applications* (pp. 167–190). Burlington, MA: Elsevier.

Wang, P. S., Lane, M., Olfson, M., Pincus, H. A., Wells, K. B., & Kessler, R. C. (2005). Twelve-month use of mental health services in the United States: Results from the National Comorbidity Survey Replication. *Archives of General Psychiatry, 62*, 629–640.

Watson, D., Clark, L. A., & Tellegen, A. (1988). Development and validation of brief measures of positive and negative affect: The PANAS scales. *Journal of Personality and Social Psychology, 6*, 1063–1070.

Wegner, D. M. (1994). Ironic processes of mental control. *Psychological Review, 101*, 34–52.

Wegner, D. M., & Zanakos, S. (1994). Chronic thought suppression. *Journal of Personality, 62*, 615–640.

Wells, A. (1995). Meta-cognition and worry: A cognitive model of generalized anxiety disorder. *Behavioural and Cognitive Psychotherapy, 23*, 301–320.

Wells, A., & Davies, M. I. (1994). The Thought Control Questionnaire: A measure of individual differences in the control of unwanted thoughts. *Behaviour Research and Therapy, 32*, 871–878.

Williams, J. M. G., Teasdale, J. D., Segal, Z. V., & Kabat-Zinn, J. (2007). *The mindful way through depression: Freeing yourself from chronic unhappiness.* New York: Guilford Press.

Williams, K. A., Kolar, M. M., Reger, B. E., & Pearson, J. C. (2001). Evaluation of a wellness-based mindfulness stress reduction intervention: A controlled trial. *American Journal of Health Promotion, 15*, 422–432.

Williams, K. E., Chambless, D. L., & Ahrens, A. (1997). Are emotions frightening?: An extension of the fear of fear construct. *Behaviour Research and Therapy, 35*, 239–248.

Wilson, K. G., & Murrell, A. R. (2004). Values work in acceptance and commitment therapy: Setting a course for behavioral treatment. In S. C. Hayes, V. M. Follette, & M. M. Linehan (Eds.), *Mindfulness and acceptance: Expanding the cognitive-behavioral tradition* (pp. 120–151). New York: Guilford Press.

Witkiewitz, K., Marlatt, G. A., & Walker, D. D. (2005). Mindfulness-based relapse prevention for alcohol use disorders: The meditative tortoise wins the race. *Journal of Cognitive Psychotherapy, 19*, 221–228.

Woods, D. W., Wetterneck, C. T., & Flessner, C. A. (2006). A controlled evaluation of acceptance and commitment therapy plus habit reversal for trichotillomania. *Behaviour Research and Therapy, 44*, 639–656.

Woody, S. R., Detweiler-Bedell, J., Teachman, B. A., & O'Hearn, T. (2003). *Treatment planning in psychotherapy: Taking the guesswork out of clinical care.* New York: Guilford Press.

Wilson, K. G., & Groom, J. (2002). *The Valued Living Questionnaire.* University: Department of Psychology, University of Mississippi.

Zettle, R. D., & Hayes, S. C. (1987). Component and process analysis of cognitive therapy. *Psychological Reports, 61*, 939–953.

Zettle, R. D., & Rains, J. C. (1989). Group cognitive and contextual therapies in treatment of depression. *Journal of Clinical Psychology, 45*, 436–445.

Zohar, D., Tzischinsky, O., Epstein, R., & Lavie, P. (2005). The effects of sleep loss on medical residents' emotional reactions to work events: A cognitive-energy model. *Sleep: Journal of Sleep and Sleep Disorders Research, 28*, 47–54.

Index

Page numbers followed by *f* indicate figure, *t* indicate table.